AF539651

Integrative Rheumatology

Weil Integrative Medicine Library

Published and Forthcoming Volumes

SERIES EDITOR

ANDREW T. WEIL, MD

Donald I. Abrams and Andrew T. Weil: *Integrative Oncology*
Timothy P. Culbert and Karen Olness: *Integrative Pediatrics*
Victoria Maizes and Tieraona Low Dog: *Integrative Women's Health*
Randy Horwitz and Daniel Muller: *Integrative Rheumatology*
Daniel A. Monti and Bernard Beitman: *Integrative Psychiatry*
Stephen Devries and James Dalen: *Integrative Cardiology*

Integrative Rheumatology

EDITED BY

Randy Horwitz, MD, PhD
Medical Director, Arizona Center for Integrative Medicine
Assistant Professor of Clinical Medicine
University of Arizona College of Medicine

Daniel Muller, MD, PhD
Associate Professor of Medicine
Section of Rheumatology
University of Wisconsin School of
Medicine and Public Health

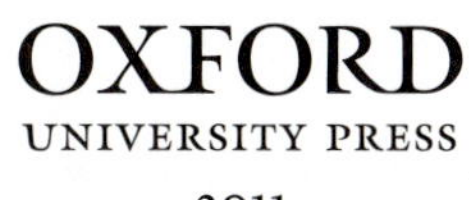

OXFORD
UNIVERSITY PRESS
2011

OXFORD
UNIVERSITY PRESS

Oxford University Press, Inc., publishes works that further
Oxford University's objective of excellence
in research, scholarship, and education.

Oxford New York
Auckland Cape Town Dar es Salaam Hong Kong Karachi
Kuala Lumpur Madrid Melbourne Mexico City Nairobi
New Delhi Shanghai Taipei Toronto

With offices in
Argentina Austria Brazil Chile Czech Republic France Greece
Guatemala Hungary Italy Japan Poland Portugal Singapore
South Korea Switzerland Thailand Turkey Ukraine Vietnam

Published by Oxford University Press, Inc.
198 Madison Avenue, New York, New York 10016
www.oup.com

Library of Congress Cataloging-in-Publication Data

Integrative rheumatology / edited by Randy Horwitz, Daniel Muller.
p. ; cm. — (Weil integrative medicine library)
Includes bibliographical references.
Summary: "In this volume in the series, the authors describe a rational and evidence-based approach to the integrative therapy of rheumatologic, allergic, and autoimmune disorders, integrating the principles of alternative and complementary therapies into the principles and practice of conventional medical therapy"—Provided by publisher.
ISBN 978-0-19-531121-1 (hardback : alk. paper) 1. Rheumatism—Alternative treatment.
2. Autoimmune diseases—Alternative treatment. 3. Allergy—Alternative treatment.
4. Rheumatology. I. Horwitz, Randy. II. Muller, Daniel, 1953- III. Series:
Weil integrative medicine library.
[DNLM: 1. Rheumatic Diseases—therapy. 2. Autoimmune Diseases—therapy.
3. Integrative Medicine. WE 544 I5805 2011]
RC927.I55 2011
616.7'23—dc22

2010007434

ISBN 978-0-19-531121-1

---

1 3 5 7 9 8 6 4 2

Printed in the United States of America
on acid-free paper

PREFACE

"Integrative Medicine is healing-oriented medicine that takes account of the whole person (body, mind, and spirit), including all aspects of lifestyle.

It emphasizes the therapeutic relationship and makes use of all appropriate therapies, both conventional and alternative."

The term *integrative medicine* connotes a separate field of medicine to many patients and practitioners. Most associate integrative medicine with complementary and alternative (CAM) approaches to disease management. In reality, integrative medicine represents a unique approach to patients and to patient care. Its practitioners are rooted in Western medicine, yet utilize traditional and complementary healing techniques and modalities in an effort to help the body to heal. The value of such an approach becomes apparent when confronted with chronic conditions for which inadequate therapy exists, or when the use of such therapy is associated with considerable adverse consequences. Thus, the field of Rheumatology is ideal for integrative interventions.

This text is designed to introduce the reader to some integrative approaches that may be clinically helpful in patients who are dealing with rheumatologic disorders. Early chapters introduce these modalities and interventions, and later chapters provide recommendations for specific rheumatologic conditions. Some of these deserve a preview.

Dietary therapy is a cornerstone of the practice of integrative medicine. Hippocrates is credited with stating that patients should "Let your food be your medicine, and your medicine be your food." No other medicine is taken with such regularity (and gusto) in the Western world as food. Patients who might normally miss afternoon doses of medications rarely forget to eat lunch. In Chapter 2, Johnson describes the potential impact of various food choices upon systemic inflammation. Though we routinely classify foods as "proinflammatory" and "anti-inflammatory," it is truly the composite of the diet that contributes to health and healing. Years of clinical experience have documented the impact of dietary choices upon clinical outcomes, whether studying the Mediterranean diet in cardiology, or the gluten-free diet in patients with celiac disease. The heterogeneity of clinical rheumatology conditions (even in those with the same diagnosis) may preclude large-scale definitive trials, yet dietary changes can be made with small numbers of patients in a clinical practice, with surprisingly good results.

In Chapter 3, Calder discusses the importance of omega-3 fatty acids in the diet (and as supplements)—a concept that has been popularized recently in the lay press, yet is based upon sound nutritional science. The choice of dietary fatty acids can have a significant impact upon both the *de novo* production of inflammatory mediators following a provocative trigger, and upon the host immune response. Many of our pharmaceutical interventions for rheumatological diseases are designed to block the formation or the effects of inflammatory mediators deep in their biosynthetic pathway. Increased intake of omega-3 fatty acids provides less substrate for the initial formation of these mediators, thus dampening the host inflammatory response. Neutrophil membrane fatty acid composition can be measurably altered in as little as 6 weeks. Daily servings of fatty fish, or fish oil, also produce a modest attenuation of host immune function (e.g., cytokine production) with no side effects. The addition of omega-3 fats to the diet is routinely used in our practice for all inflammatory conditions.

Exercise is also an important component of lifestyle management for the patient with arthritis (as it is for anyone). It is important to stress to the patient all of the benefits of a regular exercise program. Many patients with arthritis, particularly osteoarthritis, are reluctant to exercise owing to the widely held belief that such activity will hasten the deterioration of the affected joints. As pointed out by Yocum (Chapter 4), the use of appropriate fitness professionals (athletic trainers and physical therapists) with skill in dealing with joint disorders is crucial. These professionals will be able to suggest an exercise program that will reduce direct stress on the joints, while providing benefit to the cardiovascular system, muscles, and bones. Classes also provide the peer-group motivation needed to develop lifelong habits. Finally, adequate pain relief is essential prior to beginning any exercise regimen. In concert with dietary recommendations, exercise offers both physical and psychological benefits for all rheumatology patients.

Integrative medicine is a comprehensive approach to patient care. Although many modalities are employed, the use of **botanicals and dietary supplements** are most frequently identified with the practice. Many of our current pharmaceuticals have been isolated from botanicals, and herbal medicine relies upon the fact that many of these herbs have been safely used for generations. In addition, naturallyrmaceutical therapies or alternative modalities are used. Many of the therapeutic trials described, especially those involving glucosamine and chondroitin sulfate, provide some documentation as to the relative safety of these compounds for chronic use. Empirical evidence from clinical observations may warrant a trial of these agents.

The benefits of **manual medicine** (Chapter 7) in dealing with chronic pain have withstood the test of time in our own clinic. Although they cannot repair joint erosions or regrow cartilage, we find that most patients benefit from gentle osteopathic manipulation, massage therapy, or other manual modalities. We are fortunate to work with Dr. Harmon Myers, an osteopathic physician who has studied and taught the Counterstrain technique for several decades, and who has provided outstanding results (and relief) for our patients. The key in properly using manual medicine in your practice is to find trusted and experienced practitioners. We urge rheumatologists to experience the manual therapies firsthand prior to referring patients.

The field of **Mind-Body Medicine** (MBM) is gaining prominence in conventional medical practices, and is central to the practice of integrative medicine. As more studies are published, more information regarding the central role of the mind in the course of chronic conditions is emerging. The development of psychoneuroimmunology as a distinct discipline is evidence of the strong links between the mind and immune function. Mind-body interventions can be as simple as a breathing exercise, or as complex as a session of hypnotherapy. The techniques can be taught easily and, unlike pharmaceuticals or supplements, are quite affordable. In addition, they are safe to use, with an enviable safety profile. We urge all healthcare practitioners to consider introducing such techniques to their patients with chronic conditions. MBM modalities can greatly affect pain sensation and symptoms, but can also mitigate the immunological effects of inflammation. In Chapter 8, Broderick explores the variety of MBM interventions that have demonstrated efficacy in the care of the patient who is dealing with rheumatological disorders, and why such recommendations should be an integral part of your patient care.

The vast majority of our patients with (and without) rheumatological conditions report sleep disruptions—often severe in nature. This is particularly problematic in patients with fibromyalgia. We typically begin our evaluation with a careful sleep history, then focus our initial efforts upon the restoration of adequate sleep quality. The botanicals and supplements described in Chapter 9 are useful as gentle hypnotics, but are always combined with "sleep hygiene" interventions and mind-body relaxation techniques for maximal effect.

The text then explores various non-Western systems of medicine. **Acupuncture** is one of the oldest systems of medicine still being practiced. As a distinct system of medicine, as opposed to an adjunct therapy, it is difficult to find valid experimental trials comparing it to Western therapies. Further, many published trials are fraught with methodological challenges. In our clinic, we recommend traditional Chinese medicine (TCM) therapy to many patients with rheumatologic conditions—especially (but not limited to) patients with OA. In cases of severe OA, symptomatic control is central, and we have found acupuncture to be very effective in this regard. Any modality that allows the patient to decrease potentially harmful medications, while permitting more activity with less pain, is beneficial. While effectiveness is not guaranteed for all patients, a trial of therapy with a TCM practitioner or medical acupuncturist is always worthwhile. In patients who are unable to tolerate narcotic drugs or NSAIDs, acupuncture provides an important therapeutic alternative. The modality is very well tolerated, and uses an approach that has withstood the test of time. In China, true integration and respect for traditional and Western healing practices routinely occurs.

Energy Medicine, as described by Chiasson (Chapter 11), encompasses many diverse forms of therapy—both hands-on and distance healing. This modality is one of the more difficult ones to explain to a conventional healthcare practitioner. In most cases, the "energy" that is being manipulated is impossible to objectively measure and track. In addition, there are few studies to support its use. In our clinic, we see many patients who report benefits from such therapy. This may be related to an unmeasurable energy that is transferred, or perhaps it is a result of the practitioner's attention and the "laying on of hands" from a caring individual with good intent. In either case, the modality is very safe, has the potential for easing pain and/or anxiety, and is worth considering as adjunctive therapy.

Other approaches are important to learn about, as many patients will be using these as complementary therapies. The **Ayurvedic** approach, used by millions of individuals in India and elsewhere, has been popularized in this country by well-known practitioners, such as Deepak Chopra, MD, and many patients may ask about the suitability for such an approach in the treatment of rheumatological conditions. Chapter 12 provides a rudimentary explanation of the Ayurvedic system and provides guidelines for the rheumatologist who wishes to introduce this approach to patients, or at least to be able to answer questions regarding the Ayurvedic treatment of rheumatological disease.

Homeopathy is one of the oldest forms of medicine practiced in the United States. Until recently, one of our allopathic medical schools bore the name of the father of homeopathy, Samuel Hahnemann. Since the release of the Flexner report in 1910, however, the practice has fallen out of favor among conventional Western practitioners. Few practices of medicine elicit as much controversy and vitriol as that of homeopathy. In Chapter 13, Bell, an allopathic and homeopathic physician and researcher, presents many cogent arguments for reconsidering the use of homeopathy in patients with rheumatological conditions. An overwhelmingly positive safety profile combined with a high degree of patient satisfaction and clinical improvement, especially among patients with hard-to-treat conditions (e.g., fibromyalgia), makes this choice a viable option for many patients.

The text closes by exploring the use of Integrative modalities in the care of specific clinical conditions, including osteoarthritis (OA), rheumatoid arthritis (RA), fibromyalgia, and systemic lupus erythematosus (SLE). In addition, we address the special concerns of the pediatric rheumatology patient. These chapters are authored by respected rheumatologists, and provide guidelines and evidence for the incorporation of complementary therapies into the care plans for patients dealing with these conditions. The amount of research performed often relates to the prevalence of the condition. For example, existing literature tells us that many patients with SLE are using complementary and alternative treatments. Unfortunately, except for a few studies with DHEA, there is little or no published research to support the use of these therapies. We have to remember that there are 10-fold fewer patients with SLE compared to those with rheumatoid arthritis, which is about 1% of the population. This relative scarcity of patients makes studies more difficult to perform. Nonetheless, we can use our rational as well as intuitive skills and apply a range of integrative methods to SLE. Just as in rheumatoid arthritis, we do not want to forego the lifesaving allopathic treatments. Yet, just as we use similar allopathic treatments for both rheumatoid arthritis and SLE, we can use anti-inflammatory supplements, herbals, and mind-body techniques for patients with SLE.

Finally, of all demographic groups that suffer from rheumatological conditions, none deserves more attention than the pediatric patient. Potentially life-threatening therapies are used chronically, and for more years in the young person with arthralgias and chronic pain. It behooves the pediatric rheumatologist to investigate every and all potential therapeutic interventions in an attempt to avoid the long-term complications commonly seen with the use of conventional pharmacotherapy. Any intervention that will help control pain and allow for a dose reduction in analgesic and immunosuppressive therapy should be viewed as beneficial. Often, potent therapy is required to control acute flares; however, during periods of quiescence, other modalities (such as acupuncture or mind-body relaxation interventions) should be used to safely allow reduction of standard therapies to the lowest possible dosages.

This text is to inform, and hopefully to stimulate the clinician to investigate aspects of care that are usually not emphasized during a conventional residency and fellowship. Patients are seeking effective yet safe therapies for chronic conditions that they will be dealing with for many years. Many are not willing to risk the rarer complications of many therapies, which include overwhelming infections and perhaps even malignancies. Many of the approaches discussed in this book can be used in concert with conventional therapies in order to provide symptomatic relief, and hopefully a more quiescent disease course.

Randy Horwitz, MD, PhD

CONTENTS

FOREWORD I

Rheumatological disorders all but call out for integrative medical management. They are systemic diseases, whose course and severity are strongly affected by diet and other aspects of lifestyle. They have a high potential for remission, even for complete disappearance. Their ups and downs often correlate with mental/emotional changes. Many of us have seen the first sudden appearance of rheumatoid arthritis in young women who are in the midst of emotional trauma. I have seen several cases of systemic lupus erythematosus go into complete remission when patients fell in love. (I wish I could arrange for more patients to fall in love.)

Conventional treatment for these disorders is suppressive, not curative, and the powerful drugs used often produce serious side effects; moreover, suppression of autoimmune inflammatory conditions may decrease the probability of remission. Conventional treatment is absolutely necessary to deal with severe exacerbations. The challenge is to keep the disease process under control without creating long-term dependence on suppressive drugs.

In fact, there are many strategies for managing these disorders. Because inappropriate inflammation is responsible for the pain and tissue damage associated with them, it is important to teach patients how dietary choices affect inflammatory status. Simply following an anti-inflammatory diet—not onerous, since it is based on the Mediterranean diet—may enable many to use lower doses of less toxic medication. Additional benefit may result from adding natural products with significant anti-inflammatory effects (ginger and turmeric, for example).

The mind/body interactions that are so evident in rheumatological disorders can be turned to advantage with simple, inexpensive, low-tech interventions like journaling, hypnosis, guided imagery, breath work, and mindfulness training. My colleagues and I have seen good results in patients who have worked with practitioners of Chinese medicine and Ayurvedic medicine, whole systems that rely on dietary change, botanical remedies, body and energy work, and specialized techniques like acupuncture. Usually, the patients were under the care of rheumatologists as well; lucky ones worked with rheumatologists open to integrative treatment.

Although I am trained and licensed as a general practitioner, I hold an endowed chair in Integrative Rheumatology at the University of Arizona, where I also direct the Arizona Center for Integrative Medicine (AzCIM). In these positions, I am working with my colleagues to develop a robust field of integrative rheumatology. AzCIM counts several rheumatologists among our graduate fellows, offers scholarships for rheumatologists, and is designing a specialized curriculum in integrative rheumatology.

Sadly, rheumatology has been one of the more resistant specialties to the growing influence of integrative medicine, probably because it has stronger ties to the basic sciences than other medical specialties, and takes on their prejudices against complementary and alternative therapies, tending to dismiss them as "unscientific." I hope this attitude will soon be gone, because it weakens clinical practice and impedes patients from receiving optimum care. Too often today, patients are offered only the narrow treatment options of conventional medicine and get no support, or worse, when they inquire about other therapeutic options.

Publication of this volume is a big step in the right direction. Drs. Horwitz and Muller have drawn on the expertise of diverse contributors to compile a wealth of practical information about the integrative management of rheumatological disease, and the benefits and limitations of therapeutic approaches not currently included in medical school curriculums, residencies, and fellowship training. I am confident that *Integrative Rheumatology* will help clinicians expand and enhance their practices, and ultimately enable more patients to receive optimum care.

Andrew Weil, MD
Series Editor
Tucson, Arizona

FOREWORD II

"Cure when possible, but care, always" is an important tenet of medicine but, unfortunately, it is more and more a remnant of the past. Just as society has become enamored of the 15-second sound bite, medicine is often focused on quick fixes for long-term problems. Ongoing relationships between patients and their physicians, and continuity of care, are less and less frequently seen in health care today. The emphasis on technical solutions for acute episodes of long-term disease has brought our health care system close to financial collapse, and has resulted in an ineffective approach to the bane of our nation's health—chronic disease that is ineffectively prevented and inefficiently cared for, despite our ability to do far better.

During the past decade, rheumatology has developed and incorporated powerful therapeutics to modify potentially life-threatening or crippling diseases. Nonetheless, even with the best our specialty has to offer, we rarely cure. Rheumatic diseases, by their nature, are almost always chronic, debilitating, and painful. The responsibility of our specialty is to abate or minimize rheumatic disease, while enhancing our patient's quality of life regardless of the level of ongoing disease or disability. Unfortunately, as in all other areas of medicine, rheumatologists' approach to patients is more often directed to using the newest therapies to modify the disease, while overlooking the broad needs of the person they are treating. The modalities needed to specifically inhibit the joint-destructive processes of rheumatoid arthritis are clearly different than those needed to allow a patient with rheumatic arthritis to lead a good life. The latter is benefited, of course, by disease ameliorating therapies, but more is required. Additionally, the approaches needed to improve the quality of life are far more heterogeneous and individualized than those needed to alter the pathogenesis of the disease. For this reason, I have become a strong advocate of integrative medicine in general and, as a component of it, integrative rheumatology.

In my view, integrative medicine is an approach to the delivery of health care which draws upon the best of the scientific approach to medicine, but refocuses on:

- The responsibility of the provider to partner with the patient to improve the latter's health, recognizing the comprehensive and ongoing nature of health care;
- the importance of compassion and caring;
- the willingness to entertain nonconventional modalities with scientific evaluation; and
- the recognition of the importance of the mind-body relationship in wellbeing.

Above all, integrative medicine encompasses the long-term caring bond between the patient and the caregiver, and the responsibility of the latter to enable the patient to benefit from the full array of modalities which can be shown to improve health.

Integrative Rheumatology provides a comprehensive overview of approaches that can potentially benefit the millions who suffer with rheumatic diseases. Clearly, integrative strategies are requisite for the best treatment of chronic illnesses. Hopefully, the integrative approaches described herein will soon become part of the routine practice of rheumatology. Integrative approaches, when applied to rheumatology, assume that patients will be afforded the best proven therapies to modify the disease progress and relieve pain and disability. In addition to standard approaches, however, the integrative rheumatologist believes and commits to being the patient's mentor and partner, and to providing access to complementary and alternative therapies which are known to be helpful and otherwise harmless. While understanding the importance of science and the clinical evidence of its benefit, the integrative rheumatologist should have the humility needed to understand that many beneficial therapies began as unproven remedies. He or she will also understand the power of the patient's capacity to heal themselves, and the importance of hope and empowerment in coping with serious illness. The partnership of the rheumatologist with the patient to attain these ends forges a powerful bond, too often missing in today's medical practice. Such approaches are not only likely to achieve better clinical outcome, but they will assure greater satisfaction and feelings of accomplishment on the part of both the physician and the patient. Delivering compassionate care is deeply rewarding for the physician, who is often inundated by the otherwise tedious burdens of their practice. Some will say integrative rheumatology is nothing more than what conventional rheumatology should be. To this I say amen! Hopefully this will soon be the case.

Ralph Snyderman MD
Chancellor Emeritus
James B Duke Professor of Medicne
Duke University

CONTRIBUTORS

Paul D. Abramson, MD
Medical Director at My Doctor Medical Group
Clinical Faculty at University of California, San Francisco
Medical Staff, Hospitalist at California Pacific Medical Center
San Francisco, CA

Iris R. Bell, MD, MD(H), PhD
Professor
Departments of Family and Community Medicine, Psychiatry, Psychology, Medicine, and Public Health
College of Medicine
University of Arizona
Tucson, AZ

Joan E. Broderick, PhD
Associate Professor
Department of Psychiatry and Behavioral Science
Stony Brook University
Stony Brook, NY

Philip C. Calder, PhD
Institute of Human Nutrition
School of Medicine
University of Southampton
United Kingdom

Ann Marie Chiasson, MD, MPH
Clinical Assistant Professor
Arizona Center for Integrative Medicine
University of Arizona
Medical Director, The Haven, Addiction Recovery for Women
Tucson, AZ

Karen M. Cooper, RN, BSN, MA
Izumi Joi, LLC
Triage Nurse, Group Health Cooperative
Madison, WI

Randy Horwitz, MD, PhD
Medical Director,
Arizona Center for Integrative Medicine
Assistant Professor of Clinical Medicine
University of Arizona
College of Medicine

Julia B. Jernberg, MD
Clinical Assistant Professor of Medicine
University of Wisconsin School of Medicine and Public Health
Madison, WI

Kathleen Johnson, MS, RD
Nutrition Consultant
Tucson, AZ

Doerte U. Junghaenel, PhD
Assistant Professor of Psychiatry
Department of Psychiatry and Behavioral Science
Stony Brook University
Stony Brook, NY

Sharon L. Kolasinski, MD
Professor of Clinical Medicine
Division of Rheumatology
University of Pennsylvania
Philadelphia, PA

George Lewith, MA, MD, FRCP, MRCGP
Professor of Health Research
Complementary and Integrated Medicine Research Unit
University of Southampton
United Kingdom

Tieraona Low Dog, MD
Fellowship Director,
Arizona Center for Integrative Medicine
Clinical Associate Professor of Medicine
University of Arizona Health Sciences Center
Tucson, AZ

Nisha Manek, MD, MRCP
Assistant Professor
Department of Medicine
Division of Rheumatology
Mayo Clinic
Rochester, MN

Daniel Muller, MD, PhD
Associate Professor of Medicine
Section of Rheumatology
University of Wisconsin School of Medicine and Public Health
Madison, WI

Rubin R. Naiman, PhD
Director of Circadian Health Associates
Sleep Specialist and Clinical Assistant Professor of Medicine
Center for Integrative Medicine
University of Arizona
Tucson, AZ

Michelle Petri, MD, MPH
Professor
Division of Rheumatology
Department of Medicine
Co-Director
Hopkins Lupus Pregnancy Center
Johns Hopkins University
Baltimore, MD

Deborah Jane Power, DO
Physician
Catalina Pointe
Arthritis and Rheumatology Specialists, PC
Tucson, AZ

Anastasia Rowland-Seymour, MD
Assistant Professor of Medicine
Division of General Internal Medicine
Department of Medicine
Johns Hopkins University
Baltimore, MD

Nancy J. Selfridge, MD
Associate Professor
Department of Integrative Medicine
Ross University School of Medicine
Freeport, Grand Bahama

Malynn Utzinger, MA, MD
Assistant Clinical Professor
Department of Family Medicine
University of Wisconsin
Founder, LifeWorks Integral and Doctor Malynn
Madison, WI

Peter White, PhD, BSc, MCSP
School of Health Sciences
University of Southampton
United Kingdom

David E. Yocum, MD
Adjunct Clinical Professor of Medicine
Stanford University Medical Center
Senior Director
US Head of Safety
Global Safety Head, Inflammation and Ophthalmology
Genentech, Inc.
South San Francisco, CA

Integrative Rheumatology

1

The Use of CAM Therapies in Integrative Rheumatology

DANIEL MULLER, MD, PhD

What are complementary and alternative medicine (CAM) therapies? Usually we think of these in the negative; i.e., whatever is not allopathic, or conventional, therapy. However, as soon as we start using these therapies in the majority of conventional practices, do they then become allopathic? Perhaps we can consider only those therapies that are not paid for by insurance companies. However, that also is a moving target, since many of these therapies are indeed paid for by third-party payers, depending on what company is involved. So maybe we just have to use that apocryphal remark by Justice Potter Stewart about pornography: "I can't define it, but I know it when I see it."

When we practice integrative rheumatology we use the science and art of medicine to help the patient, without regard for labels such as "allopathic," "conventional," or "CAM." In these chapters you will find recommendations for therapy that are, more often than not, supported by traditional scientific double-blinded studies. On other occasions, recommendations will be put forth that enjoy less support from traditional scientific investigations. In all cases the practitioner needs to weigh the risks, potential benefits, and economics of any therapeutic modality.

We traditionally regard the "placebo effect" with disdain. Perhaps we need to redefine this placebo effect as the "activation of the natural healing powers" of an individual, with part of our job being to find the best ways to stimulate this healing. Barrett and colleagues proposed eight specific clinical actions: speak positively about treatments, provide encouragement, develop trust, provide reassurance, support relationships, respect uniqueness, explore values, and create ceremony.[1] To support these recommendations, a recent article directly relates practitioner empathy to decreases in duration of the common cold, and to salutary immune activity.[2]

On the other hand, we also cannot be complacent about the possible risks of CAM therapies. Supplements and herbals from Third World countries have been contaminated by heavy metals. Domestic preparations have been found to have too much or too little of the proposed therapeutic agent. Some CAM practitioners may not be competent. By the same token, there are many allopathic practitioners of borderline competence, and more patients have been hurt by allopathic medications than by CAM supplements and herbals.

As a practitioner, you will decide at what level you will use whatever you identify as CAM therapies. At the most basic level, you will know enough to discuss what the patient is using and make recommendations about possible risks and benefits. At the next level, you will work with CAM practitioners either as outside referrals or directly within your office. Finally, you might choose to learn some of these modalities and use them in your practice. Perhaps you might learn guided visualization or acupuncture, while also realizing that just because you are skilled in that modality, not every patient may be a candidate.

Here is a broad list of recommendations that I think about when a patient enters my clinic, all discussed further in individual chapters:

Mind/Meditation

1. Breath exercises, relaxation, mindfulness, paying attention
2. See the big picture, reduce "reactivity"
3. Learn your personality type, get into balance
4. *Metta, tonglen*, any form of prayer
5. Creativity
6. Laughter

Body/Diet

1. Healthy high-fiber fillers – grapefruit, carrots, celery, green lettuces
2. Good quality protein – nuts, fish, beans – especially needed with exercise
3. Low-glycemic carbohydrates, no high-fructose corn syrup
4. Good fats, reduce transfats (no partially hydrogenated oils)
5. Supplements – Calcium, Magnesium, Selenium, Zinc, Omega-3-FA, Vitamins C, D, E

Body/Exercise

1. Aerobic
2. Strength – light weights, high repetition
3. Stretching

4. CORE exercises – abdominal and back
5. Combinations of meditation and exercise – Eastern (yoga, tai chi) and Western (Alexander, Feldenkrais)
6. Walk in nature

Spirit/Next Steps

1. Your job – right work, do no harm
2. Your relationships – play with positive people, avoid abusers
3. Find hope, meaning, purpose – volunteer

Treatment/CAM

1. Passive methods – massage, acupuncture, herbals
2. Psychotherapy – deal with the shadow (what do you dislike or hate?)
3. Guided imagery
4. Eye-movement desensitization and reprocessing, emotional freedom technique

REFERENCES

1. Barrett B, Muller D, Rakel D, Rabago D, Marchand L, Scheder J. Placebo, meaning, and health. *Perspect Biol Med.* 2006;49(2):178–198.
2. Rakel D, Hoeft T, Barrett B, Chewning B, Craig B, Niu M. Practitioner empathy and the duration of the common cold. *Fam Med.* 2009;41(7):494–501.

2

Nutritional Interventions in Rheumatology

KATHLEEN JOHNSON, MS, RD

KEY CONCEPTS

- The primary effect of diet and nutrition on rheumatic diseases is on the inflammatory process.
- Intestinal inflammation increases intestinal permeability, which is associated with the systemic inflammation of some rheumatic diseases. Plant-based, dairy and gluten-free diets that are individualized for other food sensitivities are often effective in improving the state of rheumatoid arthritis.
- The Mediterranean diet pattern includes most of the nutritional factors described in the anti-inflammatory diet, has been associated with reduced risk of rheumatoid arthritis, and has been used to treat rheumatoid arthritis.
- Increasing omega-3 fatty acids, particularly EPA and DHA, is the most globally effective single nutritional strategy for rheumatic diseases, having a measurable impact on inflammation.
- Many of the dietary strategies used with rheumatic diseases are complicated. Patients may benefit from consultation with a professional nutritionist familiar with these concepts to clarify food choices and help plan meals.

■

Introduction

It is not surprising that a variety of nutritional and dietary interventions have been explored for the complex array of rheumatologic diseases; these have met with varying degrees of success. Some rheumatic conditions are common: symptoms of arthritis affect many adults. A recent study on food and health trends found that one-third of Americans report that someone in their household is trying to manage or treat arthritis or joint pain.[1] In a recent Finnish study, 40% of female patients diagnosed with rheumatoid arthritis believed diet contributed to their disease and 51% tried dietary changes to treat their disease after diagnosis.[2]

The complex disease processes and etiologies of rheumatic diseases involve inflammation, the autoimmune response, trauma, aging and endocrine dysregulation. The evidence that has accumulated from well-designed trials of nutritional approaches to rheumatological diseases (including rheumatoid arthritis, systemic lupus erythematosus, ankylosing spondylitis, osteoarthritis, and fibromyalgia) has helped further an understanding of these processes.

Although some rheumatic diseases are considered to be noninflammatory, inflammation is a predominant feature in most. Even fibromyalgia, not generally considered an inflammatory disease, is characterized by increased levels of inflammatory mediators.

The primary effect of nutrition and diet on rheumatic diseases is seen in the inflammatory process. The nutritional and dietary factors involved in these diseases will be discussed here, along with descriptions of the most effective interventions.

Inflammation, Immune Function, and the Gut

The inflammatory processes that are characteristic of many rheumatic diseases may begin in the digestive tract.[18] The lining of the gut is the most significant interface between "self" and "non-self" in the body and, as such, is a critical venue for immune activity. Inflammation in the gut, long associated with arthritis,[3] is characterized by increased intestinal permeability, which allows greater migration of food antigens, bacteria, bacterial remnants or other substances into the bloodstream. Rheumatoid arthritis and ankylosing spondylitis have both been associated with increased intestinal permeability.[4] Non-steroidal anti-inflammatory drugs (NSAIDs) are frequently used with rheumatic diseases. Although they block inflammation and ameliorate rheumatic symptoms, they can increase inflammation in the gut.[5]

Decreasing Antigen Load

Various dietary strategies that decrease ingestion of the most common food allergens have been associated with significant improvement in subjective and objective parameters of disease status in patients with rheumatoid arthritis.[6] Improvement has been seen with fasting, elimination diets, and vegetarian diets. The precise mechanisms for the improvements are unknown, but the experience from one Norwegian study has begun to clarify the factors involved.[7]

THE NORWEGIAN STUDY

Patients with rheumatoid arthritis were randomized to either an experimental diet group (N=27) or a control group (N=26). The experimental group was sent to a health farm where they fasted for 7–10 days on a diet of herbal teas, garlic, and vegetable broths and juices. After the fast, subjects received a basic vegan diet consisting of the fasting regimen plus the vegetables used for the broth and juice. New foods consistent with a vegan, gluten-free diet were introduced one at a time, but eliminated permanently if they exacerbated symptoms. The diet also excluded refined sugar, salt, alcohol, citrus fruit, tea, coffee and preservatives. This individualized diet was followed for three and a half months, after which a lactovegetarian diet was begun. Milk, other dairy products, and gluten-containing foods were introduced, again being eliminated if they caused symptoms. The resulting individualized diet was followed for an additional eight months. Members of the control group followed their own typical diets for the course of the trial.

Individuals in the experimental group were classified as either diet responders (12 of 27) or non-responders, on the basis of improvement in disease parameters. Several observations from the study are notable. A range of antibodies against food antigens was measured, but, interestingly, there was no correlation with the foods that caused symptoms for the responders. Fatty acid levels, which might also influence inflammation, were not different between responders and non-responders, nor was weight change different between responders and non-responders. However, two differences between the groups were noted. The first was that although compliance is a common problem in similar intervention studies, a year after the completion of the study, all of the responders had elected to continue the diet. Secondly, antibody activity against

Proteus mirabilis was found in all subjects, but decreased significantly only in the diet responders. This may indicate a role of intestinal flora in dietary control of rheumatoid arthritis symptoms.

Intestinal Microflora

Antibodies against *Proteus mirabilis* have been documented in rheumatoid arthritis patients in many other studies.[8–10] *Proteus* spp. are a normal component of intestinal microflora and are often implicated in urinary tract infections. An amino acid sequence found on the surface membrane of the bacteria closely resembles a sequence on the b-chain of the human leukocyte antigen (HLA) DR1 molecule and on the HLA–DR4 subtypes, which are both associated with rheumatoid arthritis.[11] Higher autoantibody titers against both haplotypes have been documented in patients with rheumatoid arthritis relative to controls.[12] Controversy continues in the literature over whether or not the presence of anti-*Proteus* antibodies influences the disease process in rheumatological conditions.

Also of interest is the coexistence of small intestine bacterial overgrowth (SIBO) as well as irritable bowel syndrome (IBS) in individuals with fibromyalgia.[13] SIBO refers to the migration of large intestine bacteria into the small intestine, leading to inflammation and increased permeability. In two clinical trials, patients with fibromyalgia improved on a "living" or raw diet rich in lactobacilli.[14,15] Although no trials to date have studied food allergies and fibromyalgia, patients with irritable bowel syndrome have shown improvement with an elimination diet.[16]

Higher levels of antibodies to *Klebsiella* strains have been found in patients with ankylosing spondylitis compared to controls,[17] raising the possibility that bacteria-specific immune responses may play a role in the pathogenesis of many rheumatological conditions. More research is needed before this can be substantiated, however.

OTHER DIET TRIALS

Other experimental diet trials in patients with rheumatoid arthritis have used a variety of specialized diets, including: elemental diets containing no whole proteins; a restricted elimination diet; a vegan, gluten-free diet; a raw vegan diet rich in *lactobacilli*; and fasting followed by a lactovegetarian diet. These studies were of much shorter duration than the Norwegian study, lasting from 2 weeks to 24 weeks and resulting in varying degrees of improvement in disease status.[14,18–25] In general, treatment groups improved more than placebo groups, but not all subjects in treatment groups responded similarly. In addition, several case reports in the literature demonstrate improvement in individual patients with rheumatoid arthritis when specific foods were eliminated based upon a positive IgE or IgG antibody titer.[6]

The important question that arises from these studies is whether positive results are due to eliminating specific food antigens, or from attenuating the inflammation and increased intestinal permeability that might be secondary to dysbiosis or antigenic load. The latter explanation is favored, although other explanations are considered, such as bowel improvement secondary to reduced disease activity.[7] Continued research will help clarify this question.

As an example, in a recent trial, patients with either rheumatoid arthritis or fibromyalgia were assigned to either a Mediterranean diet or a modified fast regimen. Fasting resulted in improvements with both groups, but was more significant for those with rheumatoid arthritis.[26] Intestinal flora was unchanged for both groups. Of note, neither intervention limited dairy and gluten.

The results of these experimental approaches are compelling, but compliance with the complicated and restricted diets is an issue for patients. Nonetheless, some version of a vegetarian and gluten/dairy-free diet with a lead-in period of fasting should be considered.

Finally, the use of probiotic supplementation is worth considering. Probiotics are live, nonpathogenic microorganism that have the potential to change the balance of microflora in the intestinal tract. Dysbiosis, an imbalance of intestinal microflora, can affect localized immune reactions and inflammation

Table 2.1.

Gluten-free grains	*Gluten-containing grains*
Oats (if labeled "certified gluten-free")	Wheat
Rice	Spelt or farro
Wild rice	Triticale
Millet	Kamut
Quinoa	Barley
Buckwheat	Rye
Amaranth	
Corn	

in the gut, as well as intestinal permeability. Increased intestinal permeability is thought to influence the systemic inflammation of some rheumatic diseases. Clinical trials generally use specific strains or combinations of bacteria and/or yeast. Not all strains have the same effects on all conditions. General recommendations for practitioners interested in recommending probiotics include researching the strains used in treating specific diseases, and choosing brands with greater than 1 billion Colony Forming Units or CFU's from a reputable company.

Treating Inflammation with Nutrients

The addition of "anti-inflammatory nutrients," which act through mechanisms similar to medications such as NSAIDs and cortisol, is also an effective intervention. These dietary additions include fatty acids, vitamins E, B6 and D, flavonoids, and those dietary factors that influence blood sugar levels and insulin sensitivity. A closer examination of these nutrients will allow the practitioner to make specific, evidence based dietary recommendations.

FATTY ACIDS

The influence of dietary fatty acids on rheumatic diseases is represented in a large body of published evidence. Fatty acids in the omega-6 and omega-3 families play primary roles in inflammation, and are discussed in detail in Chapter 3.

Table 2.2.

The anti-inflammatory diet
Increase
Omega-3 fatty acids, especially EPA and DHA
GLA
Dietary flavonoids
Vitamin E (especially gamma-tocopherol)
Anti-inflammatory spices - ginger, turmeric
Low glycemic index
Reduce
Linoleic acid
Arachidonic acid
Trans fats

The proportion of fatty acids present in adipose tissue and in cell membrane phospholipids reflects, in a broad way, the proportions in the diet.[27] Their influence on inflammatory processes arises from their presence in the cell membranes of immune cells, where they influence physical characteristics of the membrane such as fluidity and thickness, function as ligands for various nuclear receptors that regulate gene expression, and serve as substrates for the production of eicosanoids.

Omega-6 Fatty Acids

The omega-6 (n-6) family of polyunsaturated fatty acids (PUFAs) is the most predominant type of fatty acid in the human diet. The dietary n-6 fatty acids of most interest are the 18:2 linoleic acid (LA), the 18:3 gamma-linolenic acid (GLA), and the 20:4 arachidonic acid (ARA). LA is very common in the Western diet, and is found in seed oils such as corn, safflower, and sunflower, as well as whole grains.[28] GLA occurs naturally in the oils of evening primrose, borage, and blackcurrant, and as such is primarily consumed as a dietary supplement. ARA is found in animal products and is most abundant in beef from cattle fed a diet of grain, and in conventionally produced eggs.

In general, the eicosanoids produced from ARA are proinflammatory and stimulate the production of the inflammatory cytokines, chiefly TNF-a and interleukin-1b. The n-6 family of fatty acids does have some anti-inflammatory activity as well. The eicosanoids synthesized from di-homo-gamma-linolenic acid, a metabolite of GLA, have anti-inflammatory effects that are well documented.[29–31] Lipoxins synthesized from ARA have anti-inflammatory effects and play a role in the resolution of inflammation.[32]

Omega-3 Fatty Acids

The omega-3 (n-3) family of PUFAs is less plentiful in a typical Western diet than the n-6 family. The dietary n-3 fatty acids of interest are the 18:3 alpha-linolenic acid (ALA), the 20:5 eicosapentaenoic acid (EPA), and the 22:6 docosahexaenoic acid (DHA). ALA is found in flaxseed, flaxseed oil, canola oil, walnuts, walnut oil, soybeans, purslane, and pumpkin seeds. It is also rich in grasses. EPA and DHA are found in algae, fish that feed on algae, and in wild game and livestock that feed on grasses.[33]

The prostaglandins, leukotrienes, and thromboxanes produced from EPA and DHA are not anti-inflammatory *per se*, but exhibit far less potent inflammatory activity than those from ARA. They also reduce inflammatory ARA eicosanoids by competitive substrate binding of the COX 1 and 2 enzymes. Molecules named resolvins and protectins are synthesized from EPA and DHA and demonstrate anti-inflammatory properties.[34]

Healthy adults given supplements of flaxseed oil (rich in ALA) experience an increase in leukocyte EPA and a decrease in inflammatory cytokines.[35] Delta-6-desaturase, the first enzyme in the conversion of the 18-carbon fatty acids to the 20- and 22-carbon fatty acids, however, has variable activity in humans, and is limited in those with rheumatoid arthritis and insulin resistance, so ALA-rich foods are not a reliable way to increase longer-chain fatty acids and decrease inflammation.[36] Stearidonic acid, a 20:5 n-3 fatty acid, occurs downstream of the delta-6-desaturase enzyme, in approximately the same position as GLA. It occurs naturally in echium oil and may be an effective plant-based alternative to EPA and DHA for reducing inflammation.[36] Further details regarding this fatty acid pathway can be found in Chapter 5.

GLA is an n-6 metabolite that occurs downstream of delta-6-desaturase, which, as discussed earlier, is an immediate precursor to a less inflammatory family of eicosanoids. Sources of GLA have been shown to ameliorate symptoms of rheumatoid arthritis. GLA certainly has the potential to be converted to ARA, but an adequate concurrent intake of EPA and DHA appear to prevent that conversion.[37]

Fish oil is the most popular source of n-3 fatty acids in the consumer marketplace. A large number of studies have shown the effectiveness of fish oil supplements in reducing the inflammation and symptoms of rheumatoid arthritis, as well as reducing requirements for NSAIDs.[38] The minimal effective dose is considered to be 2.6–4 gm or more daily of EPA plus DHA.[6] Until recently, intervention studies employed increasing n-3 fatty acid intake against a background of a typical Western diet high in n-6 fatty acids. However, n-3

A very low fat diet (10–25% calories from fat) is not generally recommended to reduce inflammation. A total fat intake of 30–40% of calories is more desirable, but care should be taken in choosing the fats ingested. A very low fat diet will, by definition, be high in protein and/or carbohydrate, and run the risk of worsening either blood sugar control or immune over-stimulation. Healthy oils such as expeller-pressed canola and extra virgin olive (which are relatively low in linoleic acid), mayonnaise and salad dressings made from these oils, as well as nuts and fatty fish are all sources of anti-inflammatory fatty acids. Other nutrients found in these foods include gamma-tocopherol, polyphenols and plant sterols - all beneficial in managing inflammatory disorders.

supplementation seems to be even more effective against a background of low n-6 fatty acid intake.[39]

Supplementation with n-3 fatty acids provides symptomatic relief in patients with systemic lupus erythematosus and ankylosing spondylitis.[40,41] There is also evidence that n-3 fatty acids affect both inflammation and cartilage degradation in patients with osteoarthritis.[42]

DIETARY FLAVONOIDS

Flavonoids are a large family of polyphenolic substances found in plants. There are many categories of flavonoids, including flavanones (citrus bioflavonoids), flavones (quercetin) and flavanols (tea flavonoids). Related polyphenols are also found in extra virgin olive oil. Flavonoids are extremely bioactive and are primarily known for their antioxidant capabilities. In this capacity, they are thought to help protect against the oxidative damage that accompanies inflammation. They are also now recognized for distinct anti-inflammatory properties.[43] Research continues to clarify their roles in a wide range of other cellular functions, including platelet aggregation, the inflammatory cascade, nitric oxide synthesis, inhibiting angiogenesis, inhibiting cell proliferation, stimulating apoptosis, inhibiting mast cell degranulation, and enhancing cP450 enzyme activity in the liver. Flavonoids inhibit the liberation of fatty acids from membrane phospholipids, an initial step in the inflammatory cascade, by inhibiting phospholipase activity.[44] They also protect against cellular damage caused by TNF-alpha.[45]

Consumption of dark cherries by humans, and a polyphenol-enriched virgin olive oil by rats, have both been shown to reduce inflammatory markers of inflammation.[46,47]

Mediterranean diet pattern

The classic Mediterranean diet pattern described frequently in the literature and in clinical trials includes many of the characteristics of the anti-inflammatory diet, including high intake of canola and olive oil, increased fish intake, reduced red meat intake, and increased vegetable and fruit intake with generous intake of flavonoids. It has been associated with reduced risk of rheumatoid arthritis, reduced levels of inflammatory cytokines, and reduced risk of cardiovascular disease—a common risk among patients with rheumatoid arthritis. Remember that a Mediterranean diet pattern needn't include only the foods of the Mediterranean region, but it should focus on the nutritional factors found in those foods.

VITAMIN E

Vitamin E is a potent antioxidant. Studies that have examined the effects of vitamin E supplements on patients with rheumatoid arthritis have generally had mixed results, but have almost exclusively used dl-alpha-tocopherol or d-alpha-tocopherol rather than mixed isomer supplements.[6] One vitamin E isomer, gamma-tocopherol, is capable of potent anti-inflammatory activity by inhibiting cyclooxygenase activity and decreasing proinflammatory eicosanoid production.[48,49] Gamma-tocopherol is the primary form of vitamin E found in foods, and is rich in nuts and unprocessed oils.[50,51] Supplements of alpha-tocopherol, the most common supplemental form, appear to reduce serum gamma-tocopherol levels, an important factor that may account for the limited success of the vitamin E clinical trials that used alpha-tocopherol.[52]

Nutritional Factors Associated with Insulin Resistance

Insulin resistance and the resultant metabolic syndrome and diabetes all result in increased systemic inflammation. All three conditions, as well as hypoglycemia, have been observed in individuals with rheumatoid arthritis, gout and fibromyalgia.[53–55] It is believed that managing serum glucose and insulin levels can help lower inflammation. Several nutritional interventions have been useful in managing insulin resistance by lowering and stabilizing blood sugar levels and improving insulin sensitivity. They include adopting a dietary pattern moderately high in carbohydrates with a focus on low-glycemic index foods, a minimal intake of fructose, avoiding saturated and trans fats, and insuring adequate magnesium intake.[56,57]

Insulin resistance is not only a common comorbidity with rheumatoid arthritis and systemic lupus erythematosus, it is also associated with elevated uric acid levels, and is now thought to be a primary cause of gout. Reducing fructose and sugar-sweetened beverages has been shown to be effective in treating gout.[58]

Nutrients Best Addressed Through Supplementation

Other nutritional factors influencing inflammation lead to recommendations for supplementation. Many of these are detailed in Chapter 6. Vitamin B6 status is independently associated with inflammation, as well as playing a role in hyperhomocysteinemia, a condition that is also associated with inflammation.[59] Elevated homocysteine is also worsened by inadequate folic acid, vitamin B12 (cyanocobalamin), choline and betaine. The dietary pattern described above is rich in all these nutrients, but to insure optimal status, supplementation is recommended.

Inadequate vitamin D intake has recently been associated with increased risk of autoimmune diseases and inflammatory diseases. The most recent discussions of this nutrient suggest that the RDA is insufficient for optimal vitamin D status. The current recommendations suggest 1000–2000 IU of vitamin D daily. This intake is impossible to achieve through food, and requires supplementation. Because environmental and genetic factors influence vitamin D status, measuring serum levels of 25-OH vitamin D may help define which patients will benefit from higher supplemental doses of vitamin D. Currently optimal serum levels of 25-OH-D are thought to be 75–80 nmol/L.[60]

Weight Loss

Weight loss has long been recommended for patients suffering from osteoarthritis, particularly of the knee. The recommendations to exercise and lose weight, however, are infrequently followed.[61] The recent recognition of adipose tissue as an endocrine and inflammatory organ lends more importance to weight loss as a strategy. Not only can loss of adipose tissue reduce inflammatory cytokines, but can also lessen the biomechanical load on arthritic knee joints. Recent trials on weight loss for subjects with osteoarthritis of the knee have found improvement in objective and subjective parameters with as little as 5.7% loss of total body weight.[62,63]

Translating Nutrient Learning into Food Advice

Patients with arthritis are exposed to a great deal of advice in the lay literature about what to eat and what supplements to take. These are often isolated and brief reports on research studies that focus on one food or nutrient. Human nutrition reflects a system of complex interactions, and although much is clarified by double blind, placebo-controlled studies on individual nutrients, the overall effect of a dietary pattern can be more illuminating. Good examples include the Norwegian trial (above), which used an individualized vegetarian diet, and trials using a Mediterranean diet.[7,64,65] Both strategies utilize a combination of factors likely to influence inflammation and disease. The most effective advice for patients, although the most time consuming, is comprehensive and individualized.

To maximize patient compliance, however, the research findings discussed here need to be translated into practical strategies for dietary choices. Additionally, a nutrition professional who understands these principles and has a good knowledge of food and eating behaviors can help patients develop healthy patterns that will be effective and sustainable.

The following practical nutritional guidelines for patients with rheumatological diseases include components from the Mediterranean diet pattern, recommendations for insulin resistance, specific supplement advice inspired by clinical trials, and advice about elimination diets. Remember that any one piece of advice from this list will not be as effective as a pattern established by following most or all of the advice. However, if a patient's ability to make dietary changes is limited, the most effective strategy is probably the addition of omega-3 fatty acids.

DIETARY RECOMMENDATIONS FOR PATIENTS WITH RHEUMATOLOGICAL CONDITIONS

- Consider either an elimination/challenge diet or a gluten and dairy-free diet.
- Focus on a balanced diet rich in plant foods including vegetables, fruits, whole grains, legumes, and nuts.
- Eat two to four servings of coldwater fish (e.g., sardines or salmon) per week. Choose wild-caught salmon when possible. Farmed salmon tends to have less omega-3 fatty acids than wild caught. If eating a vegetarian diet, consider a supplement of long-chain omega-3 fatty acids derived from algae, rather than relying upon other plant sources of omega-3 fatty acids.
- Eat other n-3 rich foods daily - omega-3 eggs, walnuts, flaxseed, and soybeans.
- Use expeller-pressed canola oil and extra virgin olive oil in cooking, food preparation, and as ingredients in mayonnaise and salad dressings. Avoid corn, safflower and sunflower oils.
- Avoid foods with hydrogenated or partially hydrogenated oils as ingredients.
- Avoid or minimize red meat and poultry, but when eaten, choose grass-fed beef, lamb and wild game, rather than conventionally produced beef. Choose eggs laid by hens fed an omega-3 rich diet.

- Choose foods rich in flavonoids every day. Choose from cherries, berries, pomegranates, grapes and other dark red fruits, apples, citrus fruit and juice, onions, dark chocolate and green tea.
- Avoid sugar, sugary foods and beverages, foods with high-fructose corn syrup as a primary ingredient, and high-fructose fruits and juices.
- Choose low-glycemic index carbohydrate rich foods rather than high-glycemic index foods, and whole grains and wholegrain products rather than refined.
- Consider supplements containing GLA—oil of borage, blackcurrant oil, or evening primrose oil.
- Consider supplements containing high gamma-tocopherol vitamin E.
- Consider vitamin B6 (pyridoxine) and vitamin D (cholecalciferol) supplementation.
- Consider a probiotic.

REFERENCES

1. Sloan AE. The top ten functional food trends. *Food Technol.* 2000;54(4):33–62.
2. Salminen E, Heikkila S, Poussa T, Lagstrom H, Saario R, Salminen S. Female patients tend to alter their diet following the diagnosis of rheumatoid arthritis and breast cancer. *Prev Med.* 2002;34(5): 529–535.
3. Rooney PJ, et al. A short review of the relationship between intestinal permeability and inflammatory joint disease. *Clin and Exper Rheumat.* 1990;8:75–83.
4. Smith MD, Gibson RA, Brooks PM. Abnormal bowel permeability in ankylosing spondylitis and rheumatoid arthritis. *J Rheumatol,* 1985;12(2):299–305.
5. Bjarnason I, et al. Intestinal permeability and inflammation in rheumatoid arthritis: effects of non-steroidal anti-inflammatory drugs. *Lancet.* 1984;324(8413): 1171–1173.
6. Stamp KL, James JM, Cleland LG. Diet and rheumatoid arthritis: a review of the literature. *Semin Arthritis and Rheum.* 2005;35(2):77–94.
7. Kjeldsen-Kragh J. Rheumatoid arthritis treated with vegetarian diets. *Am J Clin Nutr.* 1999;70(Suppl):594S–600S.
8. Ebringer A, Ptaszynska T, Corbett M, et al. Antibodies to *proteus* in rheumatoid arthritis. *Lancet.* 1985;2:305–307.
9. Deighton CM, Gray JW, Bint AJ, Walker DJ. Anti-*Proteus* antibodies in rheumatoid arthritis same-sexed sibships. *Br J Rheumatol.* 1992;31:241–245.
10. Rashid T, Ebringer A. Rheumatoid arthritis is linked to Proteus—the evidence. *Clin Rheumatol.* 2007;26(7):1036–1043.
11. Wilson C, Tiwana H, Ebringer A. Molecular mimicry between HLA-DR alleles associated with rheumatoid arthritis and Proteus mirabilis as the aetiological basis for autoimmunity. *Microbes Infect.* 2000;2(12):1489–1496.

12. Rashid T, Jayakumar KS, Binder A, Ellis S, Cunningham P, Ebringer A. Rheumatoid arthritis have elevated antibodies to cross-reactive and non cross-reactive antigens from Proteus microbes. *Clin Exp Rheumatol.* 2007;25(2):259–267.
13. Pimentel M, Wallace D, Hallegua D, Chow E, Kong Y, Park S, Lin HC. A link between irritable bowel syndrome and fibromyalgia may be related to findings on lactulose breath testing. *Ann Rheum Dis.* 2004;63, (4):450–452.
14. Kaartinen K, Lammi K, Hypen M, Nenonen M, Hanninen O, Rauma AL. Vegan diet alleviates fibromyalgia symptoms. *Scand J Rheumatol.* 2000;29(5):308–313.
15. Donaldson MS, Speight N, Loomis S. Fibromyalgia syndrome improved using a mostly raw vegetarian diet an observational study. *BMC Complement Altern Med.* 2001;1:7.
16. Atkinson W, Sheldon TA, Shaath N, Whorwell PJ. Food elimination based on IgG antibodies in irritable bowel syndrome: a randomised controlled trial. *Gut.* 2004;53:1459–1464.
17. Tiwana H, Wilson C, Walmsley RS, Wakefield AJ, Smith MS, Cox NL, Hudson MJ, Ebringer A. Antibody responses to gut bacteria in ankylosing spondylitis, rheumatoid arthritis, Crohn's disease and ulcerative colitis. *Rheumatol Int.* 1997;17(1):11–16.
18. Podas T, Nightingale J, Oldham R, Roy S, Sheehan NJ, Mayberry JF. Is rheumatoid arthritis a disease that starts in the intestine? A pilot study comparing an elemental diet with oral prednisolone. *Postgrad Med J.* 2006;83:128–131.
19. van der Laar MA, van der Korst JK. Food intolerance in rheumatoid arthritis. I. A double blind, controlled trial of the clinical effects of elimination of milk allergens and azo dyes. *Ann Rheum Dis.* 1992;51:298–302.
20. Skoldstam L, Larsson L, Lindstrom F. Effects of fasting and lactovegetarian diet on rheumatoid arthritis. *Scand J Rheumatol.* 1979;8:249–255.
21. Darlington LG, Ramsey NW, Mansfield JR. Placebo-controlled, blind study of dietary manipulation therapy in rheumatoid arthritis. *Lancet.* 1986;327:236–238.
22. Beri D, Malaviya AN, Shandilya R, Singh RR. Effect of dietary restrictions on disease activity in rheumatoid arthritis. *Ann Rheum Dis.* 1988;47:69–72.
23. Hafstrom I, Ringertz B, Spangberg A, von Zweigbergk L, Brannemark S, Nylander I, Ronnelid J, Laasonen L, Klareskog L. A vegan diet free of gluten improves the signs and symptoms of rheumatoid arthritis: the effects on arthritis correlate with a reduction in antibodies to food antigens. *Rheumatology.* 2001;40:1175–1179.
24. Panush R, Carter R, Katz P, Kowsari B, Longley S, Finnie S. Diet therapy for rheumatoid arthritis. *Arthritis Rheum.* 1983;26:462–471.
25. Peltonen R, Nenonen M, Helve T, Hanninen O., Toivanen P, Eerola E. Faecal microbial flora and disease activity in rheumatoid arthritis during a vegan diet. *Br J Rheumatol.* 1997;86:64–68.
26. Michalsen A, Riegert M, Ludtke R, Backer M, Langhorst J, Schwickert M, Dobos GJ. Mediterranean diet or extended fasting's influence on changing the intestinal microflora, immunoglobulin A secretion and clinical outcome in patients with rheumatoid arthritis and fibromyalgia: an observational study. *BMC Complement Altern Med.* 2005;5:22.
27. Arterburn LM, Hall EB, Oken H. Distribution, interconversion, and dose response of n-3 fatty acids in humans. *Am J Clin Nutr.* 2006;83(Suppl),1467S–1476S.

28. Moshregh A, Goldman J, Cleveland L. What we eat in America, NHANES 2001–2002: Usual nutrient intakes from food compared to dietary reference intakes. U.S. Department of Agriculture, Agricultural Research Service; 2005.
29. Levin G, Duffin KL, Obukowicz MG, Hummert SL, Fujiwara H, Needleman P, Raz A. Differential metabolism of dihomo-gamma-linolenic acid and arachidonic acid by cyclo-oxygenase-1 and cyclo-oxygenase-2: implications for cellular synthesis of prostaglandin E1 and prostaglandin E2. *Biochem J.* 2002;365:489–496.
30. Belch JJF, Hill A. Evening primrose oil and borage oil in rheumatologic conditions. *Am J Clin Nutr.* 2000;71(Suppl):352S–356S.
31. Johnson MM, Swan DD, Surette ME, Stegner J, Chilton T, Fonteh AN, Chilton FH. Dietary supplementation with gamma-linolenic acid alters fatty acid content and eicosanoid production in healthy humans. *J Nutr.* 1997;127(8):1435–1444.
32. Calder PC. (2006). n-3 Polyunsaturated fatty acids, inflammation, and inflammatory diseases. *Am J Clin Nutr.* 83(Suppl):1505S–1519S.
33. Knight TW, Knowles S, Death AF, West J, Agnew M, Morris CA, Purchas RW. Factors affecting the variation in fatty acid concentrations in lean beef from grass-fed cattle in New Zealand and the implications for human health. *New Zealand J of Ag Research.* 2003;46:83–95.
34. Yacoubian S, Serhan CN. New endogenous anti-inflammatory and proresolving lipid mediators: implications for rheumatic diseases. *Nat Clin Pract Rheumatol.* 2007;3(10):570–579.
35. James MJ, Gibson RA, Cleland LG. Dietary polyunsaturated fatty acids and inflammatory mediator production. *Am J Clin Nutr.* 2000;71(Suppl):343S–348S.
36. Chilton FH, Rudel LL, Parks JS, Arm JP, Seeds MC. Mechanisms by which botanical lipids affect inflammatory disorders. *Am J Clin Nutr.* 2008;87(Suppl): 498S–503S.
37. Barham JB, Edens MB, Fonteh AN, Johnson MM, Easter L, Chilton FH. Addition of eicosapentaenoic acid to gamma-linolenic acid-supplemented diets prevents serum arachidonic acid accumulation in humans. *J Nutr.* 2000;130(8):1925–1931.
38. Kremer JM. (2000). n-3 fatty acids supplements in rheumatoid arthritis. *Am J Clin Nutr.* 71 (Suppl): 349S–351S.
39. Adam O, Beringer C, Kless T, Lemmen C, Adam A, Wiseman M, Adam P, Klimmek R, Forth W. Anti-inflammatory effects of a low arachidonic acid diet and fish oil in patients with rheumatoid arthritis. *Rheumatol Int.* 2003;23(1):27–36.
40. Simopoulos AP. (2002). Omega-3 fatty acids in inflammation and autoimmune diseases. *J Am Coll Nutr.* 21(6): 495–505.
41. Sundstrom B, Stainacke K, Hagfors L, Johansson G. Supplementation of omega-3 fatty acids in patients with ankylosing spondylitis. *Scand J Rheumatol.* 2006;35(5):359–362.
42. Curtis CL, Rees SG, Cramp J, Flannery CR, Hughes CE, Little CB, Williams R, Wilson C, Dent CM, Harwood JL, Caterson B. Effects of n-3 fatty acids on cartilage metabolism. *Proc Nutr Soc.* 2002;61(3):381–389.
43. González-Gallego J, Sánchez-Campos S, Tuñón MJ. Anti-inflammatory properties of dietary flavonoids. *Nutr Hosp.* 2007;22(3):287–293.
44. Lattig J, Bohl M, Fischer P, Tischer S, Tietbohl C, Menschikowski M, Gutzeit, Metz P, Pisabarro MT. Mechanism of inhibition of human secretory phospholipase

A2 by flavonoids: rationale for lead design. *J Comput Aided Mol Des.* 2007;21(8): 473–483.

45. Kumazawa Y, Kawaguchi K, Takimoto H. Immunomodulating effects of flavonoids on acute and chronic inflammatory responses caused by tumor necrosis factor alpha. *Curr Pharm Des.* 2006;12(32):4271–4279.
46. Kelly DS. Consumption of bing cherries lowers circulating concentrations of inflammation markers in healthy men and women. *J Nutr.* 2006;136(4):981–986.
47. Martinez-Dominguez E, de la Puerta R, Ruiz-Gutierrez V. Protective effects upon experimental inflammation models of a polyphenol-supplemented virgin olive oil diet. *Inflamm Res.* 2001;50(2):102–106.
48. Jiang Q, Elson-Schwab I, Courtemanche C, Ames BN. Gamma-tocopherol and its major metabolite, in contrast to alpha-tocopherol, inhibit cyclooxygenase activity in macrophages and epithelial cells. *Proc Natl Acad Sci USA.* 2000;97(21): 11494–11499.
49. Jiang Q, Ames BN. Gamma-tocopherol, but not alpha-tocopherol, decreases proinflammatory eicosanoids and inflammation damage in rats. *FASEB J.* 2003; 17(8): 816–822.
50. Fan Y, Chapkin RS. Importance of dietary gamma-linolenic acid in human health and nutrition. *J Nutr.* 1998;128(9):1411–1414.
51. Jiang Q, Christen S, Shigenaga MK, Ames BN. Gamma-tocopherol, the major form of vitamin E in the US diet, deserves more attention. *Am J Clin Nutr.* 2001;74:714–722.
52. Huang HY, Appel LJ. Supplementation of diets with alpha-tocopherol reduces serum concentrations of gamma- and delta-tocopherol in humans. *J Nutr.* 2003; 133(10):3137–3140.
53. Karvounaris SA, Sidiropoulos PI, Papadakis JA, Spanakis EK, Bertsias GK, Kritikos HD, Ganotakis ES, Boumpas DT. Metabolic syndrome is common among middle-to-older aged Mediterranean patients with rheumatoid arthritis and correlates with disease activity: a retrospective, cross-sectional, controlled study. *Ann Rheum Dis.* 2007;66:28–33.
54. Choi HK, Ford ES, Li C, Curhan G. Prevalence of the metabolic syndrome in patients with gout: the Third National Health and Nutrition Examination Survey. *Arthritis Rheum.* 2007;15(1):109–115.
55. Buskila D. Fibromyalgia, chronic fatigue syndrome, and myofascial pain syndrome. *Curr Opin Rheumatol.* 2000;12(2):113–123.
56. Bulló M, Casas-Agustench P, Amigó-Correig P, Aranceta J, Salas-Salvadó J. Inflammation, obesity and comorbidities: the role of diet. *Public Health Nutr.* 2007; 10(10A):1164–1172.
57. Riccardi G, Rivellese AA, Giacco R. Role of glycemic index and glycemic load in the healthy state, in prediabetes, and in diabetes. *Am J Clin Nutr.* 2008;87(1): 269S–274S.
58. Choi HK, Curhan G. Soft drinks, fructose consumption, and the risk of gout in men: prospective cohort study. *BMJ.* 2008;336(7639):3099–12.
59. Friso S, Jacques PF, Wilson PW, Rosenberg IH, Selhub J. Low circulating vitamin B(6) is associated with elevation of the inflammation marker C-reactive protein independently of plasma homocysteine levels. *Circulation.* 2001;103(23):2788–2791.

60. Nieves JW. Osteoporosis: the role of micronutrients. *Am J Clin Nutr.* 2005;81(Suppl): 1232S–1239S.
61. Porcheret M, Jordan K, Jinks C, Croft P. Primary care treatment of knee pain—a survey in older adults. *Rheumatology.* 2007;46(11):1694–1700.
62. Miller GD, Nicklas BJ, Davis C, Loeser RF, Lenchik L, Messier SP. Intensive weight loss program improves physical function in older obese adults with knee osteoarthritis. *Obesity.* 2006;14(7):1219–1230.
63. Christensen R, Bartels EM, Astrup A, Bliddal H. Effect of weight reduction in obese patients diagnosed with knee osteoarthritis: a systematic review and meta-analysis. *Ann Rheum Dis.* 2007;66(4):433–439.
64. McKellar G, Morrison E, McEntegart A, Hampson R, Tierney A, Mackle G, Scoular J, Scott JA, Capell HA. A pilot study of a Mediterranean-type diet intervention in female patients with rheumatoid arthritis living in areas of social deprivation in Glasgow. *Ann Rheum Dis.* 2007;66(9):1239–43.
65. Choi HK. Dietary risk factors for rheumatic diseases. *Curr Opin Rheumatol.* 2005;17:141–146.

3

Polyunsaturated Fatty Acids, Inflammatory Processes and Rheumatoid Arthritis

PHILLIP C. CALDER, PhD

KEY CONCEPTS

- There is a shorthand notation that describes the structural characteristics of fatty acids. This allows grouping of fatty acids into families and aids understanding of their metabolism, their relationships with one another, and of their biological functions
- There are two main families of polyunsaturated fatty acids (PUFAs): the omega-6 (or n-6) and the omega-3 (or n-3) families. The simplest members of these families are found in foods of plant origin like seed oils, nuts, and green tissues. In most Western diets, the intake of n-6 PUFAs is greater than that of n-3 PUFAs. The simple n-6 and n-3 PUFAs can be metabolized to more complex derivatives, which have biological activity.
- Arachidonic acid is the most biologically active n-6 PUFA. It is found in inflammatory cell membranes, from where it can be released and subsequently converted to prostaglandins and thromboxanes by cyclooxygenase enzymes, and to leukotrienes by lipoxygenase enzymes. These mediators are involved in inflammatory processes, and cyclooxygenases are targets for existing anti-inflammatory drugs.
- The complex n-3 PUFAs are found in oily fish and fish oils. When consumed in sufficiently high quantities, they partly replace arachidonic acid in inflammatory cell membranes, and they inhibit arachidonic acid metabolism. One of these n-3 PUFAs, eicosapentaenoic acid (EPA), gives rise to prostaglandins and leukotrienes with weak inflammatory activity, while EPA and another n-3 PUFA, docosahexaenoic acid, produce resolvins, a family of potent anti-inflammatory mediators. Thus, n-3 PUFAs are considered to be anti-inflammatory.

- At sufficiently high intakes, n-3 PUFAs also inhibit inflammatory cytokine production, T-cell reactivity, and antigen presentation via major histocompatibility complex II.
- N-3 PUFAs, in the form of fish oil, have been trialed many times in rheumatoid arthritis, usually with some clinical benefit.
- Meta-analyses reveal a significant beneficial impact of n-3 PUFAs on patient-assessed pain, duration of morning stiffness, number of painful and/or tender joints, and consumption of non-steroidal anti-inflammatory drugs (NSAIDs).
- There is a role for n-3 PUFAs in the form of fish oil, or similar, in therapy of rheumatoid arthritis.

■

Introduction

This chapter will describe the anti-inflammatory effects of so-called long-chain omega-3 (n-3) polyunsaturated fatty acids (PUFAs) and the evidence that these fatty acids have a role in the therapy of rheumatoid arthritis (RA). The chapter begins with a description of how fatty acids are named, and of their metabolic relationships with one another, and then describes the link between fatty acid nutrition and inflammatory processes, which partly results from synthesis of inflammatory eicosanoid mediators from the n-6 PUFA, arachidonic acid. Then, the various anti-inflammatory actions of long chain n-3 PUFAs are described. Finally, the efficacy of long-chain n-3 PUFAs is evaluated by considering data from animal models and, more importantly, clinical trials. The latter are collated and their designs and findings summarized. Additionally, conclusions from meta-analyses are presented. Some of the content of this chapter is taken from Calder (2008).[1]

Fatty Acid Structure, Nomenclature, Sources, Intakes and Roles

Fatty acids are hydrocarbon chains with a carboxyl group at one end and a methyl group at the other. The carboxyl group is reactive and readily forms ester links with alcohol groups, for example those on glycerol or cholesterol, in turn forming acylglycerols (e.g., triacylglycerols, phospholipids) and cholesteryl esters. The most abundant fatty acids have straight chains of an even number of carbon atoms. Fatty acid chain lengths vary from 2 to 30 or more, and the chain may contain double bonds. Fatty acids containing double bonds in the acyl chain are referred to as *unsaturated fatty acids;* a fatty acid containing two or more double bonds is called a *polyunsaturated fatty acid,* or PUFA. Saturated fatty acids do not contain double bonds in the acyl chain.

The systematic name for a fatty acid is determined simply by the number of carbons and the number of double bonds in the acyl chain (Table 3.1). There are multiple possibilities for the position of double bonds within the hydrocarbon chain, and each double bond may be in the *cis* or *trans* configuration. Therefore, when naming an unsaturated fatty acid it is important that the exact positions of double bonds and their configurations be clearly identified. Traditionally, the position of double bonds was identified by naming the

Table 3.1 Fatty acid nomenclature.

Systematic name	*Trivial name*	*Shorthand notation*
Octanoic	Caprylic	8:0
Decanoic	Capric	10:0
Dodecanoic	Lauric	12:0
Tetradecanoic	Myrsitic	14:0
Hexadecanoic	Palmitic	16:0
Octadecanoic	Stearic	18:0
cis 9-Hexadecenoic	Palmitoleic	16:1n-7
cis 9-Octadecenoic	Oleic	18:1n-9
cis 9, *cis* 12-Octadecadienoic	Linoleic	18:2n-6
All *cis* 9, 12, 15-Octadecatrienoic	α-Linolenic	18:3n-3
All *cis* 6, 9, 12-Octadecatrienoic	γ-Linolenic	18:3n-6
All *cis* 8, 11, 14-Eicosatrienoic	Dihomo-γ-linolenic	20:3n-6
All *cis* 5, 8, 11, 14-Eicosatetraenoic	Arachidonic	20:4n-6
All *cis* 5, 8, 11, 14, 17-Eicosapentaenoic	Eicosapentaenoic	20:5n-3
All *cis* 7, 10, 13, 16, 19-Docosapentaenoic	Docosapentaenoic	22:5n-3
All *cis* 4, 7, 10, 13, 16, 19-Docosahexaenoic	Docosahexaenoic	22:6n-3

carbon number (from carbon 1 [the carboxyl carbon]) on which each double bond occurs. Thus, octadecadienoic acid, an 18-carbon fatty acid with *cis* double bonds between carbons 9 and 10 and carbons 12 and 13 is correctly denoted as *cis* 9, *cis* 12-octadecadienoic acid, or as *cis*, *cis*, 9,12-octadecadienoic acid. More recently, an alternative shorthand notation for fatty acids has come into frequent use. This relies upon identifying the number of carbon atoms in the chain, and the number of double bonds and their position. Thus, octadecanoic acid is notated as 18:0, indicating that it has an acyl chain of 18 carbons and does not contain any double bonds. Unsaturated fatty acids are named simply by identifying the number of double bonds and the position of the first double bond counted from the methyl terminus (with the methyl, or ω, carbon as number 1) of the acyl chain. The first double bond is identified as ω-x, where x is the carbon number on which the double bond occurs. Therefore *cis*, *cis*, 9,12-octadecadienoic acid is also known as 18:2ω-6. The ω-x nomenclature is sometimes referred to as omega x (e.g., 18:2 omega 6) or n-x (e.g., 18:2n-6).

In addition to these nomenclatures, fatty acids are often described by their common names (Table 3.1). Figure 3.1 shows the structure of several 18-carbon fatty acids indicating the position of the double bonds in the chain and how this is reflected in their naming. Most common unsaturated fatty acids contain *cis* rather than *trans* double bonds. *Trans* double bonds do occur, however, as intermediates in the biosynthesis of fatty acids, in ruminant fats (e.g., cow's milk), in plant lipids, and in some seed oils.

There are two principal families of PUFAs: the n-6 (or omega-6) and the n-3 (or omega-3) families. The simplest members of each family—linoleic acid (18:2n-6) and α-linolenic acid (18:3n-3)—cannot be synthesized by mammals.

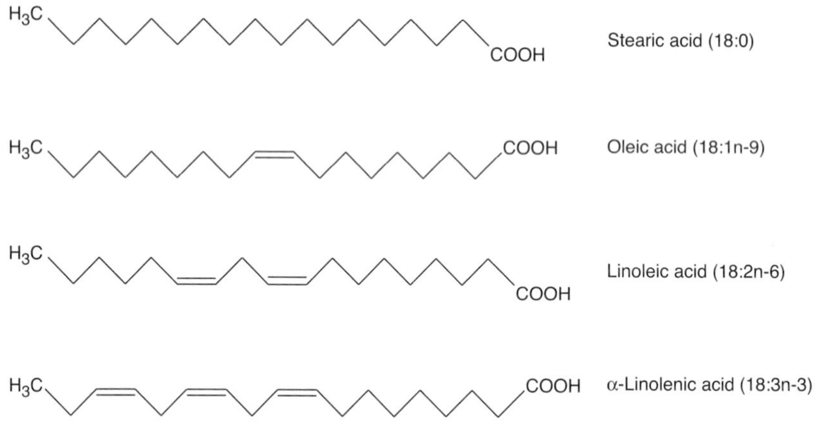

H_3C COOH Stearic acid (18:0)

H_3C COOH Oleic acid (18:1n-9)

H_3C COOH Linoleic acid (18:2n-6)

H_3C COOH α-Linolenic acid (18:3n-3)

FIGURE 3.1. The structure and naming of selected 18 carbon fatty acids.

Linoleic acid is found in significant quantities in many vegetable oils, including corn, sunflower and soybean oils, and in products made from such oils, such as margarines.[2,3] α-Linolenic acid is found in green plant tissues, in some common vegetable oils, including soybean and rapeseed oils, in some nuts, and in flaxseeds (also known as linseeds) and flaxseed oil. Between them, linoleic and α-linolenic acids contribute over 95%, and perhaps as much as 98% of dietary PUFA intake in most Western diets.[2,3] The intake of linoleic acid in Western countries increased greatly in the second half of the 20th Century, following the introduction and marketing of cooking oils and margarines. Typical intakes of both essential fatty acids are in excess of requirements. However, the changed pattern of consumption of linoleic acid has resulted in a marked increase in the ratio of n-6 to n-3 PUFAs in the diet. This ratio is typically between 5 and 20 in most Western populations.[4]

Although linoleic and α-linolenic acids cannot be synthesized by humans, they can be metabolized to other fatty acids (Figure 3.2). This is achieved by the insertion of additional double bonds into the acyl chain (i.e., unsaturation) and by elongation of the acyl chain. Thus, linoleic acid can be converted via γ-linolenic acid (18:3n-6) and dihomo-γ-linolenic acid (20:3n-6) to arachidonic

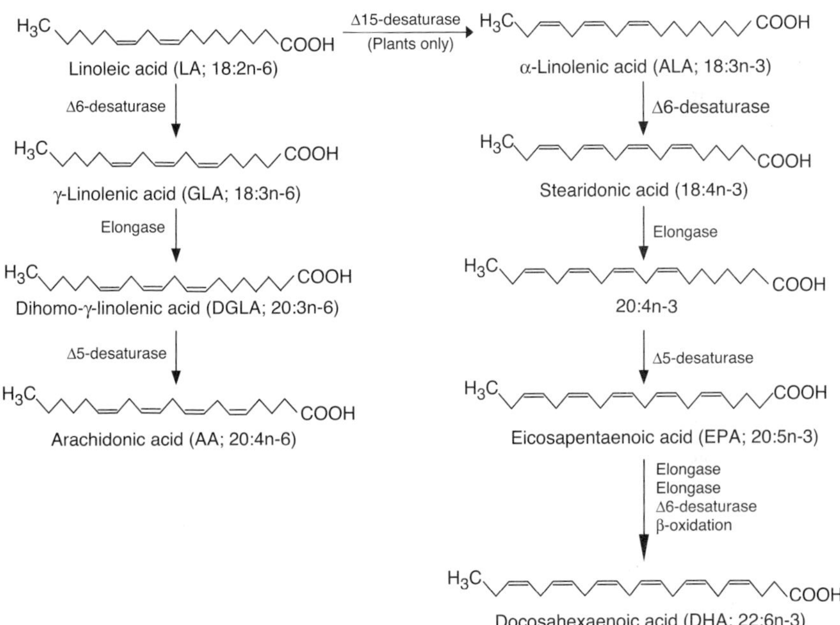

FIGURE 3.2. The biosynthesis of polyunsaturated fatty acids. AA, arachidonic acid; ALA, α-linolenic acid; DGLA, dihomo-γ-linolenic acid; DHA, docosahexaenoic acid; EPA, eicosapentaenoic acid; GLA, γ-linolenic acid; LA, linoleic acid.

acid (20:4n-6) (Figure 3.2). By an analogous set of reactions catalyzed by the same enzymes, α-linolenic acid can be converted to eicosapentaenoic acid (20:5n-3; EPA). Both arachidonic acid and EPA can be further metabolized, EPA giving rise to docosapentaenoic acid (22:5n-3; DPA) and docosahexaenoic acid (22:6n-3; DHA) (Figure 3.2).

Dietary intakes of the longer-chain, more unsaturated PUFAs, are typically much lower than of linoleic and α-linolenic acids. Some plant oils contain γ-linolenic acid, dihomo-γ-linolenic acid, and stearidonic acid, but typical intakes of these fatty acids from the diet are likely to be < 10 mg/day. Arachidonic acid is found in meats, and intakes are estimated at 50 to 500 mg/day.[3] EPA, DPA, and DHA are found in fish, especially so-called "oily" fish (tuna, salmon, mackerel, herring, sardine). One oily fish meal can provide between 1.5 and 3.5 g of these long-chain n-3 PUFAs.[5] The commercial products known as "fish oils" also contain these long-chain n-3 PUFAs, which typically will contribute about 30% of the fatty acids present. Thus, consumption of a typical 1 g fish oil capsule per day can provide about 300 mg of these fatty acids. In the absence of oily fish or fish oil consumption, intake of long-chain n-3 PUFAs is likely to be < 100 mg/day,[5] although foods fortified with these fatty acids are now available in many countries.

PUFAs are important constituents of cells, where they play roles assuring the correct environment for membrane protein function, maintaining membrane fluidity, and regulating cell signaling, gene expression, and cellular function.[3] In addition, some PUFAs, particularly arachidonic acid, act as substrates for synthesis of eicosanoids, which are involved in regulation of many cell and tissue responses.

Arachidonic Acid, Eicosanoids and the Link with Inflammation

Eicosanoids are key mediators and regulators of inflammation[6,7] and are generated from 20 carbon PUFAs. Because inflammatory cells typically contain a high proportion of the n-6 PUFA arachidonic acid, and low proportions of other 20-carbon PUFAs, arachidonic acid is usually the major substrate for eicosanoid synthesis. Eicosanoids, which include prostaglandins (PGs), thromboxanes, leukotrienes (LTs) and other oxidized derivatives, are generated from arachidonic acid by the metabolic processes summarized in Figure 3.3. They are involved in modulating the intensity and duration of inflammatory responses,[6,7] have cell- and stimulus-specific sources, and frequently have opposing effects. Expression of both isoforms of cyclooxygenase is increased in the synovium of RA patients, and in joint tissues in rat models of arthritis.[8]

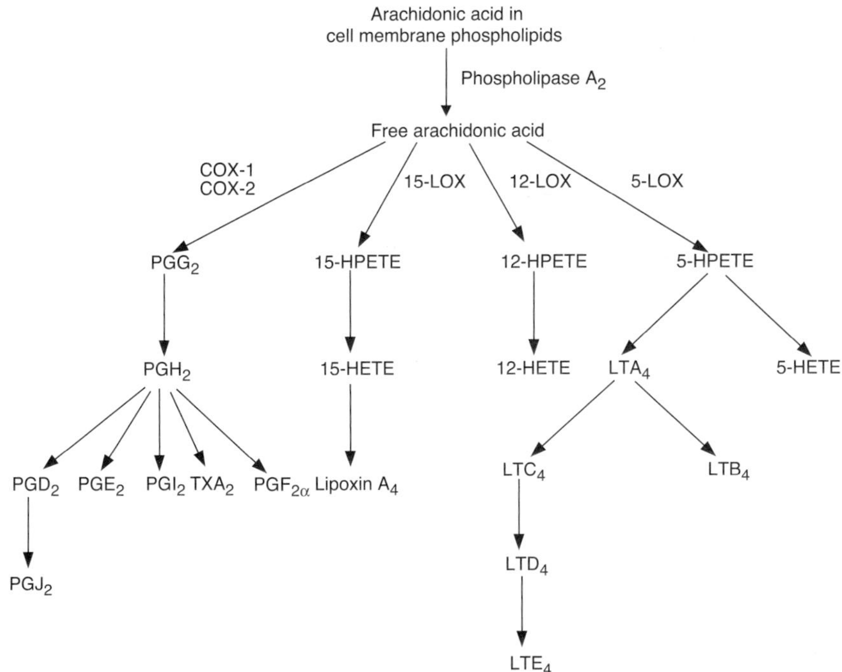

FIGURE 3.3. Outline of the pathway of eicosanoid synthesis from arachidonic acid. COX, cyclooxygenase; HETE, hydroxyeicosatetraenoic acid; HPETE, hydroperoxyeicosatetraenoic acid; LOX, lipoxygenase; LT, leukotriene; PG, prostaglandin; TX, thromboxane.

PGE_2, LTB_4 and 5-hydroxyeicosatetraenoic acid are found in the synovial fluid of patients with active RA.[9]

Infiltrating leukocytes such as neutrophils, monocytes, and synoviocytes are important sources of eicosanoids in RA. PGE_2 has a number of proinflammatory effects including increasing vascular permeability, vasodilation, blood flow and local pyrexia, and potentiation of pain caused by other agents. It also promotes the production of some matrix metalloproteinases and stimulates bone resorption. The efficacy of non-steroidal anti-inflammatory drugs (NSAIDs), which act to inhibit cyclooxygenase activity in RA, indicates the importance of this pathway in the pathophysiology of the disease. However, although these drugs provide rapid relief of pain and stiffness by inhibiting joint inflammation, they do not influence the course of the disease. LTB_4 increases vascular permeability, enhances local blood flow, is a potent chemotactic agent for leukocytes, induces release of lysosomal enzymes, and enhances release of reactive oxygen species and inflammatory cytokines like tumor necrosis factor (TNF)-α, interleukin (IL)-1β, and IL-6.

Very Long Chain n-3 PUFAs and Inflammatory Processes

Increased consumption of EPA and DHA from oily fish or from fish oils results in their incorporation into immune cell phospholipids,[10–13] which occurs in a dose-response fashion and is partly at the expense of arachidonic acid. The changed membrane fatty acid composition is believed to influence immune cell function and inflammatory processes[14] (Figure 3.4). The influence of n-3 PUFAs on many aspects of immune function has been reviewed many times previously,[10–27] and the reader is referred to these articles for details beyond those provided in the following sections.

ANTIGEN-PRESENTING CELL FUNCTION

There have been several studies of the effects of n-3 PUFAs on major histocompatibility class (MHC) II or human leukocyte antigen (HLA) expression,

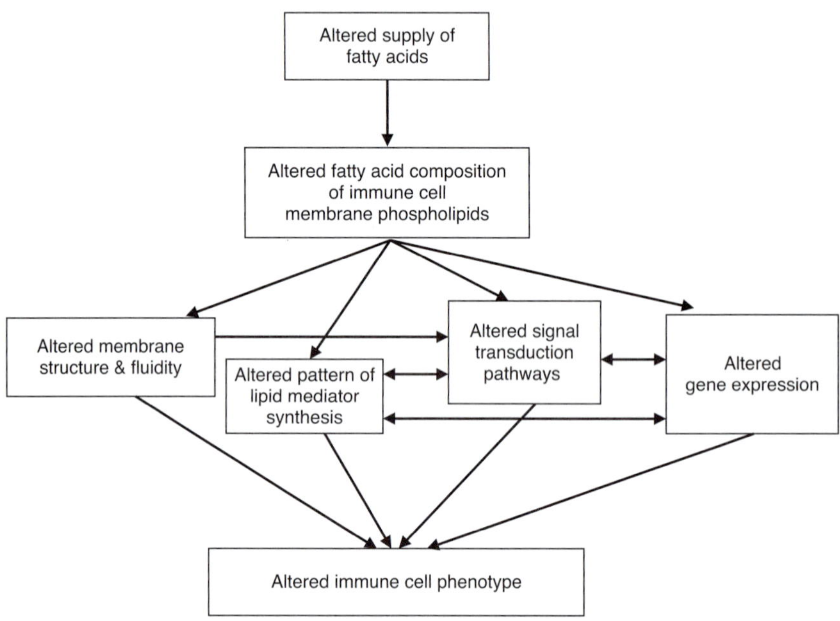

FIGURE 3.4. Outline of the mechanisms by which fatty acids can influence immune cell function.

or antigen presentation via class II.[28] These studies have typically found that class II expression and antigen presentation via class II are decreased by n-3 PUFAs. An in vitro study in which spleen cells were incubated with EPA reported decreased ability of those cells to present antigen.[29] This study did not report class II expression. Incubating murine macrophages with DHA decreased expression of the class II molecules (called Ia in mice).[30] Likewise, incubating mouse macrophages with EPA or DHA decreased interferon-γ-induced upregulation of class II,[31] and incubating mouse dendritic cells with DHA decreased endotoxin-induced class II upregulation.[32] Hughes et al.[33] reported that EPA and DHA treatment could diminish the upregulation of HLA-DR and HLA-DP that is seen with interferon (IFN)-γ stimulation of human monocytes. It was later demonstrated that these fatty acids decreased the ability of human monocytes to present antigen.[34] Three studies, one in mice,[35] one in rats,[36] and one in humans,[37] have reported effects of dietary n-3 PUFAs on class II expression. Feeding mice fish oil, which contains EPA and DHA, resulted in a reduction in MHC II expression on peritoneal cells (mainly B lymphocytes and macrophages).[35] A human supplementation study with fish oil reported decreased expression of HLA-DR, -DP and -DQ on IFN γ stimulated blood monocytes,[37] with similar effects to those seen with n-3 PUFAs in vitro.[33] These studies did not examine antigen presentation activity. However, a study that involved feeding an EPA-rich oil to mice showed decreased antigen (keyhole limpet hemocyanin) presentation by spleen cells to T cell clones.[29] Perhaps the most thorough study of this type to date is that of Sanderson et al.[36] Feeding a fish-oil-rich diet to rats resulted in decreased expression of MHC II on dendritic cells. These cells had a much reduced capacity to present antigen (keyhole limpet hemocyanin) to antigen-sensitized spleen T cells. The reduction in antigen presentation was probably much greater than could be explained by the reduction in class II expression, suggesting that other interactions between antigen-presenting cells and T lymphocytes were affected by dietary n-3 PUFAs. Sanderson et al.[36] reported that levels of the co-stimulatory molecules CD2, CD11a and CD18 were also decreased on dendritic cells from rats fed fish oil.

T Lymphocyte Reactivity

In vitro studies demonstrate that EPA and DHA decrease T cell proliferation[38–41] and the production of Th1 type cytokines like IL-2.[38,39,42] Feeding studies in rodents and supplementation studies in humans also show that fish oil decreases T cell proliferation[43–48] and production of Th1-type cytokines like IL-2[42,43,46,48] and IFN-γ,[42,48] although it is important to note that not all human studies report such an effect.[11] The reason for these discrepancies in the literature is not entirely clear, but the likely contributing factors are dose of n-3 PUFA used, technical factors, and differences among subjects studied.

The mechanism by which long-chain n-3 PUFAs affect T-cell reactivity was initially thought to relate to altered patterns of eicosanoid synthesis, but this mechanism was shown to be unlikely through the use of eicosanoid synthesis inhibitors and pure eicosanoids in vitro.[40] Studies over the last few years have demonstrated that the inhibitory effects of n-3 PUFAs in general, and of EPA in particular, relate to membrane-mediated effects that impact on the early stages of cell signaling.[49–52]

Inflammatory Mediator Production

EICOSANOIDS Increased consumption of very-long-chain n-3 PUFAs, such as EPA and DHA, results in decreased amounts of arachidonic acid in immune cell membranes, and available for synthesis of eicosanoids.[10–13] Thus, feeding fish oil to laboratory rodents, or supplementing the diet of humans with fish oil, has been reported to result in decreased production by inflammatory cells of a range of eicosanoids including PGE_2, thromboxane B_2, LTB_4, 5-hydroxyeicosatetraenoic acid and LTE_4.[10–13] A recent study demonstrated the dose-response effect to dietary EPA of PGE_2 production by endotoxin-stimulated human mononuclear cells, and suggests that an EPA intake of more than 2 g/d is required to be effective.[53]

EPA is also able to act as a substrate for both cyclooxygenase and 5-lipoxygenase, giving rise to eicosanoids with a slightly different structure to those formed from arachidonic acid. Thus, fish oil supplementation of the human diet has been shown to result in increased production by inflammatory cells of LTB_5, LTE_5 and 5-hydroxyeicosapentaenoic acid.[10–13] The functional significance of this is that the mediators formed from EPA are frequently less potent than those formed from arachidonic acid; for example, LTB_5 is less potent than LTB_4 as a neutrophil chemotactic agent.[54,55]

RESOLVINS AND RELATED COMPOUNDS – NOVEL EPA- AND DHA-DERIVED ANTI-INFLAMMATORY MEDIATORS Recent studies have identified a novel group of trihydroxyeicosapentaenoic acid mediators, termed *E-series resolvins*, formed from EPA by a series of reactions involving cyclooxygenase-2 (acting in the presence of aspirin) and 5-lipoxygenase. These mediators appear to exert potent anti-inflammatory actions.[56–58] In addition, DHA-derived trihydroxydocosahexanoic acid mediators termed D-series resolvins are produced by a similar series of reactions, and these too are anti-inflammatory.[59,60] Metabolism of DHA via a series of steps, several involving

5-lipoxygenase, generates a dihydroxydocosatriene termed *neuroprotectin D1*, again a potent anti-inflammatory molecule.[61] The identification of these novel EPA- and DHA-derived mediators is an exciting new area of n-3 fatty acids and inflammatory mediators, and the implications to a variety of conditions may be of great importance.[62,63]

INFLAMMATORY CYTOKINES Cell culture studies demonstrate that EPA and DHA can inhibit the production of IL-1β and TNF-α by monocytes,[64] and the production of IL-6 and IL-8 by venous endothelial cells.[65] Fish-oil feeding decreased *ex vivo* production of TNF-α, IL-1β and IL-6 by rodent macrophages.[67–69] Supplementation of the diet of healthy human volunteers with fish oil decreased production of TNF, or IL-1 or IL-6, by mononuclear cells in some studies,[10–13] although a number of other studies show little effect of n-3 PUFAs on production of inflammatory cytokines in humans.[11] The reason for these discrepancies in the literature is not entirely clear, but dose of n-3 PUFA used, technical factors, and differences among subjects studied, including genetic differences,[70,71] are likely to be contributing factors.

N-3 PUFAs and Animal Models of RA

The effects of n-3 PUFAs from fish oil on antigen presentation, T-cell reactivity and inflammatory lipid and peptide mediator production (Table 3.2), suggest that these fatty acids might have a role both in decreasing the risk of development of RA and in decreasing severity in those patients with the disease. Indeed, dietary fish oil has been shown to have beneficial effects in animal models of arthritis. For example, compared with vegetable oil, feeding mice fish oil delayed the onset (mean 34 days vs. 25 days), and reduced the incidence (69% vs. 93%) and severity (mean peak severity score 6.7 vs. 9.8) of type II collagen-induced arthritis.[72] In another study, both EPA and DHA suppressed Streptococcal cell-wall-induced arthritis in rats, but EPA was more effective.[73]

Trials of N-3 PUFAs in RA

Several studies report anti-inflammatory effects of fish oil in patients with RA, such as decreased LTB_4 production by neutrophils[74–77] and monocytes,[76,78] decreased PGE_2 production by mononuclear cells,[79] decreased IL-1 production by monocytes,[80] decreased plasma IL-1β concentrations,[81] decreased serum C-reactive protein concentrations,[74,82] and normalization of the neutrophil chemotactic response.[83] A number of randomized, placebo-controlled,

Table 3.2. Summary of the anti-inflammatory effects of long chain n-3 PUFAs.

Effect	*Mechanism of action*
Decreased production of arachidonic acid-derived mediators (PGE_2 etc.)	Decreased arachidonic acid content of inflammatory cells; Inhibition of arachidonic acid metabolism by EPA and DHA
Production of EPA-derived eicosanoids with low inflammatory potential	Increased EPA content of inflammatory cells
Production of anti-inflammatory E- and D-series resolvins	Increased EPA and DHA content of inflammatory cells
Decreased production of inflammatory cytokines (TNF-α etc.)	Inhibition of inflammatory signalling (inhibition of nuclear factor K B activation; activation of peroxisome proliferator activated receptor γ)
Decreased T cell reactivity; Deceased production of Th1-type cytokines (IFN-γ etc.)	Inhibition of T cell signalling (disruption of membrane rafts)
Decreased MHC II expression and antigen presentation	Not known

double-blind studies of fish oil in rheumatoid arthritis have been reported.[74–78,80–82,84–94] The characteristics and findings of these trials are summarized in Table 3.3. The dose of long-chain n-3 PUFAs used in these trials was between 1.6 and 7.1 g/day and averaged about 3.5 g/day (see Table 3.3). Almost all of these trials showed some benefit of long-chain n-3 PUFAs (Table 3.3). Such benefits include reduced duration of morning stiffness, reduced number of tender or swollen joints, reduced joint pain, reduced time to fatigue, increased grip strength and decreased use of non-steroidal anti-inflammatory drugs (Table 3.3). A number of reviews of these trials have been published,[95–101] and each has concluded that there is benefit from fish oil. In an editorial commentary discussing the use of fish oil in rheumatoid arthritis, it was concluded that "the findings of benefit from fish oil in rheumatoid arthritis are robust," "dietary fish oil supplements in rheumatoid arthritis have treatment efficacy," and "dietary fish oil supplements should now be regarded as part of the standard therapy for rheumatoid arthritis."[102]

A meta-analysis that included data from nine trials published between 1985 and 1992 inclusive, and from one unpublished trial, has been conducted.[103] This concluded that "dietary fish oil supplementation for three months significantly reduced tender joint count (mean difference -2.9; P = 0.001) and

Table 3.3. Summary of the results of placebo-controlled studies using dietary long chain n-3 PUFAs (in the form of fish oil) in patients with rheumatoid arthritis. Taken from Calder, 2008.

Reference	*Dose of EPA+ DHA (g/day)*	*Duration (wk)*	*Placebo*	*Clinical outcomes improved with long chain n-3 PUFAs*
Kremer et al., 1985	1.8 + 1.2	12	Paraffin oil	Number of tender joints; Duration of morning stiffness
Kremer et al., 1987	2.7 + 1.8	14	Olive oil	Number of tender joints; Number of swollen joints; Time to fatigue; Physician's global assessment
Cleland et al., 1988	3.2 + 2.0	12	Olive oil	Number of tender joints; Grip strength
van der Tempel et al., 1990	2.0 + 1.3	12	Coconut oil	Number of swollen joints; Duration of morning stiffness
Kremer et al., 1990	1.7 + 1.2	24	Olive oil	Number of tender joints; Number of swollen joints; Grip strength; Physician's global assessment
Kremer et al., 1990	3.5 + 2.4	24	Olive oil	Number of tender joints; Number of swollen joints; Grip strength; Physician's global assessment; Duration of morning stiffness
Tullekan et al., 1990	2.0 + 1.3	12	Coconut oil	Number of swollen joints; Joint pain index
Skoldstam et al., 1992	1.8 + 1.2	24	Mixed oils	Number and severity of tender joints; Physician's global assessment; Use of NSAIDs
Esperson et al., 1992	2.0 + 1.2	12	Mixed oils	Number and severity of tender joints
Nielsen et al., 1992	2.0 + 1.2	12	Vegetable oil	Number of tender joints; Duration of morning stiffness
Kjedsen-Kragh et al., 1992	3.8 + 2.0	16	Corn oil	Number and severity of tender joints; Duration of morning stiffness
Lau et al., 1993	1.7 + 1.1	52	Air	Use of NSAIDs

(continued)

Table 3.3. (Continued)

Reference	*Dose of EPA+ DHA (g/day)*	*Duration (wk)*	*Placebo*	*Clinical outcomes improved with long chain n-3 PUFAs*
Geusens et al., 1994	1.7 + 0.4	52	Olive oil	Physician's pain assessment; Patient's global assessment; Use of NSAIDs &/or Disease modifying anti-rheumatic drugs
Kremer et al., 1995	4.6 + 2.5	26 to 30	Corn oil	Number of tender joints; Duration of morning stiffness; Physician's assessment of pain; Physician's global assessment; Patient's global assessment
Volker etal., 2000	Total 40 mg/kg (Approx. 2.2 to 3.0)	15	Mixed oils	Number of swollen joints; Duration of morning stiffness; Patient's assessment of pain; Patient's global assessment; Physician's global assessment; Health assessment by questionnaire
Adam et al., 2003	Approx 2.4 + 1.8	12	Corn oil	Number of swollen joints; Number of tender joints; Patient's global assessment; Physician's global assessment; Patient's assessment of pain
Remans et al., 2004	1.4 + 0.2 (+ 0.5 γ-linolenic acid) in a liquid supplement	16	Liquid supplement without added PUFA	None
Berbert et al., 2005	Total 3.0	24	Soybean oil	Duration of morning stiffness; Joint pain; Time to onset of fatigue; Ritchie's articular index; Grip strength, Patient's global assessment
Sundrarjun et al., 2004	1.9 + 1.5	24	Not stated	None
Galarraga et al., 2008	1.5 + 0.7	36	Air	Use of NSAIDs; Patient's assessment of pain

morning stiffness (mean difference -25.9 minutes; P = 0.01)." A more recent meta-analysis that included data from trials published between 1985 and 2002 was conducted,[104] although this included one study of flaxseed oil, one study that did not use a control for fish oil, and one study in which transdermal administration of n-3 PUFAs by ultrasound, rather than the oral route, was used. This meta-analysis analysis concluded that fish oil supplementation has no effect on "patient report of pain, swollen joint count, disease activity, or patient's global assessment." However, this conclusion may be flawed, because of the inappropriate manner in which studies were combined (see above) and because of a poor understanding of the study designs used. For example, the meta-analysis fails to recognize that patients' ability to reduce the need for using NSAIDs, or their ability to be withdrawn from NSAID use, as was done in some designs, must indicate a reduction in pain with n-3 PUFA use. This meta-analysis does state that "in a qualitative analysis of seven studies that assessed the effect of n-3 fatty acids on anti-inflammatory drug or corticosteroid requirement, six demonstrated reduced requirement for these drugs," and concluded that "n-3 fatty acids may reduce requirements for corticosteroids."[104] The effects of long-chain n-3 PUFAs on tender joint count was not assessed by this meta-analysis, which reiterated the findings of the earlier meta-analysis[103] that "n-3 fatty acids reduce tender joint counts." Recently, a new meta-analysis of n-3 PUFAs and was published;[105] this included data from 17 trials, including one trial in RA with flaxseed oil and two trials of fish oil—not in RA patients, but in patients reporting joint pain. Data on six outcomes was analyzed. These are summarized in Table 3.4. This meta-analysis provides further evidence of the robustness of the efficacy of n-3 PUFAs in RA.

Table 3.4. Summary of the findings of the meta-analysis of Goldberg and Katz, 2007. Taken from Calder, 2008.

Outcome	*Number of studies*	*Number of patients (control; n-3 PUFA)*	*Significance of effect of n-3 PUFAs (P)*
Patient assessed pain	13	247; 254	0.03
Physician assessed pain	3	61; 62	0.45
Duration of morning stiffness	8	150; 156	0.003
Number of painful and/or tender joints	10	210; 215	0.003
Ritchie articular index	4	68; 67	0.40
NSAID consumption	3	79; 77	0.01

Several other studies also provide information about the benefits of n-3 PUFAs in RA. For example, Cleland et al[79] compared outcomes among patients with RA who did not consume fish oil supplements and those who did. They found that fish oil users were more likely to reduce use of NSAIDs and were more likely to be in remission.

Summary

The primary fatty acid of interest in most inflammatory processes is the n-6 polyunsaturated fatty acid (PUFA) arachidonic acid, which is the precursor of inflammatory eicosanoids like prostaglandin E_2 and leukotriene B_4, and the n-3 PUFAs eicosapentaenoic acid (EPA) and docosahexaenoic acid (DHA). EPA and DHA are found in oily fish and fish oils. Eicosanoids derived from the n-6 PUFA arachidonic acid play a role in rheumatoid arthritis (RA), and the efficacy of non-steroidal antiinflammatory drugs in RA indicates the importance of pro-inflammatory cyclooxygenase pathway products of arachidonic acid in the pathophysiology of the disease. EPA and DHA inhibit arachidonic acid metabolism to inflammatory eicosanoids. EPA also gives rise to eicosanoid mediators that are less inflammatory than those produced from arachidonic acid, and both EPA and DHA give rise to resolvins that are anti-inflammatory and inflammation-resolving. In addition to modifying the lipid mediator profile, n-3 PUFAs exert effects on other aspects of immunity relevant to RA, like antigen presentation, T-cell reactivity and inflammatory cytokine production. Fish oil has been shown to slow the development of arthritis in an animal model, and to reduce disease severity. Randomized clinical trials have demonstrated a range of clinical benefits in patients with RA, including reducing pain, duration of morning stiffness, and reducing use of non-steroidal anti-inflammatory drugs.

Overall Conclusions

Eicosanoids derived from the n-6 PUFA arachidonic acid play a role in RA, and the efficacy of NSAIDs in RA indicates the importance of pro-inflammatory cyclooxygenase pathway products in the pathophysiology of the disease. At sufficiently high intakes, long-chain n-3 PUFAs decrease the production of inflammatory eicosanoids from arachidonic acid, and promote the production of less inflammatory eicosanoids from EPA, and of anti-inflammatory resolvins and similar mediators from EPA and DHA. Long-chain n-3 PUFAs have other anti-inflammatory actions including decreasing antigen presentation via MHC II, decreasing T-cell reactivity and Th1-type cytokine production, and decreasing inflammatory cytokine production by monocyte/macrophages. Work with animal models of RA has demonstrated efficacy of fish oil. There have been a number of clinical trials of fish oil in patients with RA. Most of these trials report clinical improvements (e.g., improved patient-assessed pain, decreased morning stiffness, fewer painful or tender joints, decreased use of NSAIDs), and when the trials have been pooled in meta-analyses, statistically significant clinical benefit has emerged.

REFERENCES

1. Calder PC. Polyunsaturated fatty acids, inflammatory processes and rheumatoid arthritis. *Proc Nutr Soc.* 2008;67:409–418.
2. British Nutrition Foundation. *Unsaturated Fatty Acids.* London: Chapman & Hall; 1992.
3. Calder PC and Burdge GC. Fatty acids. In: Nicolaou A & Kokotos G, eds. *Bioactive Lipids.* Bridgewater: The Oily Press; 2004:1–36.
4. Burdge GC & Calder PC. Dietary α-linolenic acid and health related outcomes: a metabolic perspective. *Nutr Res Rev.* 2006;19:26–52.
5. British Nutrition Foundation. *Briefing Paper: n-3 fatty acids and health.* London: British Nutrition Foundation; 1999.
6. Lewis RA, Austen KF & Soberman RJ. Leukotrienes and other products of the 5-lipoxygenase pathway: biochemistry and relation to pathobiology in human diseases. *N Engl J Med.* 1990;323:645–655.
7. Tilley SL, Coffman TM & Koller BH. Mixed messages: modulation of inflammation and immune responses by prostaglandins and thromboxanes. *J Clin Invest.* 2001;108:15–23.
8. Sano H, Hla T, Maier JAM, Crofford LJ, Case JP, Maciag T & Wilder RL. In vivo cyclooxygenase expression in synovial tissues of patients with rheumatoid arthritis and osteoarthritis and rats with adjuvant and streptococcal cell wall arthritis. *J Clin Invest.* 1992;89:97–108.
9. Sperling RI. Eicosanoids in rheumatoid arthritis. *Rheum Dis Clin North Am.* 1995;21:741–758.
10. Calder PC. N-3 fatty acids and mononuclear phagocyte function. In: Kremer JM, ed. *Medicinal Fatty Acids.* Basel: Birkhauser; 1998:1–27.
11. Calder PC. n-3 Polyunsaturated fatty acids, inflammation and immunity: pouring oil on troubled waters or another fishy tale? *Nutr Res.* 2001;1:309–341.
12. Calder PC. N-3 polyunsaturated fatty acids, inflammation, and inflammatory diseases. *Am J Clin Nutr.* 2006;83:1505S–1519S.
13. Calder PC. Immunomodulation by omega-3 fatty acids. *Prostaglandins Leukot Essent Fatty Acids.* 2007;77:327–335.
14. Calder PC. Polyunsaturated fatty acids and inflammation. *Prostaglandins Leukot Essent Fatty Acids.* 2006;75:197–202.

15. Calder PC. Sir David Cuthbertson Medal Lecture: Immunomodulatory and anti-inflammatory effects of omega-3 polyunsaturated fatty acids. *Proc Nutr Soc.* 1996;55:737–774.
16. Calder PC. N-3 polyunsaturated fatty acids and cytokine production in health and disease. *Ann Nutr Metab.* 1997;41:203–234.
17. Calder PC. Dietary fatty acids and lymphocyte functions. *Proc Nutr Soc.* 1998;57:487–502.
18. Calder PC. Polyunsaturated fatty acids, inflammation and immunity. *Lipids.* 2001;36:1007–1024.
19. Calder PC. N-3 polyunsaturated fatty acids and inflammation: from molecular biology to the clinic. *Lipids.* 2003;38:342–352.
20. Calder PC, Yaqoob P, Thies F, Wallace FA & Miles EA. Fatty acids and lymphocyte functions. *Br J Nutr.* 2002;87:S31–S48.
21. Miles EA & Calder PC. Modulation of immune function by dietary fatty acids. *Proc Nutr Soc.* 1998;57:277–292.
22. Kelley DS. Modulation of human immune and inflammatory responses by dietary fatty acids. *Nutrition.* 2001;17:669–673.
23. Yaqoob P. Fatty acids as gatekeepers of immune cell regulation. *Trends Immunol.* 2003;24:639–645.
24. Switzer KC, McMurray DN & Chapkin RS. Effects of dietary n-3 polyunsaturated fatty acids on T-cell membrane composition and function. *Lipids.* 2004;39:1163–1170.
25. Fritsche K. Fatty acids as modulators of the immune response. *Annu Rev Nutr.* 2006;26:45–73.
26. Sijben JWC & Calder PC. Differential immunomodulation with long-chain n-3 PUFA in health and disease. *Proc Nutr Soc.* 2007;66:237–259.
27. Yaqoob P & Calder PC. Fatty acids and immune function: new insights into mechanisms. *Br J Nutr.* 2007;98:S41–S45.
28. Calder PC. Polyunsaturated fatty acids alter the rules of engagement. *Future Lipidol.* 2007;2:27–30.
29. Fujikawa M, Yamashita N, Yamazaki K, Sugiyama E, Suzuki H & Hamazaki T. Eicosapentaenoic acid inhibits antigen-presenting cell function of murine splenocytes. *Immunology.* 1992;75:330–335.
30. Khair-el-Din TA, Sicher SC, Vazquez MA & Lu CY. Inhibition of macrophage nitric-oxide production and Ia-expression by docosahexaenoic acid, a constituent of fetal and neonatal serum. *Am J Reprod Immunol.* 1996;36:1–10.
31. Khair-el-Din TA, Sicher SC, Vazquez MA, Wright WJ & Lu CY. Docosahexaenoic acid, a major constituent of fetal serum and fish oil diets, inhibits IFN gamma-induced Ia-expression by murine macrophages in vitro. *J Immunol.* 1995;154:1296–1306.
32. Weatherill AR, Lee JY, Zhao L, Lemay DG, Youn HS & Hwang DH. Saturated and polyunsaturated fatty acids reciprocally modulate dendritic cell functions mediated through TLR4. *J Immunol.* 2005;174:5390–5397.
33. Hughes DA, Southon S & Pinder AC. (n-3. Polyunsaturated fatty acids modulate the expression of functionally associated molecules on human monocytes in vitro. *J Nutr.* 1996;126:603–610.

34. Hughes DA & Pinder AC. N-3 polyunsaturated fatty acids modulate the expression of functionally associated molecules on human monocytes and inhibit antigen-presentation in vitro. *Clin Exp Immunol.* 1997;110:516–523.
35. Huang SC, Misfeldt ML & Fritsche KL. Dietary fat influences Ia antigen expression and immune cell populations in the murine peritoneum and spleen. *J Nutr.* 1992;122:1219–1231.
36. Sanderson P, MacPherson GG, Jenkins CH & Calder PC. Dietary fish oil diminishes the antigen presentation activity of rat dendritic cells. *J Leukoc Biol.* 1997; 62:771–777.
37. Hughes DA, Pinder AC, Piper Z, Johnson IT & Lund EK. Fish oil supplementation inhibits the expression of major histocompatibility complex class II molecules and adhesion molecules on human monocytes. *Am J Clin Nutr.* 1996;63:267–272.
38. Calder PC & Newsholme EA. Unsaturated fatty acids suppress interleukin-2 production and transferin receptor expression by concanavalin A-stimulated rat lymphocytes. *Mediators Inflamm.* 1992;1:107–115.
39. Calder PC & Newsholme EA. Polyunsaturated fatty acids suppress human peripheral blood lymphocyte proliferation and interleukin-2 production. *Clin Sci.* 1992;82:695–700.
40. Calder PC, Bevan SJ & Newsholme EA. The inhibition of T-lymphocyte proliferation by fatty acids is via an eicosanoid-independent mechanism. *Immunology.* 1992;75:108–115.
41. Calder PC, Yaqoob P, Harvey DJ, Watts A & Newsholme EA. The incorporation of fatty acids by lymphocytes and the effect on fatty acid composition and membrane fluidity. *Biochem J.* 1994;300:509–518.
42. Wallace FA, Miles EA, Evans C, Stock TE, Yaqoob P & Calder PC. Dietary fatty acids influence the production of Th1. but not Th2-type cytokines. *J Leukoc Biol.* 2001;69:449–457.
43. Meydani SN, Endres S, Woods MM, Goldin BR, Soo C, Morrill-Labrode A, Dinarello CA & Gorbach SL. Oral (n-3) fatty acid supplementation suppresses cytokine production and lymphocyte proliferation: comparison between young and older women. *J Nutr.* 1991;121:547–555.
44. Yaqoob P, Newsholme EA & Calder PC. The effect of dietary lipid manipulation on rat lymphocyte subsets and proliferation. Immunology. 1994;82:603–610.
45. Yaqoob P & Calder PC. The effects of dietary lipid manipulation on the production of murine T-cell-derived cytokines. *Cytokine.* 1995;7:548–553.
46. Jolly CA, Jiang YH, Chapkin RS & McMurray DN. Dietary (n-3) polyunsaturated fatty acids suppress murine lymphoproliferation, interleukin-2 secretion, and the formation of diacylglycerol and ceramide. *J Nutr.* 1997;127:37–43.
47. Peterson LD, Jeffery NM, Thies F, Sanderson P, Newsholme EA & Calder PC. Eicosapentaenoic and docosahexaenoic acids alter rat spleen leukocyte fatty acid composition and prostaglandin E_2 production but have different effects on lymphocyte functions and cell-mediated immunity. *Lipids.* 1998;33:171–180.
48. Trebble TM, Wootton SA, Miles EA, Mullee M, Arden NK, Ballinger AB, Stroud MA & Calder PC. Prostaglandin E_2 production and T-cell function after fish-oil

supplementation: response to antioxidant co-supplementation. *Am J Clin Nutr.* 2003;78:376–382.

49. Sanderson P & Calder PC. Dietary fish oil appears to inhibit the activation of phospholipase C- in lymphocytes. *Biochim Biophys Acta.* 1998;1392:300–308.
50. Stulnig TM, Huber J, Leitinger N, Imre EM, Angelisova P, Nowotny P, & Waldhausl W. Polyunsaturated eicosapentaenoic acid displaces proteins from membrane rafts by altering raft lipid composition. *J Biol Chem.* 2001;276:37335–37340.
51. Zeyda M, Staffler G, Horejsi V, Waldhausl W & Stulnig TM. LAT displacement from lipid rafts as a molecular mechanism for the inhibition of T cell signaling by polyunsaturated fatty acids. *J Biol Chem.* 2002;277:28418–28423.
52. Zeyda M, Szekeres AB, Säemann MD, Geyeregger R, Stockinger H, Zlabinger GJ, Waldhäusl W & Stulnig TM. Suppression of T cell signaling by polyunsaturated fatty acids: selectivity in inhibition of mitogen-activated protein kinase and nuclear factor activation. *J Immunol.* 2003;170:6033–6039.
53. Rees D, Miles EA, Banerjee T, Wells SJ, Roynette CE, Wahle KWJW & Calder PC. Dose-related effects of eicosapentaenoic acid on innate immune function in healthy humans: a comparison of young and older men. *Am J Clin Nutr.* z2006;83:331–42.
54. Goldman DW, Pickett WC & Goetzl EJ. Human neutrophil chemotactic and degranulating activities of leukotriene B_5 (LTB_5) derived from eicosapentaenoic acid. *Biochem Biophys Res Commun.* 1983;117:282–288.
55. Lee TH, Mencia-Huerta JM, Shih C, Corey EJ, Lewis RA & Austen KF. Characterization and biologic properties of 5,12-dihydroxy derivatives of eicosapentaenoic acid, including leukotriene-B5 and the double lipoxygenase product. *J Biol Chem.* 1984;259:2383–2389.
56. Serhan CN, Clish CB, Brannon J, Colgan SP, Chiang N & Gronert K. Novel functional sets of lipid-derived mediators with antinflammatory actions generated from omega-3 fatty acids via cyclooxygenase 2-nonsteroidal antiinflammatory drugs and transcellular processing. *J Exp Med.* 2000;192:1197–1204.
57. Serhan CN, Clish CB, Brannon J, Colgan SP, Gronert K & Chiang N. Anti-microinflammatory lipid signals generated from dietary n-3 fatty acids via cyclooxygenase-2 and transcellular processing: a novel mechanism for NSAID and n-3 PUFA therapeutic actions. *J Physiol Pharmacol.* 2000;4:643–654.
58. Serhan CN, Hong S, Gronert K, Colgan SP, Chiang N, Devchand PR, Mirick G & Moussignac RL. Resolvins: a family of bioactive products of omega-3 fatty acid transformation circuits initiated by aspirin treatment that counter pro-inflammation signals. *J Exp Med.* 2002;196:1025–1037.
59. Hong S, Gronert K, Devchand P, Moussignac R-L & Serhan CN. Novel docosatrienes and 17S-resolvins generated from docosahexaenoic acid in murine brain, human blood and glial cells: autocoids in anti-inflammation. *J Biol Chem.* 2003;278:14677–14687.
60. Marcheselli VL, Hong S, Lukiw WJ & Hua Tian X. Novel docosanoids inhibit brain ischemia reperfusion-mediated leukocyte infiltration and pro-inflammatory gene expression. *J Biol Chem.* 2003;278:43807–43817.

61. Mukherjee PK, Marcheselli VL, Serhan CN & Bazan NG. Neuroprotectin D1. A docosahexaenoic acid-derived docosatriene protects human retinal pigment epithelial cells from oxidative stress. *Proceedings of the National Academy of Sciences of the USA* 2004;101:8491–8496.
62. Serhan CN, Arita M, Hong S & Gotlinger K. Resolvins, docosatrienes, and neuroprotectins, novel omega-3-derived mediators, and their endogenous aspirin-triggered epimers. *Lipids.* 2004;39:1125–1132.
63. Serhan CN. Novel eicosanoid and docosanoid mediators: resolvins, docosatrienes, and neuroprotrectins. *Curr Opin Clin Nutr Metab Care.* 2005;8:115–121.
64. Babcock TA, Novak T, Ong E, Jho DH, Helton WS & Espat NJ. Modulation of lipopolysaccharide-stimulated macrophage tumor necrosis factor-α production by G-3 fatty acid is associated with differential cyclooxygenase-2 protein expression and is independent of interleukin-10. *J Surg Res.* 2002;107:135–139.
65. de Caterina R, Cybulsky MI, Clinton SK, Gimbrone MA & Libby P. The omega-3 fatty acid docosahexaenoate reduces cytokine-induced expression of proatherogenic and proinflammatory proteins in human endothelial cells. *Arterioscler Thromb.* 1994;14:1829–1836.
66. Khalfoun B, Thibault F, Watier H, Bardos P & Lebranchu Y. Docosahexaenoic and eicosapentaenoic acids inhibit in vitro human endothelial cell production of interleukin-6. *Adv Exp Med Biol.* 1997;400:589–597.
67. Billiar T, Bankey P, Svingen B, Curran RD, West MA, Holman RT, Simmons RL & Cerra FB. Fatty acid uptake and Kupffer Cell function: fish oil alters eicosanoid and monokine production to endotoxin stimulation. *Surgery.* 1988;104: 343–349.
68. Renier G, Skamene E, de Sanctis J & Radzioch D. Dietary n-3 polyunsaturated fatty acids prevent the development of atherosclerotic lesions in mice: modulation of macrophage secretory activities. *Arterioscler Thromb.* 1993;13:1515–1524.
69. Yaqoob P & Calder PC. Effects of dietary lipid manipulation upon inflammatory mediator production by murine macrophages. *Cell Immunol.* 1995;163:120–128.
70. Grimble RF, Howell WM, O'Reilly G, Turner SJ, Markovic O, Hirrell S, East JM & Calder PC. The ability of fish oil to suppress tumor necrosis factor-α production by peripheral blood mononuclear cells in healthy men is associated with polymorphisms in genes that influence tumor necrosis factor α production. *Am J Clin Nutr.* 2002;76:454–459.
71. Shen J, Arnett DK, Peacock JM, Parnell LD, Kraja A, Hixson JE, Tsai MY, Lai CQ, Kabagambe EK, Straka RJ & Ordovas JM. Interleukin1beta genetic polymorphisms interact with polyunsaturated fatty acids to modulate risk of the metabolic syndrome. *J Nutr.* 2007;137:1846–1851.
72. Leslie CA, Gonnerman WA, Ullman MD, Hayes KC, Franzblau C & Cathcart ES. Dietary fish oil modulates macrophage fatty acids and decreases arthritis susceptibility in mice. *J Exp Med.* 1985;162:1336–1349.
73. Volker DH, FitzGerald PEB & Garg ML. The eicosapentaenoic to docosahexaenoic acid ratio of diets affects the pathogenesis of arthritis in Lew/SSN rats. *J Nutr.* 2000;130:559–565.

74. Kremer JM, Bigauoette J, Michalek AV, Timchalk MA, Lininger L, Rynes RI, Huyck C, Zieminski J & Bartholomew LE. Effects of manipulation of dietary fatty acids on manifestations of rheumatoid arthritis. *Lancet*. 1985;184–187.
75. Kremer JM, Jubiz W, Michalek A, Rynes RI, Bartholomew LE, Bigouette J, Timchalk M, Beller D & Lininger L. Fish-oil supplementation in active rheumatoid arthritis. *Ann Intern Med*. 1987;106:497–503.
76. Cleland LG, French JK, Betts WH, Murphy GA & Elliot MJ. Clinical and biochemical effects of dietary fish oil supplements in rheumatoid arthritis. *J Rheumatol*. 1988;15:1471–1475.
77. van der Tempel H, Tullekan JE, Limburg PC, Muskiet FAJ & van Rijswijk MH. Effects of fish oil supplementation in rheumatoid arthritis. *Ann Rheum Dis*. 1990;49:76–80.
78. Tullekan JE, Limburg PC, Muskiet FAJ & van Rijswijk MH. Vitamin E status during dietary fish oil supplementation in rheumatoid arthritis. *Arthritis Rheum*. 1990;33:1416–1419.
79. Cleland LG, Caughey GE, James MJ & Proudman SM. Reduction of cardiovascular risk factors with longterm fish oil treatment in early rheumatoid arthritis. *J Rheumatol*. 2006;33:1973–1979.
80. Kremer JM, Lawrence DA, Jubiz W, DiGiacomo R, Rynes R, Bartholomew LE & Sherman M. Dietary fish oil and olive oil supplementation in patients with rheumatoid arthritis. *Arthritis Rheum*. 1990;33:810–820.
81. Esperson GT, Grunnet N, Lervang HH, Nielsen GL, Thomsen BS, Faarvang KL, Dyerberg J & Ernst E. Decreased interleukin-1 beta levels in plasma from rheumatoid arthritis patients after dietary supplementation with n-3 polyunsaturated fatty acids. *Clin Rheumatol*. 1992;11:393–395.
82. Sundrarjun T, Komindr S, Archararit N, Dahaln W, Puchaiwatananon O, Angthararak S, Udomsuppayakui U & Chuncharunee S. Effects of n-3 fatty acids on serum interleukin-6. tumour necrosis factor-alpha and soluble tumour necrosis factor receptor p55 in active rheumatoid arthritis. *J Int Med Res*. 2004; 32:443–454.
83. Sperling RI, Weinblatt M, Robin JL, Ravalese J, Hoover RL, House F, Coblyn JS, Fraser PA, Spur BW & Robinson DR. Effects of dietary supplementation with marine fish oil on leukocyte lipid mediator generation and function in rheumatoid arthritis. *Arthritis Rheum*. 1987;30:988–997.
84. Skoldstam L, Borjesson O, Kjallman A, Seiving B & Akesson B. Effect of six months of fish oil supplementation in stable rheumatoid arthritis: a double blind, controlled study. *Scand J Rheumatol*. 1992;21:178–185.
85. Nielsen GL, Faarvang KL, Thomsen BS, Teglbjaerg KL, Jensen LT, Hansen TM, Lervang HH, Schmidt EB, Dyerberg J & Ernst E. The effects of dietary supplementation with n-3 polyunsaturated fatty acids in patients with rheumatoid arthritis: a randomized, double blind trial. *Eur J Clin Invest*. 1992;22:687–691.
86. Kjeldsen-Kragh J, Lund JA, Riise T, Finnanger B, Haaland K, Finstad R, Mikkelsen K & Forre O. Dietary omega-3 fatty acid supplementation and naproxen treatment in patients with rheumatoid arthritis. *J. Rheumatol*. 1992;19:1531–1536.

87. Lau CS, Morley KD & Belch JJF. Effects of fish oil supplementation on non-steroidal anti-inflammatory drug requirement in patients with mild rheumatoid arthritis. *Brit J Rheumatol.* 1993;32:982–989.
88. Geusens P, Wouters C, Nijs J, Jiang Y & Dequeker J. Long-term effect of omega-3 fatty acid supplementation in active rheumatoid arthritis. *Arthritis Rheum.* 1994;37:824–829.
89. Kremer JM, Lawrence DA, Petrillo GF, Litts LL, Mullaly PM, Rynes RI, Stocker RP, Parhami N, Greenstein NS & Fuchs BR. Effects of high-dose fish oil on rheumatoid arthritis after stopping nonsteroidal antiinflammatory drugs: clinical and immune correlates. *Arthritis Rheum.* 1995;38:1107–1114.
90. Volker D, Fitzgerald P, Major G & Garg M. Efficacy of fish oil concentrate in the treatment of rheumatoid arthritis. *J Rheumatol.* 2000;27:2343–2346.
91. Adam O, Beringer C, Kless T, Lemmen C, Adam A, Wiseman M, Adam P, Klimmek R & Forth W. Anti-inflammatory effects of a low arachidonic acid diet and fish oil in patients with rheumatoid arthritis. *Rheumatol Internat.* 2003;23:27–36.
92. Remans PH, Sont JK, Wagenaar LW, Wouters-Wesseling W, Zuijderduin WM, Jongma A, Breedveld FC & van Laar JM. Nutrient supplementation with polyunsaturated fatty acids and micronutrients in rheumatoid arthritis: clinical and biochemical effects. *Eur J Clin Nutr.* 2004;58:839–845.
93. Berbert AA, Kondo CR, Almendra CL, Matsuo T & Dichi I. Supplementation of fish oil and olive oil in patients with rheumatoid arthritis. *Nutrition* 2005;21: 131–136.
94. Galarraga B, Ho, M, Youssef HM, Hill A, McMahon H, Hall C, Ogston S, Nuki G & Belch JJF. Cod liver oil (n-3 fatty acids) as an non-steroidal anti-inflammatory drug sparing agent in rheumatoid arthritis. *Rheumatol.* 2008;47:665–669.
95. Volker D & Garg M. Dietary n-3 fatty acid supplementation in rheumatoid arthritis – mechanisms, clinical outcomes, controversies, and future directions. *J Clin Biochem Nutr.* 1996;20:83–87.
96. James MJ & Cleland LG. Dietary n-3 fatty acids and therapy for rheumatoid arthritis. *Seminars in Arthritis Rheum.* 1997;27:85–97.
97. Geusens PP. N-3 fatty acids in the treatment of rheumatoid arthritis. In: Kremer JM, ed. *Medicinal Fatty Acids in Inflammation.* Basel: Birkhauser Verlag; 1998:111–123.
98. Kremer JM. N-3 fatty acid supplements in rheumatoid arthritis. *Am J Clin Nutr.* 2000;71:349S–351S.
99. Calder PC. The scientific basis for fish oil supplementation in rheumatoid arthritis. In: Ransley JK, Donnelly JK & Read NW, eds. *Nutritional Supplements in Health and Disease.* London: Springer Verlag; 2001:175–197.
100. Calder PC & Zurier RB. Polyunsaturated fatty acids and rheumatoid arthritis. *Curr Opin Clin Nutr Metab Care.* 2001;4:115–121.
101. Cleland LG, James MJ & Proudman SM. The role of fish oils in the treatment of rheumatoid arthritis. *Drugs.* 2003;63:845–853.
102. Cleland LG & James MJ. Fish oil and rheumatoid arthritis: antiinflammatory and collateral health benefits. *J Rheumatol.* 2000;27:2305–2307.

103. Fortin PR, Lew RA, Liang MH, Wright EA, Beckett LA, Chalmers TC & Sperling RI. Validation of a meta-analysis: The effects of fish oil in rheumatoid arthritis. *J Clin Epidemiol.* 1995;48:1379–1390.
104. MacLean CH, Mojica WA, Morton SC, Pencharz J, et al. Effects of omega-3 fatty acids on inflammatory bowel disease, rheumatoid arthritis, renal disease, systemic lupus erythematosus, and osteoporosis, Evidence Report/Technical Assessment No. 89. AHRQ Publication No. 04-E012-2, 2004. Agency for Healthcare Research and Quality, Rockville.
105. Goldberg RJ & Katz J. A meta-analysis of the analgesic effects of omega-3 polyunsaturated fatty acid supplementation for inflammatory joint pain. *Pain.* 2007;129:210–233.

4

Physical Activity and Arthritis

DAVID E. YOCUM, MD

KEY CONCEPTS

- Exercise can reduce pain and improve function in individuals with arthritis. The benefits transcend physical and functional improvement, positively affecting mental health and psychosocial measures, with results equal to or exceeding approved medications.
- The most important factor in ensuring lifelong adherence to an exercise regimen is to be sure that it is tailored to the individual to maximize enjoyment and compliance.
- Recent studies suggest that people who exercise regularly have thicker cartilage with more proteoglycan, a major component of cartilage.
- The most effective exercise programs combine a well-designed strengthening program for all muscle groups, in addition to regular aerobic activity performed at least 3 days per week. For more severe forms of arthritis, input from physician and physical therapist will help to maximize success.

■

Introduction

Over 20% of Americans have been diagnosed with arthritis, and 50% of individuals over the age of 65 have some form of arthritis.[1] There are over 100 forms of arthritis, of which rheumatoid arthritis (RA) and osteoarthritis (OA) are by far the most common. RA is an autoimmune inflammatory disease that can affect almost any joint in the body. Similarly, OA can occur in any joint, but appears most frequently in the knee and hip joints. Both cause pain and impairment in body functions, such as muscle strength, range of joint motion, and joint stability. Furthermore, both also have a major impact on physical functioning in daily life, and frequently lead to moderate or severe limitations in participation and a decreased quality of life.[2–4] Based upon published evidence, it is clear that exercise can reduce pain and improve function in individuals with arthritis. The benefits transcend physical and functional improvement, positively affecting mental health and psychosocial measures.

Exercise and Arthritis

In the past, exercise was felt to be detrimental to people with inflammatory forms of arthritis, such as RA, perhaps owing to increased wear and tear on the affected joints. However, recent studies demonstrate a positive benefit, sometimes similar to the drugs used to treat the disease itself.[5,6,9] The best outcome appears to be associated with a combination of strengthening and aerobic exercise.

Therapeutic exercise is recommended in several recent treatment guidelines for patients with OA of the hip or knee.[7,8] A lack of regular physical activity is a risk factor for functional decline, and is associated with increased health care costs among patients with arthritis.[9] Regular exercise aims to improve overall function and to help meet the physical demands of daily living. Exercise is typically defined as a range of activities involving muscular contraction and bodily movement, but, in actuality, is a modality that can be delivered in many ways. The most important factor in ensuring lifelong adherence to an exercise regimen is to be sure that it is tailored to the individual to maximize enjoyment and compliance.

Many systematic reviews have outlined the effectiveness of exercise therapy in patients with arthritis,[2,7,8,10] specifically demonstrating beneficial effects on pain, physical function, and patient overall wellbeing. Interestingly, most of these studies focus on short-term results, and there are few studies examining long-term effects. Because arthritis is a progressive disease with long-term effects, it is important that beneficial post-treatment results are sustained in the long term. A recent review of long-term studies supports the sustained benefits of exercise in OA.[7]

DIRECT BENEFITS OF EXERCISE ON THE JOINT

Regular exercise is routinely recommended for people with diabetes and coronary artery disease, owing to many improved outcome parameters. However, the effect of regular exercise on the outcome of arthritis, especially in those who are overweight, is unclear. Cartilage loss is the pathologic hallmark of OA, but the disease affects all components of the joint, especially as it progresses. Dynamic loading has a trophic effect on cartilage, and with frequent dynamic loading, especially in a healthy range, cartilage might be induced to become thicker. If, in fact, the rate of cartilage loss slows, OA progression might be slowed, perhaps leading to decreased disease incidence in those individuals engaging in regular activity.[11,12] This has been documented in animal models of OA.

In most animal studies, weight-bearing exercise has been shown to protect against the development of OA.[13,14] Studies on cartilage thickness in exercising versus non-exercising humans have reported varied results. In a recent short-term trial, Roos and Dahlberg[15] reported that individuals without OA who were randomized to an exercise regimen had a healthier distribution of proteoglycans within cartilage as demonstrated by imaging studies, compared with sedentary individuals not participating in exercise. This finding suggests an overall protective effect on the development of OA over a longer period. Triathletes have thicker cartilage in their patellae (but thinner cartilage in their medial femoral condyles) than do age-matched inactive study volunteers.[16] In children, vigorous self-reported activity over a 2-week period was associated with an accretion of cartilage when compared with children with no reports of vigorous activity.[17] Obesity is a major risk factor for knee OA, and its effect is thought to be due to increased loading. Weight bearing activity and recreational activity may be injurious to the knees of persons who are overweight, but this issue has not been well studied.[18] The use of an exercise program to reduce weight, thus lowering OA risk, is highly recommended.

EFFECT OF EXERCISE ON THE DEVELOPMENT AND PROGRESSION OF ARTHRITIS

Although many studies have attempted to determine whether physical activity prevents (or causes) knee OA, the answer is not known, in part because of inherent limitations in addressing this issue. Some studies used a cross-sectional analysis, with individuals providing recalled exercise activity.[19] Other studies using prospective designs have relied upon self-reported arthritis symptoms,[20] an entity with questionable validity at best. Individuals who are healthy may exercise more, may visit doctors for health problems less, and may not get the opportunity to have their OA diagnosed.

Few prospective studies exist in which persons have been surveyed about activity and then followed to see who develops OA. Follow-up needs to be long enough for OA to develop. In the few studies using this approach, the results have been conflicting. One study tracked young and middle-aged runners for up to 10 years and found no increase in knee OA by serial radiographic evaluation.[16] Interestingly, in the most recent follow-up, runners did not show joint space loss, whereas non-runners did—a difference that was not statistically significant, but suggested that running may help to preserve cartilage thickness. Another study was unable to demonstrate an association between physical activity on disease occurrence in middle-aged women.[21] However, while the numbers were small, follow-up was short (4 years), and confidence limits were wide, results of the study did suggest that regular walking protected against joint space loss. Therefore, these two studies, in markedly different populations, not only found no increased risk of OA with regular exercise, but suggested the possibility of disease protection.

In contrast, another study found that elderly patients who self-reported high levels of heavy physical activity had an increased risk of radiographic knee OA.[22] In this study, with a large number of overweight persons, body mass index (BMI) above the median was found to further increase the risk of knee OA among those who exercised. Finally, a large elderly cohort followed for the development of hip OA[23] demonstrated that elderly women who had been more active in middle age had more hip OA by radiograph.

Discordance of study results has arisen in part because studies are often small and follow insufficient numbers of overweight elderly adults. In addition, many studies use suboptimal questionnaires asking about specific physical activities, so that the relationship to knee OA of popular physical activities, such as recreational walking, remains unknown. The studies are also fraught with ambiguity, using different definitions of OA, or even focusing upon different, less affected joints. For example, studies examining OA of the knee often focus on tibiofemoral disease, whereas much symptomatic disease occurs in the patellofemoral compartment, an area that is not well studied.

There are relatively few studies examining the effect of exercise upon inflammatory arthritis. Studies can be especially challenging due to the fact that patients often suffer flares that can severely limit the individual's ability to exercise. One study, however, has shown significant benefits to exercise in patients with RA.[6]

Psychosocial Effects of Exercise on the Outcome of Arthritis

There is considerable evidence linking psychosocial factors with arthritis activity. Interpersonal stress and depression have been shown to be associated with increased pain and arthritis activity.[24] Both can work together synergistically to further enhance disease activity.[25] Depression is also one of the many negative outcomes associated with arthritis. For example, the presence of OA is associated with greater emotional distress, poor sleep quality, greater numbers of sick days, more fatigue, and more visits to the primary health care provider. Depression, outlook on life, and use of coping mechanisms all influence the degree of success and quality of life following a total joint replacement. Poor interpersonal relationships have been shown to have a negative effect on arthritis activity.[26] In contrast, good interpersonal relationships have been shown to have nearly the same benefit to improving function in a person with RA as that of an anti-arthritis drug.[27,28] Regular exercise has been shown to be helpful with respect to psychological wellbeing.

There have been many studies examining the positive psychological effects of exercise. In one study, both aerobic exercise and strengthening programs had positive effects on depression, especially in those individuals with a high compliance.[28] Programs combining exercise and stress management are associated with enhanced coping mechanisms, decreased pain, and in one study, evidence of improved immune function.[29,30] Another study using patients with RA who were taking biologic therapies demonstrated that a combination of aerobic exercise and muscle strengthening enhanced the outcome of the patient over the benefits of the pharmaceutical treatment alone.[6] Studies have routinely demonstrated the need for interventions that provide a combination of exercise, education, and self-help management in the care of chronic rheumatologic diseases. Interestingly, little is known about whether reversing depression has beneficial effects on arthritis.

Clinical Guidelines

Based upon the published evidence, exercise can reduce pain and improve function for people with arthritis. Additional benefits include better coping skills and improved psychosocial interactions. Initial professional instruction from an appropriate physician, a physical therapist and an exercise trainer, as well as periodic review, may be needed to achieve an effective exercise program.

Studies have demonstrated that merely telling patients to exercise and letting them go about their business is not likely to achieve the desired results. Individualization of exercise regimens at the outset, especially in people with inflammatory arthritis, may improve the effectiveness of the overall program. In addition, a physical therapist who understands the pathophysiology of arthritis can be a great help in focusing on individual joints or total body mechanics. It is important to remember that flares of disease may affect the individual's response to exercise.

The most effective exercise programs provide the combination of a well-designed strengthening program for all muscle groups, along with regular aerobic activity performed at least 3 days per week. This can be accomplished with exercise sessions of up to one hour. For people with arthritis, especially those with inflammatory forms and those who are more sedentary, programs should start at lower levels and progressively increase, slowly, as tolerated. When an individual is unable to progress after a few months, the overall situation may need to be reexamined. For example, a patient may need their medications adjusted to lower pain, especially prior to exercise. One must also consider the stage of the arthritis before starting exercise. A joint that is far advanced may need to be replaced. However, exercise and strengthening in other areas of the body prior to joint replacement can have a positive effect on the outcome of the surgery.

Age, beginning activity level, and existing joint deformities are just some of the factors that need to be taken into account when initiating an exercise program. Family and social support can be major factors in determining success. Involving partners can often be very helpful. There are also community-based programs run by organizations such as the Arthritis Foundation that not only provide group support, but are often associated with pools or other exercise facilities that offer participation at a lower cost.

Case Studies

To illustrate the proper use of exercise in the patient with arthritis, here are two typical cases that we see in clinic.

CASE NUMBER 1

Jim recently lost his wife, is moderately overweight, and has not been active due to pain in his right knee. He noticeably limps, and only takes an occasional pain pill as he does not like drugs. Radiographs of the knee demonstrate OA with adequate joint space. However, due to inactivity, there is significant muscle loss in the right leg.

First, it is important to reduce the pain that Jim is experiencing in order for him to participate in an active exercise program. In addition, Jim needs to lose weight to reduce pressure on the knee and increase the likelihood that he will be able to exercise comfortably. Several allied health practitioners would be useful here. First, a visit to a nutritionist would be useful in order to help Jim achieve some weight loss through appropriate dietary modifications. Second, a consultation by a well-trained physical therapist will help to set up a proper strengthening program. Finally, Jim's psychological state needs to be assessed, as depression over the loss of his wife may be playing a major role in his lack of activity. A support group such as those offered by the Arthritis Foundation may help, or, if his depression is more severe, Jim may need professional counseling.

CASE NUMBER 2

Jane has had RA for about 5 years, and while the disease is fairly well controlled, she notes a lot of muscle pain and a general sense of weakness with doing housework or walking more than one or two blocks. She admits that she is worried that if she does any exercise, her arthritis will flare. Examination and laboratories demonstrate that she has almost no joint inflammation and has no joint deformities. However, she has lost a great deal of muscle strength.

Jane needs an exercise trainer who is knowledgeable about inflammatory arthritis—one who can take her through a slower program at the outset, with gradual advancement to a more vigorous program. She also needs to understand that when a joint begins to hurt or become swollen, she needs to let the trainer know, and if necessary see her physician. In this situation, pain may not mean gain. The key in this case is to present the patient with the data supporting the benefits of exercise, and to educate her about the proper way to approach exercise. Most important is the reassurance that she has the power to improve her situation with exercise.

Conclusion

Arthritis is a lifelong condition that can lead to depression, disability, and even early death. An appropriate, individualized exercise program can have tremendous benefit, both physically and psychologically. To be successful, a team approach is key—combining the physician, the therapist, and the trainer.

Mental state and social support can be the difference between success and failure in the development of a lifelong exercise program.

REFERENCES

1. Centers for Disease Control and Prevention. Prevalence of arthritis. *MMWR*. 2006;55:1089.
2. Oddis C. New perspectives of osteoarthritis. *Am J Med*. 1996;100(Suppl 2A):2A–10S.
3. Hamerman D. Clinical implications of osteoarthritis and aging. *Ann Rheum Dis*. 1995;54(2):82–85.
4. Liang MH, Arson M, Thompson M et al. Cost and outcomes in rheumatoid arthritis and osteoarthritis. *Arthritis Rheum*. 1984;27(5):522–529.
5. Bulthuis Y, Mohammad S, Braakman-Jansen L et al. Cost effectiveness of intensive exercise therapy directly following hospital discharge in patients with arthritis: Results of a randomized controlled clinical trial. *Arthritis Rheum*. 2008;59(2):247–254.
6. Flint-Wagner HG, Lisse J, Lohman TG et al. Assessment of a 16-week training program on strength, pain and function in rheumatoid arthritis patients. *J Clinical Rheum*. 2009 Jun;15(4):165–71.
7. Pisters MF, Veenhof C, van Meeteren N et al. Long-term effectiveness of exercise in patients with osteoarthritis of the hip or knee: A systematic review. *Arthritis Rheum*. 2007;57(7):1245–1253.
8. Clyman B. Exercise in the treatment of osteoarthritis. *Current Rheum Reports*. 2001;3:520.
9. Hurley MV, Walsh NE, Mitchell HL et al. Economic evaluation of a rehabilitation program integration exercise, self-management and active coping strategies for chronic knee pain. *Arthritis Rheum*. 2007;57(7):1220–1229.
10. Minor M. Impact of exercise on osteoarthritis outcomes. *J Rheumatology*. 2004;31(Suppl 70):81–88.
11. Fukui N, Purple CR and Sandell LJ. Cell biology of osteoarthritis: The chondrocyte's response to injury. *Current Rheum Rep*. 2001;3:496–505.
12. Oegema TR. Molecular basis of the interaction of inflammation and exercise: Keep on walking! *Arthritis Rheum*. 2007;56(10):3176–3179.
13. Otterness IG, Eskra S, Bliven ML, Shay AK, Pelletier JP, Milici AJ. Exercise protects against articular cartilage degeneration in the hamster. *Arthritis Rheum*. 1998;41:2068–2076.
14. Galois L, Etienne S, Grossin L et al. Moderate-impact exercise associated with decreased severity of experimental osteoarthritis in rats. *Rheumatology*. 2003;42:692–693.
15. Roos EM, Dahlberg L. Positive effects of moderate exercise on glycosaminoglycan content in knee cartilage: a four-month randomized, controlled trial in patients at risk for osteoarthritis. Arthritis *Rheum*. 2005;52:3507–3514.

16. Muhlbauer R, Lukasz TS, Faber TS et al. Comparison of knee joint cartilage thickness in triatheletes and physically inactive volunteers based on magnetic resonance imaging and three-dimensional analysis. *Am J Sports Med.* 2000;28:541–546.
17. Jones G, Ding C, Glisson M, Hynes K, Ma D, Cicuttini F. Knee articular cartilage development in children: a longitudinal study of the effect of sex, growth, body composition and physical activity. *Pediatr Res.* 2003;54:230–236.
18. Targonska-Stepniak B. Obesity and osteoarthritis. *Rheumatologia.* 2003;41:366–370.
19. Cheng Y, Macera CA, Davis DR, Ainsworth BE, Troped PJ. Physical activity and self-reported, physician-diagnosed osteoarthritis: is physical activity a risk factor. *J Clin Epidemiol.* 2000;53:315–322.
20. Felson DT, Niu J, Clancy M, Sack B, Aliabadi P, Zhang Y. Effect of recreational physical activities on the development of knee osteoarthritis in older adults of different weights: the Framingham Study. *Arthritis Rheum.* 57(1):6–12.
21. Hart DJ, Doyle DV, Spector TD. Incidence and risk factors for radiographic knee osteoarthritis in middle-aged women: the Chingford Study. *Arthritis Rheum.* 1999;42:17–24.
22. McAlindon TE, Wilson PW Aliabadi P, Weissman B, Felson DT. Level of physical activity and the risk of radiographic and symptomatic knee osteoarthritis in the elderly: the Framingham study. *Am J Med.* 1999;106:151–157.
23. Lane NE, Hochberg MC, Pressman A, Scott JC, Nevitt MC. Recreational physical activity and the risk of osteoarthritis of the hip of elderly women. *J Rheumatol.* 1999;26:849–854.
24. Zautra AJ, Smith BW. Depression and reactivity to stress in older women with rheumatoid arthritis and osteoarthritis. *Psychosom Med.* 2001;63:687–696.
25. Dieppe PA, Lohmander LS. Pathogenesis and management of pain in osteoarthritis. *Lancet.* 2005;365:965–973.
26. Kasle S, Yocum DE, Wilhelm MS. Relational mutuality at baseline predicts functional status 6 months later more strongly for women in a rheumatoid arthritis sample. *Arthritis Rheum.* 2003;48:S646.
27. Swe K, Kasle S, Sheikh S et al. Comparison of ESR and marital satisfaction in predicting patient-reported health outcomes in rheumatoid arthritis. *Arthritis Rheum.* 2007;56:S279.
28. Cornett M, Yocum DE, Castro WL et al. Living healthy with arthritis: A community based pilot program focusing on wellness and preventive arthritis care through exercise, nutrition and a balanced lifestyle. *Arthritis Rheum.* 1998;41:S186.
29. Yocum DE, Castro WL, Cornett M. Exercise, education and behavioral modification as an alternative therapy for pain and stress in rheumatic disease. *Rheum Dis Clin North Am.* 2000;26(1):145–159.
30. Yocum DE, Zautra A, Matt K et al. Exercise and stress reduction result in positive changes in prolactin, cortisol, and immune function in rheumatoid arthritis. *Arthritis Rheum.* 1995;38:S384.

5

Herbal Medicine in Rheumatologic Disorders

TIERAONA LOW DOG, MD

KEY CONCEPTS

- The use of herbal products is common among people with rheumatologic conditions.
- There is a growing body of evidence demonstrating the beneficial effects of botanicals for a variety of rheumatologic conditions.
- Health care practitioners should ask patients about their use of herbal medicines and counsel appropriately.

Herbal Medicine

Herbal medicine can be defined as the use of plants for the purposes of healing and wholeness. It has been used by all cultures and peoples across the span of time, and has given birth to the modern sciences of botany, pharmacy, perfumery, and chemistry. Some of our most useful and beneficial medicines originate from plants, including aspirin (salicylic acid derivates, derived from willow bark and meadowsweet), quinine (from cinchona bark), digoxin (from foxglove) and morphine (from opium poppy). There is a distinct difference between the pharmaceutical practice of isolating plant constituents and the traditional practice of herbal medicine. Herbalists hold that the whole plant or plant part is "active" and that each medicinal plant is itself a chemically complex mixture, while the goal of pharmaceutical research has been to identify, isolate and produce single active ingredients from plants. While there is certainly a place for isolated constituents derived from plants, these are not herbal medicines.

The marketplace for herbal products continues to grow at a steady pace in the United States and abroad. Between 1990 and 1997, the use of herbal medicines increased by 380% in the US.[1] In fact, when looking across all complementary and alternative (CAM) practices, the greatest relative increase in the US between 1997 and 2002 was herbal medicine (12.1% vs.18.6%, respectively; representing 38 million adults).[2] The sale of herbal products grew by 50% in the UK during the period 1995–2000.[3] There are thousands of herbal products being sold in the marketplace, including a considerable number of questionable quality and dubious efficacy. Despite the flagrant use of the terms "natural" and "holistic" that surrounds these products, it could be argued that the marketing of prepackaged herbal formulations is, in some ways, simply applying the same reductionist, product-based approach that has characterized the pharmaceutical industry for decades—only substituting an herb in place of a drug. This is not to say we do not need high quality commercially prepared herbal products—we do—but it is important to stress that simply using devil's claw instead of a nonsteroidal anti-inflammatory drug (NSAID) is to miss the richness that herbal medicine has to offer. And if we are interested in treating the whole person, then these products must be used within a holistic context that takes into consideration all aspects of the individual, as one size seldom fits all.

The earliest evidence for the effectiveness of herbal medicines comes from direct human experience and observation that spanned across the millennia. Today, our evidence base has expanded to include pharmacological studies, case reports, uncontrolled clinical studies, as well as the "gold standard" randomized, double-blind, placebo-controlled clinical study (RDBPCT). Agreeing upon what level of evidence is necessary for making treatment decisions is a topic of debate among practitioners in both conventional and complementary medicine. Certain study designs, such as the RDBPCT, are generally more persuasive than others because they are inherently less subject to bias. Yet, specific questions regarding trial design emerge when studying herbal medicines. First, herbal preparations often vary between trials, making comparison difficult, as products may not be biologically or pharmacologically equivalent. Second, herbalists generally prescribe herbal mixtures, as opposed to single herb preparations, based upon the premise that when properly prepared, these mixtures offer greater efficacy and, to some degree, greater safety. Herbal formulations may offer additive, or even synergistic effects, and additional herbs can be included to modify potential side effects from the primary herb.

For example, some herbs can cause digestive upset or cramping—adverse effects that can be reduced or eliminated by adding gut antispasmodics or demulcents such as chamomile, licorice, or ginger. And thirdly, herbal practitioners often individualize treatment protocols based upon the unique characteristics of the patient. For instance, a woman with osteoarthritis who presents with menopausal hot flashes, irritability and insomnia may be given a formula that includes black cohosh (*Actaea racemosa*), hops (*Humulus lupulus*) and schizandra (*Schizandra chinensis*). Studies suggest that black cohosh can relieve menopause-related hot flashes and night sweats; however, one of its primary uses by indigenous Native Americans and physicians of the 19th and early 20th centuries was as an antirheumatic. Hops strobiles are phytoestrogenic, possess sedative effects, improve sleep, and contain compounds that inhibit COX-2. Schizandra berries are considered a premiere tonic used to ease palpitations, irritability and insomnia. Schizandra also contains weak phytoestrogens which can ease menopausal hot flashes.

This individualization of herbal therapies generally exists within a holistic framework that may include dietary recommendations, mind-body therapies, manual medicine, or other approaches that may promote wellness and healing in the patient. This integrated approach poses a challenge to the RDBPCT design. The difficulty may be, in part, because the herbal clinician and researcher are asking related, but different, questions. The researcher studies the efficacy and mechanism of a given therapy so that broad numbers of patients may potentially benefit from the treatment. The herbalist believes that each patient is unique, and the treatment plan must be individualized to meet his/her particular needs. Holism draws upon the concept that therapies are designed to treat and support the person—not the disease. Herbalists and researchers could benefit greatly from more extensive dialogues with each other—so that each can share their unique experiences and worldviews, learning from each other to improve both research and clinical care.

The Use of Botanicals in Rheumatology

Botanical medicines have been used since ancient times for the management of musculoskeletal and rheumatologic complaints. Indeed, aspirin and morphine both have their roots in plant medicine. Today, the popularity of herbal medicines remains prevalent in many parts of the world. In some areas this is due to cultural preference, in some there is limited access to other medicines, and for others it may be due to increasing dissatisfaction with long-term adverse effects of many of our conventional treatments. Surveys indicate that patients with arthritis are frequent users of complementary and alternative medicine,[4,5] particularly herbal therapies and chiropractic.

The role of inflammatory chemokines and cytokines such as tumor necrosis factor-alpha (TNF-α) and interleukins (IL-1β, IL-6); inflammatory enzymes such as cyclooxygenase (COX-1 and COX-2), 5-lipoxygenase (5-LOX) and matrix metalloproteinase (MMP-9) and adhesion molecules in the pathogenesis of arthritis is well documented, with most inflammatory mediators being regulated by the transcription factor nuclear factor-κB (NF-κB).[6] In vitro and animal data demonstrate that botanicals influence these mediators in a variety of ways, impacting cytokine secretion, histamine release, immunoglobulin secretion and class switching, lymphocyte proliferation, and cytotoxic activity,[7] due to the complex interplay of a wide range of plant compounds.[8] Some of these compounds include curcumin (turmeric), harpagoside (devil's claw), gingerols and shogaols (ginger), resveratrol (red grapes), tea polyphenols, genistein (soy), silymarin (milk thistle), boswellic acid (boswellia) and withanolides (ashwagandha).[6] Interestingly, many of these botanicals were traditionally used for the treatment of arthritis. (Table 5.1)

Table 5.1.

Anti-inflammatory Activity of Select Botanicals

Boswellia serrata	boswellic acid	NF-κB, COX-2, 5-LOX, ICAM-1
Curcuma longa	curcumin	NF-κB,COX-2, 5-LOX, TNF-α, IL-1β, IL-6, IL-8, MMPs, AMs
Harpagophytum procumbens	harpagoside	NF-κB, COX-2
Ocimum sanctum	ursolic acid	NF-κB, COX-2, MMP-9
Rosmarinus officinalis	rosmarinic aciid	NF-κB, COX-2, TNF-α, AMs
Silybum marianum	silymarin	NF-κB, 5-LOX
Tripterygium wilfordii	celastrol	NF- κB, COX-2, MMP-9, TNF-α, AMs
Uncaria tomentosa	oxindole alkaloids	NF- Kb, TNF- α
Vitis vinifera	*resveratrol*	NF-κB, COX-2, TNF-α, 5-LOX, AMs
Withania somnifera	withanolides	NF-κB, COX-2, MMP-9, ICAM-1
Zingiber officinale	gingerols, shogaols	COX-2, 5-LOX, TNF-α, IL-1 β

NF- κB, nuclear factor kappa-beta; COX-2, cyclooxygenase-2; 5-LOX, lipooxygenase; TNF- α, tumor necrosis factor α; IL – interleukin; MMP, matrix metalloproteinases, AM, adhesion molecule; ICAM-1, intercellular adhesion molecule-1

The Herbal Approach

The treatment goals for any rheumatologic condition are to improve overall health, relieve symptoms, delay the progression of disease, and improve the patient's quality of life. There are many considerations when creating a botanical prescription. As symptom relief is a primary goal, the selection of appropriate anti-inflammatory, analgesic herbs is the first step, and there are many to choose from. Additional herbs are selected in order to support wellbeing and improve overall health. For example, if pain interferes with sleep, sedative herbs such as valerian (*Valeriana officinalis*), hops (*Humulus lupulus*), passionflower (*Passiflora incarnata*) or ashwagandha (*Withania somnifera*) might be considered. Those with poor digestion may benefit from the addition of herbal fibers such as flax (*Linum usitatissimum*) or psyllium (*Plantago psyllium*), gut antispasmodics like chamomile (*Matricaria recutita*) or ginger (*Zingiber officinale*). Or, bitters such as dandelion (*Taraxacum officinale*) or chamomile could be used to enhance digestive function. Adaptogens, herbs that help the body cope with physical or mental stress, would likely be considered. Some of the most commonly used adaptogens include ginseng (*Panax ginseng, P. quinquefolius*), ashwagandha, and rhodiola (*Rhodiola rosea*). Many individuals benefit from the use of topical liniments or ointments, which can ease pain and reduce inflammation. Ginger, arnica and cayenne are excellent choices; in fact capsaicin ointments, made from cayenne, are available as FDA approved over-the-counter preparations. Essential oils of peppermint, rosemary or wintergreen are also commonly used in ointments, though care should be used with sensitive skin, and use should be avoided in patients having an acute inflammatory flare.

Perhaps the best way to illustrate the use of herbal medicine in rheumatology is with several brief vignettes.

CASE 1

A 62-year-old man with OA of the knee and chronic lower back pain presents looking for a more "natural approach" to managing his joint pain. He has been taking 800–1200 mg per day of ibuprofen with moderate relief, but has begun to experience worsening heartburn, which is partially relieved by the TUMS he takes several nights per week. Three months ago he was thoroughly evaluated by his physician and diagnosed with GERD, and was given a prescription for omeprazole and celecoxib, which have not been filled because he lost his job and health insurance shortly after the visit. He also seems to have an aversion to taking medications, other than his low-dose thiazide diuretic for hypertension. He is feeling quite depressed about his health and lack of employment. He denies any suicide ideation, but says he isn't sleeping well and is frustrated with his 10-pound weight gain over the past year due to lack of exercise.

So, how might an herbal practitioner sort through the options for putting together an herbal treatment plan? Let's start by examining the evidence based research:

*Devil's Claw (*Harpagophytum procumbens *[Burch.] DC ex. Meisn.)*

One herb that comes quickly to mind is devil's claw, a perennial plant native to Namibia, Botswana, and the Kalahari of South Africa, where the dried secondary tubers are traditionally used as a digestive tonic and to relieve fever and pain. The German health authorities approve devil's claw as a "supportive therapy for degenerative disorders of the locomotor system."[9] Harpagoside, an iridoid glycoside, inhibits the expression of COX-2 and inducible nitric oxide through the suppression of NF-κB activation.[10] A review of botanicals used in the treatment of painful osteoarthritis and chronic low back pain found strong evidence for the effectiveness of devil's claw preparations providing a minimum of 50 mg/d of harpagoside.[11] Devil's claw extracts are well tolerated; however, it is a potent bitter and may aggravate our patient's heartburn. A safety review of 28 clinical trials noted that the incidence of adverse events during treatment with devil's claw was no greater than placebo.[12] Safety in pregnancy is not known.

Avocado/Soybean Unsaponifiables

A product that has an excellent safety profile and good evidence of benefit is derived from the oily fractions of avocado (100 mg) and soybean (200 mg); the product is referred to as avocado/soybean unsaponifiables (ASUs). Four high-quality clinical trials demonstrated that ASUs improve the pain and stiffness of knee and hip OA, and reduce the need for NSAIDs.[13] The active components of the mixture have not been identified, and the mechanism of action is poorly understood. In vitro studies show that ASUs display anabolic, anticatabolic, and anti-inflammatory effects on chondrocytes.[14,15] There are no significant safety issues associated with the product. ASUs have a slow onset of action, requiring most patients to continue their analgesics for the first 4–6 weeks of use and then tapering the dose as tolerated. The dose is 300–600 mg per day.

Ashwagandha (Withania somnifera *Dunal*)

Ashwagandha has been used for centuries in India and the Middle East in the treatment of arthritic conditions, nervous exhaustion, anxiety and insomnia. Ashwagandha contains a number of pharmacologically complex compounds, including the steroidal lactone withanolides, which have been shown to possess significant anti-inflammatory and antioxidant activity. Withanolides inhibit the activation of NF-κB and NF-κB-regulated gene expression,[16] while the root has chondroprotective activity.[17]

There are no clinical trials evaluating ashwagandha as a single agent for arthritis, but it has been studied in a polyherbal formulation. An RDBPCT of 90 patients with OA of the knee found the combination extract RA-1 (*Withania somnifera, Boswellia serrata, Zingiberis officinale, Curcuma longa* extracts) to be superior to placebo in reducing pain as measured by the Visual Analogue Pain Scale (VAS) and Western Ontario and McMaster Universities Osteoarthritis Index (WOMAC).[18] RA-1 was shown to reduce joint swelling and rheumatoid factor levels in a randomized placebo-controlled study of 182 patients with RA; however, no significant difference was seen in the American College of Rheumatology 50% response criteria (ACR-50) between the two groups.[19]

The dose of powdered root is typically 2–3 grams per day, or equivalent in tincture. There are standardized extracts available containing 2.5% withanolides, taken at doses of 500 mg 2–3 times daily. These doses typically do not cause daytime drowsiness. Safety is good, though it should not be used during pregnancy.

Boswellia (Boswellia serrata *Roxb. ex Colebr.*)

Next we turn our focus to boswellia, given the review of the ashwagandha studies mentioned above. Boswellia is a large branching tree found in the dry hilly areas of India. When the bark is stripped away, a gummy oleoresin, known as *salai guggul*, is gathered. In vitro and animal data show that boswellic acids possess significant anti-inflammatory activity. An RDBPCT of 1000 mg/d *Boswellia serrata* extract (Cap WokVel® containing 333 mg boswellia extract per capsule with minimum 40% total boswellic acids, Pharmanza, Gujarat, India) showed significant decrease in pain intensity and improvements in knee function in 30 patients with OA ($p < 0.001$) compared to placebo.[20]

The evidence for boswellia in RA is mixed. A 1996 review[21] reported positive findings from several small studies for a particular boswellia extract (H-15: chloroform/methanol extract) in patients with rheumatoid arthritis. After this review, an RDBPCT of 78 patients with active RA (only 37 completed the trial) failed to show any significant benefit for 3600 mg/d boswellia extract (nine tablets/d each containing 400 mg chloroform/methanol extract) over placebo when given in addition to their current medical therapy.[22]

The most common side effect of boswellia is gastric irritation. Toxicity studies are very reassuring for doses up to 1000 mg/kg. The average dose is 400–1200 mg three times daily of boswellia standardized to contain 40–65% boswellic acid. Start with the lowest dose and titrate upwards as needed. Boswellia should not be used during pregnancy.

*Ginger (*Zingiber officinale *Roscoe)*

In addition to its long history of use as a spice, references to ginger as a medicinal agent can be found in ancient Chinese, Indian, Arabic and Greco-Roman texts. Ginger is chiefly known as an antiemetic, anti-inflammatory, circulatory stimulant, digestive aid, diaphoretic, and warming agent.

Ginger extract (170 mg 3 times/d EV.EXT 33; standardized ethanol extract of dry *Z. officinale* rhizomes, Eurovita A/S, Denmark) was found less effective than ibuprofen (400 mg 3 times/d), but more effective than placebo in 67 patients with OA of the hip or knee.[23] A concentrated extract of ginger and *Alpinia galanga* (255mg BID, equivalent to 4–6 grams of dried ginger and galangal) over a period of 6 weeks reduced pain in an RDBPCT of 261 patients with moderate to severe pain from OA of the knee.[24] The products used in these two studies by Bliddal and Altman are quite different, and comparisons cannot be made. Heartburn is a common, bothersome side effect for those taking higher doses of ginger, which could definitely pose a problem for our patient. Though the German Commission E contraindicates the use of ginger during pregnancy,[9] animal studies and follow-up from randomized trials using ginger for hyperemesis gravidarum have failed to show significant adverse effects on pregnancy outcomes at doses of 1.0–1.5 grams dried ginger per day.[25]

*Bromelain (*Ananas comosus *Merr.)*

Bromelain might be useful for our patient as he tapers off his ibuprofen, and for acute exacerbations of back pain. Bromelain refers to a combination of sulfur-containing proteolytic enzymes extracted from the stem and fruit of the pineapple plant. It is an effective anti-inflammatory with antiedematous, antithrombotic and fibrinolytic effects.[26] It is commonly used to aid digestion, reduce swelling in acute injury/postsurgery, and for relief of arthritis pain. A comparative study of an enzyme preparation (Phlogenzym™ contains bromelain 90 mg, trypsin 48 mg, and rutosid 100 mg in enteric coated tablets: Mucos Pharma, Geretsried; dose 1 tablet 3 times a day) and diclofenac (50 mg twice a day) found similar relief in pain and improvement in function at 6 weeks, in 73 patients with OA of the knee.[27] A randomized study of a non-enteric coated bromelain single-ingredient preparation was not superior to placebo in patients with moderate to severe OA of the knee.[28] Bromelain appears safe at the doses normally taken; i.e., 80–320 mg three times daily as an enteric coated preparation. Allergic reactions can occur. Theoretically, bromelain can increase the risk of bleeding, so it should be used in caution by those taking anticoagulant medication and should be discontinued prior to surgery. Bromelain and pineapple juice are both inhibitors of the drug metabolizing enzyme CYP2D9.[29]

Willow (Salix *spp)*

Willow is one of the herbs that gave rise to the birth of aspirin, our first effective NSAID. The analgesic and antipyretic properties of willow were well known by ancient Egyptian, Greek, Indian, and Roman civilizations. *Salix* species contain salicin, a prodrug of salicylate, and other components such as tannins, flavonoids, and salicin esters that contribute to its overall effect.[30] Willow bark extract (WBE) is recognized by the German Commission E for the treatment of "diseases accompanied by fever, rheumatic ailments and headaches"[9] in a daily dose equivalent to 60–120 mg salicin, while the European Scientific Cooperative for Phytotherapy ESCOP monograph recommends an equivalent of up to 240 mg/d salicin.[31]

Two RDBPCT trials in patients with OA were contradictory,[30,32] though each provided approximately 1360 mg of WBE standardized to 240 mg per day of salicin. A study of WBE (240 mg/d salicin) in 26 patients with rheumatoid arthritis showed a mean reduction of pain on the VAS of –8 mm (15%) in the WBE group compared with –2 mm (4%) in the placebo group. The difference was not statistically significant ($p = 0.93$).[32]

WBE is generally well tolerated. Roughly 3% of participants suffered allergic skin reactions in clinical trials, which disappeared soon after stopping treatment. The incidence of other adverse events was less than, or similar to, placebo.[33] Unlike aspirin, willow bark does not seem to be associated with gastrointestinal irritation. Theoretically, the risks of WBE may be similar to aspirin; thus, many authorities contraindicate the its use in febrile children to avoid the risk of Reye's syndrome, those with aspirin allergies, or those taking anticoagulant medications. While there is some impact on platelets, oral consumption of 240 mg/d of salicin as part of a willow bark extract was found have a lesser effect on platelet aggregation than 100 mg/d aspirin ($P = 0.001$).[34]

Back to Our Case

As one can see, there are numerous herbs to choose from—each with varying degrees of evidence to support its use. My experience with ginger is that it would definitely worsen our patient's heartburn, and boswellia would likely cause a similar problem. Willow produces less gastric irritation than ibuprofen, but offers no distinct advantage. I have found devil's claw to be a very effective analgesic, anti-inflammatory herb that will help his back pain and OA. But devil's claw is a bitter herb that could theoretically irritate his stomach (though I have not observed this in practice), and since our patient is already having some gastric distress, we would want to add a gut anti-inflammatory. Deglycyrrhizinated licorice (DGL) would be an excellent choice, as it relieves heartburn and heals the gastric mucosa—and, since it contains no glycyrrhizin (the compound in licorice responsible for elevation of blood pressure and hypokalemia) it would be safe for our patient. But there are other choices one could consider, such as gotu kola or chamomile. Gotu kola (*Centella asiatica*) has anxiolytic activity and facilitates the healing of aspirin- and ethanolic-induced gastric ulcers.[35,36] Chamomile (*Matricaria recutita*) is a mild sedative, gut anti-inflammatory, and weak COX-2 inhibitor.[37] As far as selecting an adaptogen, *Rhodiola rosea* comes quickly to mind, given its adaptogenic, anti-depressant and anxiolytic activity.[38–40]

One possible herbal formulation for this patient might be:

Devil's claw	(1:3)	45 ml
Rhodiola	(1:3)	40 ml
Gotu kola	(1:3)	35 ml
		120 ml

Take 5 ml three times daily in hot water (to dissipate alcohol) or in juice.

The notation of 1:3 in this prescription indicates that there is roughly 1 gram of herb per 3 ml of finished tincture. Thus, the total of 15 ml per day provides 5 grams of this herbal combination.

If one did not have access to an herbal pharmacy, the prescription may look like:

- **Devil's claw standardized extract: providing a minimum of 50 mg/d harpagoside. Products vary considerably in strength—read labels carefully.**
- **DGL chewable tablets: 800 mg 20–30 minutes before meals for 6 weeks, then 400 mg before meals until off ibuprofen.**
- **Rhodiola standardized extract containing 3% rosavins and 1% salidroside: 250 mg two times daily.**

OR:

- **ASU: 300–600 mg per day (products in US are often combined with glucosamine)**
- **Bromelain: 320 mg three times per day as enteric coated tablets**
- **Chamomile tincture (1:3): take 5 ml 2–3 times per day in hot water or juice, 20–30 minutes before meals (tea could be used, but the hydroethanolic extract is superior for healing the gastric mucosa)**

With any of these formulations, the patient should be able to wean off his ibuprofen within 4–6 weeks. The first prescription would cost roughly $40 per month. The other prescriptions could be purchased through reputable companies online, and would also cost approximately $40 per month. The third prescription would likely include 1500 mg glucosamine in the ASU product. If glucosamine (1500 mg/d) were added separately, this would be an additional $20–$30 per month. Herbal formulations are adjusted based upon patient response, generally within 6–8 weeks. A topical liniment would also be helpful for symptom relief, especially before and after exercise.

In addition to the herbal prescription, the herbal practitioner would likely discuss the importance of movement (e.g., swimming, Tai Chi), the role of mind-body (e.g., progressive muscle relaxation), the importance of diet (e.g., a modified DASH (Dietary Approaches to Stop Hypertension) diet could help him lose weight, reduce inflammation, and possibly eliminate his need for antihypertensive medication). The reader is directed to Chapter 19 for a more complete integrative approach to OA.

CASE 2

A 32-year-old, previously healthy woman gradually developed painful wrists over a 4-month period. She consulted her primary care physician after the pain and early morning stiffness began to interfere with her computer skills at work. On examination, the wrists and metacarpophalangeal joints of both hands were swollen and tender, but there were no nodules, vasculitic lesions or deformities. On laboratory investigation, she was noted to have an elevated C-reactive protein (CRP) level (27mg/l) (NR <10) but a normal hemoglobin and white-cell count. She was negative for rheumatoid factor and antinuclear antibodies. She was referred to a rheumatologist and was given the clinical diagnosis of early rheumatoid arthritis. She has been treated with ibuprofen for the past 2 months, but is still experiencing some swelling and pain in her hands. She is feeling anxious about her diagnosis and is concerned that she is going to become disabled. She is not sleeping well, and has cut back on her coffee due to her nervousness, though she admits she has a "horrible" diet. She wants to know if there is anything she can do besides, or in addition, to, the ibuprofen she is taking.

There is much that we can offer this young woman, starting with her diet. She should be started on an anti-inflammatory diet and tested for food allergies, as research shows marked elevation in TNF-α, IL-1β, erythrocyte sedimentation rate (ESR) and C-reactive protein, as well as disease exacerbation with dietary challenge in patients with positive skin prick tests.[41] Her nutritional status should be assessed, and supplementation recommended as appropriate. Encouraging her to engage in some form of mind-body practice could support her coping skills and help her manage her stress.

Before we address the herbal treatment protocol, we will examine the research for botanicals in RA. We have already discussed the research for some important botanicals—boswellia, ashwaganda, and willow—under Case 1 above.

Cat's Claw (Uncaria tomentosa *(Willd.) DC*, U. guianensis *(Aubl.) Gmel.)*

Cat's claw, known as *una de gato* in Spanish, is a large woody vine member of the Uncaria genus. The most heavily researched species are *Uncaria tomentosa*, found only in the tropical areas of Central and South America, and *U. guianensis*, which grows both in the Amazon and in areas of Bangladesh and Burma.[42] Indigenous peoples have long used the dried root, root bark, and stem, for the treatment of arthritis, fever, asthma, stomach ulcers and cancer.

In vitro, in vivo and gene-expression studies on extracts of this plant show that its anti-inflammatory activity is mediated through inhibition of NF-κB activation and suppression of TNF-α synthesis.[8] A small randomized study in patients with OA of the knee using 100 mg freeze-dried extract of *U. guianensis* was shown to improve pain with exercise, as compared with placebo, but there was no effect on pain at rest.[43] The lack of extract specifications limits the conclusions from the study.

More promising was the randomized clinical trial using 60 mg/d of a purified extract of *U. tomentosa* (20 mg root extract per capsule standardized to 1.3% pentacyclic oxindole alkaloids and free of tetracyclic oxindole alkaloids; IMMODAL® Pharmaka GmbH, Austria), which demonstrated moderate benefit in 40 patients with active rheumatoid arthritis, along with fewer side effects compared with those taking sulfasalazine or hydroxychloroquinine.[44]

A review of the safety data found a low potential for acute and subacute oral toxicity.[45] One case of renal failure was reported in a woman with SLE using "cat's claw" for an unknown duration of time; the product used was never analyzed for identification.[46] As a number of plants go by the common name "cat's claw," it is imperative that a standardized extract free of potentially toxic tetracyclic oxindole alkaloids be used. Safety in pregnancy is not known.

*Evening Primrose Oil (*Oenothera biennis *L.)*

Evening primrose oil (EPO) is extracted from the seeds of the evening primrose plant, a wildflower native to North America. The seed oils of evening primrose, blackcurrant, and borage are rich in gamma-linolenic acid (GLA). It is postulated that high levels of GLA act as a competitive inhibitor of PGE_2 and leukotrienes, suppressing inflammation.[47] A systematic review of clinical trials evaluating GLA for the treatment of RA concluded that the majority of the better-quality studies showed improvement in the relief of pain, morning stiffness and joint tenderness compared to placebo.[48] Studies using doses of 1.4–2.8 grams per day of GLA for 24 weeks showed far greater clinical improvement than studies using lower doses of GLA (500–600 mg/d) for shorter periods (6–12 weeks). Evening primrose oil is extremely safe. Mild nausea, diarrhea and flatulence have been reported in some individuals. The concern that evening primrose oil might cause epilepsy or seizures, or reduce the threshold for seizures, originated from two papers published in the early 1980s. The reexamination of the original reports[49] has shown that the association of evening primrose oil with seizures is spurious at best.

Instead of GLA, I often recommend omega-3s, as fish oil, in patients with RA. It is an excellent anti-inflammatory and its cardioprotective benefits are important, given that patients with RA have twice the likelihood of cardiac death compared to the general population. The dose is approximately 4 grams of combined EPA + DHA per day. Use a high-quality brand and store in the freezer to reduce fishy aftertaste.

*Thunder God Vine (*Tripterygium wilfordii *Hook)*

Thunder god vine, or *lei gong teng*, is a perennial vine that grows in China and Myanmar (formerly Burma). It has been used in traditional Chinese medicine for more than 2000 years. *T. wilfordii (TW)* extract has been shown to inhibit the production of cytokines and block the upregulation of a number of proinflammatory genes, including TNFα, COX2, interferon-γ, IL-2, prostaglandin, and iNOS.

A phase I NIH study of 13 patients with RA found improvement in both clinical response and laboratory findings in patients receiving 360 mg/d of an ethyl alcohol/ethyl acetate extract, with one patient meeting the American College of Rheumatology (ACR) criteria for remission.[50] An RDBPCT of 35 patients with longstanding RA found a therapeutic benefit in the group receiving 360 mg/d extract when compared to placebo ($P = 0.0001$). Less effectiveness was seen in the group receiving 180 mg/d extract, but it was still superior to placebo ($P = 0.0287$). Another randomized, controlled trial reported that the extract increased the efficacy of methotrexate and reduced adverse effects.[51] A 24-week randomized controlled phase II multicenter trial sponsored by the National Institute of Arthritis and Musculoskeletal and Skin Diseases (NIAMS) comparing TW extract (60 mg three times per day) with sulfasalazine (1 gram two times per day) in patients with RA reported that those taking the TW extract had a significantly greater ACR response than those in the sulfasalazine group.[52] As of April 2010, there are eight National Institutes of Health funded clinical trials evaluating the use of Tripterygium for a variety of conditions (www.clinicaltrials.gov).

The extract used in the studies by Tao, et al, was well tolerated at doses of 360 mg/d for up to 20 weeks, with diarrhea being the main side effect. However, numerous adverse effects are reported for *T. wilfordii* in the literature including nausea, vomiting, hair loss, dry mouth, headaches, leukopenia, thrombocytopenia, rash, skin pigmentation, stomatitis, gastritis, abdominal pain, weight loss, diastolic hypertension, and vaginal spotting.[53] Infertility was an unexpected side effect noted in men using *T. wilfordii,* and low doses of the extract have been shown to reduce sperm density and motility in both animals and humans.[54] In women, follicle-stimulating hormone and luteinizing hormone begin to rise within 2–3 months of use, reaching menopausal levels within 5 months, with estradiol falling to very low levels.[55] Long-term administration of *T. wilfordii* has been shown to decrease bone mineral density (BMD) in women with systemic lupus erythematosus who were treated with the extract for > 5 years.[56]

Despite its long history of use in traditional Chinese medicine and impressive preliminary research, given the potentially significant adverse effects and lack of well-characterized extracts in the marketplace, it is premature for practitioners to recommend the use of *T. wilfordii.*

Back to Our Case

As this patient has early RA and is being managed with NSAIDs, it would seem reasonable to use an herb such as boswellia, which has a good safety profile and would likely be beneficial for the continued pain and swelling in her hands. Boswellia has been studied in combination with ashwagandha, an excellent adaptogen that also exerts significant anti-inflammatory and anxiolytic activity, making it ideal for our patient. I would not consider cat's claw at this early stage. Hopefully, she will be able to decrease her use of ibuprofen, but if she continues to use it she may want to take gotu kola or chamomile throughout the day to protect the gastric mucosa. One other consideration would be to have her use bromelain for a few weeks to help decrease the swelling in her hands. A topical arnica ointment would also be likely to help reduce her pain and stiffness if applied at night before bed and again in the morning.

One herbal prescription for our patient would be:

Boswellia standardized extract (40–65% boswellic acid): 400 mg three times daily, increasing by 400 mg every 5–7 days as needed.
Ashwaganda standardized extract (2.5% with anolides): 500 mg three times daily
Boswellia: 320 mg enteric-coated tablets taken 3 times daily for 3–4 weeks
Chamomile tincture (1:3): add 5 ml to 1 cup hot chamomile tea. Let sit for a few minutes and drink several times per day.

Summary

The field of herbal medicine is ancient and new, using the best of what we have learned over the centuries and combining it with the advances of modern scientific research. Of course, herbal science is also evolving and our ability to study complex mixtures and complex systems is steadily growing. There is little question that botanicals will continue to hold a place in modern medicine, providing remedies that are effective at a lower cost and with fewer serious side effects.

REFERENCES

1. Eisenberg DM, Davis RB, Ettner SL, et al. Trends in alternative medicine use in the United States, 1990–1997: results of a follow-up national survey. *JAMA*. 1998;280(18): 1569–1175.
2. Tindle HA, Davis RB, Phillips RS, Eisenberg DM. Trends in use of complementary and alternative medicine by US adults: 1997–2002. *Altern Ther Health Med*. 2005;11(1):42–49.
3. Thomas KJ, Nicholl JP, Coleman P. Use and expenditure on complementary medicine in England: a population based survey. *Complement Ther Med*. 2001; 9(1):2–11.
4. Quandt SA, Chen H, Grzywacz JG, Bell RA, Lang W, Arcury TA. Use of complementary and alternative medicine by persons with arthritis: results of the National Health Interview Survey. *Arthritis Rheum*. 2005;53(5):748–755.
5. Rao JK, Mihaliak K, Kroenke K, Bradley J, Tierney WM, Weinberger M. Use of complementary therapies for arthritis among patients of rheumatologists. *Ann Intern Med*. 1999;131(6):409–416.
6. Khanna D, Sethi G, Ahn KS, et al. Natural products as a gold mine for arthritis treatment. *Curr Opin Pharmacol*. 2007 Jun;7(3):344–451.
7. Plaeger SF. Clinical immunology and traditional herbal medicines. *Clin Diagn Lab Immunol*. 2003;10(3):337–338.
8. Patwardhan B, Gautam M. Botanical immunodrugs: scope and opportunities. *Drug Discov Today*. 2005;10(7):495–502.
9. Blumenthal M, Busse WR, Goldberg A, et al. (eds). *The Complete German Commission E Monographs: Therapeutic Guide to Herbal Medicines*. Austin: American Botanical Council and Boston: Integrative Medicine Communications; 1998.
10. Huang TH, Tran VH, Duke RK, et al. Harpagoside suppresses lipopolysaccharide-induced iNOS and COX-2 expression through inhibition of NF-kappa B activation. *J Ethnopharmacol*. 2006;104(1–2):149–155.
11. Chrubasik JE, Roufogalis BD, Chrubasik S. Evidence of effectiveness of herbal antiinflammatory drugs in the treatment of painful osteoarthritis and chronic low back pain. *Phytother Res*. 2007;21(7):675–683.
12. Vlachojannis J, Roufogalis BD, Chrubasik S. Systematic review on the safety of Harpagophytum preparations for osteoarthritic and low back pain. *Phytother Res*. 2008;22(2):149–152.
13. Ernst E. Avocado-soybean unsaponifiables (ASU) for osteoarthritis – a systematic review. *Clin Rheumatol*. 2003;22(4–5):285–288.
14. Mauviel A, Daireaux M, Hartmann DJ, Galera P, Loyau G, Pujol JP. Effects of unsaponifiable extracts of avocado/soy beans (PIAS) on the production of collagen by

cultures of synoviocytes, articular chondrocytes and skin fibroblasts. *Rev Rhum Mal Osteoartic*. 1989;56(2):207–211.

15. Mauviel A, Loyau G, Pujol JP. Effect of unsaponifiable extracts of avocado and soybean (Piasclédine) on the collagenolytic action of cultures of human rheumatoid synoviocytes and rabbit articular chondrocytes treated with interleukin-1. *Rev Rhum Mal Osteoartic*. 1991;58(4):241–245.
16. Ichikawa H, Takada Y, Shishodia S, Jayaprakasam B, Nair MG, Aggarwal BB. Withanolides potentiate apoptosis, inhibit invasion, and abolish osteoclastogenesis through suppression of nuclear factor-kappaB (NF-kappaB) activation and NF-kappaB-regulated gene expression. *Mol Cancer Ther*. 2006;5(6):1434–1445.
17. Sumantran VN, Kulkarni A, Boddul S, et al. Chondroprotective potential of root extracts of Withania somnifera in osteoarthritis. *J Biosci*. 2007;32(2):299–307.
18. Chopra A, Lavin P, Patwardhan B, Chitre D. A 32-week randomized, placebo-controlled clinical evaluation of RA-11, an Ayurvedic drug, on osteoarthritis of the knees. *J Clin Rheumatol*. 2004;10(5):236–245.
19. Chopra A, Lavin P, Patwardhan B, Chitre D. Randomized double blind trial of an ayurvedic plant derived formulation for treatment of rheumatoid arthritis. *J Rheumatol*. 2000;27(6):1365–1372.
20. Kimmatkar N, Thawani V, Hingorani L, Khiyani R. Efficacy and tolerability of Boswellia serrata extract in treatment of osteoarthritis of knee—a randomized double blind placebo controlled trial. *Phytomedicine*. 2003;10(1):3–7.
21. Etzel R. Special extract of *Boswellia serrata* (H15) in the treatment of rheumatoid arthritis. *Phytomedicine*. 1996;3(1):91–94.
22. Sander O, Herborn G, Rau R. Is H15 (resin extract of Boswellia serrata, "incense") a useful supplement to established drug therapy of chronic polyarthritis? Results of a double-blind pilot study. *Z Rheumatol*. 1998;57(1):11–16.
23. Bliddal H, Rosetzsky A, Schlichting P, *et al.* A randomized, placebo-controlled, cross-over study of ginger extracts and ibuprofen in osteoarthritis. *Osteoarthritis Cartilage*. 2000;8(1):9–12.
24. Altman RD, Marcussen KC. Effects of a ginger extract on knee pain in patients with osteoarthritis. *Arthritis Rheum*. 2001;44(11):2531–2538.
25. Borrelli F, Capasso R, Aviello G, Pittler MH, Izzo AA. Effectiveness and safety of ginger in the treatment of pregnancy-induced nausea and vomiting. *Obstet Gynecol*. 2005;105(4):849–856.
26. Maurer HR. Bromelain: biochemistry, pharmacology and medical use. *Cell Mol Life Sci*. 2001;58(9):1234–1245.
27. Akhtar NM, Naseer R, Farooqi AZ, Aziz W, Nazir M. Oral enzyme combination versus diclofenac in the treatment of osteoarthritis of the knee—a double-blind prospective randomized study. *Clin Rheumatol*. 2004;23(5):410–415.
28. Brien S, Lewith G, Walker AF, Middleton R, Prescott P, Bundy R. Bromelain as an adjunctive treatment for moderate-to-severe osteoarthritis of the knee: a randomized placebo-controlled pilot study. *QJM*. 2006;99(12):841–850.
29. Hidaka M, Nagata M, Kawano Y, et al. Inhibitory effects of fruit juices on cytochrome P450 2C9 activity in vitro. *Biosci Biotechnol Biochem*. 2008;72(2):406–411.

30. Schmid B, Lüdtke R, Selbmann HK, et al. Efficacy and tolerability of a standardized willow bark extract in patients with osteoarthritis: randomized placebo-controlled, double blind clinical trial. *Phytother Res.* 2001;15(4):344–350.
31. European Scientific Cooperative on Phytotherapy, Salicis cortex Exeter, UK: ESCOP; 1996–1997:2. Monographs on the Medicinal Uses of Plant Drugs, Fascicule 4.
32. Biegert C, Wagner I, Lüdkte R, et al. Efficacy and safety of willow bark extract in the treatment of osteoarthritis and rheumatoid arthritis: results of 2 randomized double-blind controlled trials. *J Rheumato.* 2004;31(11):2121–2130.
33. Chrubasik S, Künzel O, Model A, Conradt C, Black A. Treatment of low back pain with a herbal or synthetic anti-rheumatic: a randomized controlled study. Willow bark extract for low back pain. *Rheumatology (Oxford).* 40(12):1388–1393.
34. Krivoy N, Pavlotzky E, Chrubasik S, Eisenberg E, Brook G. Effect of salicis cortex extract on human platelet aggregation. *Planta Med.* 2001;67(3):209–212.
35. Guo JS, Cheng CL, Koo MW. Inhibitory effects of Centella asiatica water extract and asiaticoside on inducible nitric oxide synthase during gastric ulcer healing in rats. *Planta Med.* 2004;70(12):1150–1154.
36. Sairam K, Rao CV, Goel RK. Effect of Centella asiatica Linn on physical and chemical factors induced gastric ulceration and secretion in rats. *Indian J Exp Bio.* 2001;39(2):137–142.
37. Ramadan M, Goeters S, Watzer B, et al. Chamazulene carboxylic acid and matricin: a natural profen and its natural prodrug, identified through similarity to synthetic drug substances. *J Nat Prod.* 2006;69(7):1041–1045.
38. Perfumi M, Mattioli L. Adaptogenic and central nervous system effects of single doses of 3% rosavin and 1% salidroside Rhodiola rosea L. extract in mice. *Phytother Res.* 2007;21(1):37–43.
39. Bystritsky A, Kerwin L, Feusner JD. A Pilot Study of Rhodiola rosea (Rhodax((R))) for Generalized Anxiety Disorder (GAD). *J Altern Complement Med.* 2008 Mar;14(2):175–80.
40. Darbinyan V, Aslanyan G, Amroyan E, Gabrielyan E, Malmström C, Panossian A. Clinical trial of Rhodiola rosea L. extract SHR-5 in the treatment of mild to moderate depression. *Nord J Psychiatry.* 2007;61(5):343–348.
41. Karatay S, Erdem T, Yildirim K, et al. The effect of individualized diet challenges consisting of allergenic foods on TNF-alpha and IL-1beta levels in patients with rheumatoid arthritis. *Rheumatology (Oxford).* 2004;43(11):1429–1433.
42. Heitzman ME, Neto CC, Winiarz E, Vaisberg AJ, Hammond GB. Ethnobotany, phytochemistry and pharmacology of Uncaria (Rubiaceae). *Phytochemistry.* 2005;66(1):5–29.
43. Piscoya J, Rodriguez Z, Bustamante SA, Okuhama NN, Miller MJ, Sandoval M. Efficacy and safety of freeze-dried cat's claw in osteoarthritis of the knee: mechanisms of action of the species Uncaria guianensis. *Inflamm Res.* 2001;50(9):442–448.
44. Mur E, Hartig F, Eibl G, Schirmer M. Randomized double blind trial of an extract from the pentacyclic alkaloid-chemotype of uncaria tomentosa for the treatment of rheumatoid arthritis. *J Rheumatol.* 2002;29(4):678–681.

45. Valerio LG Jr, Gonzales GF. Toxicological aspects of the South American herbs cat's claw (Uncaria tomentosa) and Maca (Lepidium meyenii): a critical synopsis. *Toxicol Rev*. 2005;24(1):11–35.
46. Hilepo JN, Bellucci AG, Mossey RT. Acute renal failure caused by 'cat's claw' herbal remedy in a patient with systemic lupus erythematosus. *Nephron*. 1997;77(3):361.
47. Belch JJ, Hill A. Evening primrose oil and borage oil in rheumatologic conditions. *Am J Clin Nutr*. 2000;71(1 Suppl):352S–356S.
48. Little C, Parsons T. Herbal therapy for treating rheumatoid arthritis. *Cochrane Database Syst Rev*. 2001;(1):CD002948.
49. Puri BK. The safety of evening primrose oil in epilepsy. *Prostaglandins Leukot Essent Fatty Acids*. 2007;77(2):101–103.
50. Tao X, Cush JJ, Garret M, Lipsky, PE. A phase I study of ethyl acetate extract of the chinese antirheumatic herb Tripterygium wilfordii hook F in rheumatoid arthritis. *J Rheumatol*. 2001;28(10):2160–2167.
51. Wu YJ, Lao ZY, Zhang ZL. Clinical observation on small doses Tripterygium wilfordii polyglycoside combined with methotrexate in treating rheumatoid arthritis. *Zhongguo Zhing Xi Yi Jie He Za Zhi*. 2001;21(12):895–896.
52. Goldbach-Mansky R, Wilson M, Fleischmann R. Comparison of Tripterygium wilfordii Hook F versus sulfasalazine in the treatment of rheumatoid arthritis: a randomized trial. *Ann Intern Med*. 2009;151(4):229–40, W49–51.
53. Setty AR, Sigal LH. Herbal medications commonly used in the practice of rheumatology: mechanisms of action, efficacy, and side effects. *Semin Arthritis Rheum*. 2005;34(6):773–784.
54. Lopez LM, Grimes DA, Schulz KF. Nonhormonal drugs for contraception in men: a systematic review. *Obstet Gynecol Surv*. 2005 Nov;60(11):746–752.
55. Gu CX. Cause of amenorrhea after treatment with tripterygium wilfordii F. *Zhongguo Yi Xue Ke Xue Yuan Xue Bao*. 1989;11(2):151–153.
56. Huang L, Feng S, Wang H. Decreased bone mineral density in female patients with systemic lupus erythematosus after long-term administration of Tripterygium wilfordii Hook. F. *Chin Med J (Eng)*. 2000;113(2):159–161.

6

Dietary Supplements in Rheumatologic Disorders

SHARON L. KOLASINSKI, MD

KEY CONCEPTS

- Dietary supplements, especially glucosamine and chondroitin sulfate, are among the most commonly used alternative interventions for arthritis and musculoskeletal complaints.
- Despite documented deficiencies of glucosamine, chondroitin and vitamins in patients with arthritis, surprisingly little data supports the routine use of supplements in arthritis treatment.
- It does appear clear after decades of study that glucosamine and chondroitin are generally safe. Therefore, many physicians feel comfortable recommending their use, particularly since currently available prescription medications used to treat osteoarthritis have considerable known side effects and offer no disease-modifying benefits.

Introduction

Dietary supplements are among the most commonly used alternative interventions for arthritis and musculoskeletal complaints, particularly due to the tremendous popularity of products containing glucosamine and chondroitin. According to the Nutrition Business Journal, a trade publication, the US nutrition industry had total consumer sales of almost $94 billion in 2007. Dietary supplements represented $22.5 billion of that market. Impressively, despite the general economic climate of 2007, the nutrition industry grew 10.7% during that year, while the supplement sector grew 5.9%, the highest growth since 1998, and continued to grow throughout 2008–2009.[1] Clearly, dietary supplements continue to comprise a significant category among alternative medicine options for consumers.

Definition of "Supplements"

Supplements include a broad variety of natural and synthetic products marketed to supplement the diet in aiding the quest for optimal health. Although the term "supplement" is used widely in the lay press and scientific literature, it was given legal meaning through the 1994 Dietary Supplement Health and Education Act (DSHEA).[2] According to DSHEA, a "dietary supplement" is a product taken by mouth that contains a "dietary ingredient" intended to supplement the diet. The "dietary ingredients" in these products can include vitamins, minerals, herbs or other botanicals, amino acids, enzymes, organ tissues, extracts or concentrates. They may take the form of tablets, capsules, softgels, gelcaps, liquids or powders.

Under DSHEA, dietary supplements are categorized as "food," not drugs, and, therefore are not required to undergo the rigorous testing that prescription drugs undergo. Although the law specifies that dietary supplement manufacturers are responsible for ensuring that a dietary supplement is safe before it is marketed, no evidence to this effect needs be provided to the Food and Drug Administration (FDA). On June 22, 2007, FDA made a long-awaited announcement of a final rule establishing regulations to require current good manufacturing practice for dietary supplements.[3]

In addition, DSHEA does not require manufacturers to receive FDA approval, or even to register their products with the FDA, before producing or selling dietary supplements. Neither are they required to prove the efficacy of their products, nor to produce evidence to support claims that their products are beneficial. However, manufacturers may not claim to treat, prevent or cure any specific disease or condition since only "drugs" are permitted to make such claims. When a manufacturer makes a structure/function claim on a dietary supplement label, they must include a disclaimer, familiar to many label-reading consumers, that the FDA has not evaluated the claim and that the product is not intended to diagnose, treat, cure or prevent any disease.

DSHEA does not require any post-marketing surveillance or reporting of side effects. Subsequent legislation, the Dietary Supplement and Nonprescription Drug Consumer Protection Act (PL 109-462)[4] enacted on December 22, 2006 amended the Federal Food, Drug and Cosmetic Act to require that manufacturers, packers or distributors of supplements submit any report received of a serious adverse event resulting from the use of their product to the FDA within 15 business days using the MedWatch form. The Act defined a serious adverse event as one resulting in death, a life-threatening experience, inpatient hospitalization, persistent or significant disability or incapacity or a birth defect. The FDA currently posts alerts and safety information regarding dietary supplements on their website.[5]

Osteoarthritis and Rheumatoid Arthritis

It is important to note that there are over 100 kinds of arthritis, and that scientific studies, clinical trials, and health benefit claims for one type of arthritis are not necessarily applicable to any other type of arthritis. The two most important categories of arthritis, for the purposes of this chapter, are osteoarthritis and rheumatoid arthritis, since most laboratory work and human studies using dietary supplements have focused on these two diseases.

Osteoarthritis (OA) is the most common form of arthritis in human beings, and is the form that is most often implied by the vernacular use of the term "arthritis." When osteoarthritis affects a joint, biomechanical and biochemical changes occur in the cartilage. Cartilage becomes damaged, in part through the actions of matrix metalloproteinases, and may even be completely degraded. Changes also occur in bone, and pain and disability result. Inflammation mediated by cytokines plays a mechanistic role in osteoarthritis, but it is generally felt that inflammation is a more significant contributor to the pathogenesis of rheumatoid arthritis. The incidence of osteoarthritis increases markedly in midlife and old age, and risk factors include trauma and obesity, in addition to complex genetics. The knees are very commonly affected, as are the hands, hips and spine. It is important to note that as of today, no therapy is known to prevent or modify the course of osteoarthritis, and it is the leading cause of joint replacement surgery. Treatment is aimed at improving pain control and improving function and mobility. Supplements used to treat osteoarthritis have generally been ones thought to affect the health of cartilage, since degradation of cartilage plays such a central role in the progression of osteoarthritis.

Rheumatoid arthritis (RA), on the other hand, is a disease of the immune system that results in damage to joints via inflammation. An unknown trigger results in the stimulation of cells of the immune system, which, subsequently, loses its normal regulation. Inflammatory tissue grows in the area of the joint with resultant swelling and pain. If left unchecked, the inflammation can lead to permanent damage to joints and bones with the potential for significant deformity and disability. Systemic complications, such as anemia, can also occur.

A number of disease-modifying therapies exist for rheumatoid arthritis, many of which are expensive and have significant potential side effects, since they suppress the immune system. Patients often require more than one medication to control their disease, and not all patients achieve the control of symptoms that they hope for. Supplements used to treat rheumatoid arthritis have generally been those thought to modulate the workings of the immune system.

GLUCOSAMINE

Glucosamine and chondroitin are the most important of the dietary supplements currently in use for arthritis. They are normal components of joint tissues and are known to be depleted in osteoarthritis. Numerous in vitro studies have suggested a variety of mechanisms by which supplementation with glucosamine might be of benefit in slowing the progression of osteoarthritis or treating its symptoms. Since glucosamine is an aminomonosaccharide involved in a rate-limiting step of proteoglycan synthesis, some have suggested a potential role in stimulating proteoglycan production. Others have noted that tissue concentrations sufficient to affect proteoglycan production may not be achievable by oral administration of glucosamine, and that its suppressive effects on interleukin 1-induced proinflammatory gene expression might be more important.[6]

Some clinical trials have supported a role in symptom and disease modification. Thus, proponents of the use of glucosamine and chondroitin can point to both the commonsense argument of supplementing normal connective-tissue building blocks that are depleted by disease, as well as a large number of laboratory and clinical studies that provide scientific evidence to support their use. Yet, glucosamine and chondroitin remain controversial. Data are sparse on the oral bioavailability of these compounds, and their metabolism and utilization in arthritis-damaged tissue in vitro. Other trials have failed to demonstrate meaningful clinical outcomes, either in terms of symptom relief or radiographic progression. Furthermore, several of the positive trials have been sponsored by the supplement manufacturers, raising potential conflict-of-interest concerns. It does appear reasonably clear after decades of study that glucosamine and chondroitin are generally safe. Therefore, many physicians feel comfortable recommending their use, particularly since currently available prescription medications used to treat osteoarthritis have considerable known side effects and offer no disease modifying benefits.

Data favoring the use of glucosamine include many trials that were of short duration and enrolled few subjects. Three studies of note included substantially more subjects and lasted longer that the smaller trials of the 1990s. One of the larger, favorable trials that had a substantial impact in the rheumatologic community was a Belgian study that included 212 subjects with knee osteoarthritis. The participants were assigned to receive either oral glucosamine sulfate at a dose of 1500 mg daily, or placebo, for three years. The Western Ontario and McMaster Universities Osteoarthritis Index (WOMAC) and weight-bearing anteroposterior view radiographs were used as outcome measures. WOMAC is a questionnaire instrument assessing pain, stiffness and function in those with osteoarthritis. Subjects treated with glucosamine had an average 11.7% improvement in their total WOMAC score compared to baseline. Those in the placebo group had an average 9.8% worsening in their WOMAC score. Radiographs suggested that the treatment group had less cartilage loss over the three years. In the intention-to-treat analysis, those on glucosamine sulfate had a mean joint space narrowing of 0.06 mm compared to 0.31 mm mean joint space narrowing in the placebo group. Adverse effects and early withdrawals from the trial did not differ between the glucosamine sulfate and placebo groups.[7]

A trial similar in size and design, results of which were published the following year, replicated the findings of the Belgian study. Glucosamine sulfate 1500 mg daily or placebo was given for three years to 202 Czech subjects with knee osteoarthritis, and WOMAC scores and radiographs were assessed. The investigators found that there was a 27% improvement in total WOMAC score in those treated with glucosamine sulfate, and a 16% improvement in those receiving placebo, a statistically significant difference. Anteroposterior, weight-bearing radiographs obtained in full extension showed that joint space narrowing differed between the treatment groups, again favoring glucosamine. Subjects taking glucosamine sulfate increased their joint space width by 0.04 mm at three years while subjects on placebo lost 0.19 mm, a statistically significant difference. There was no difference in the frequency or severity of adverse events in those exposed to glucosamine sulfate.[8]

A more recent favorable trial, the Glucosamine Unum In Die Efficacy (GUIDE) trial, compared glucosamine sulfate 1500 mg daily to both placebo and to acetaminophen 3 gm daily. The investigators recruited 318 subjects in Spain and Portugal and divided them evenly among the treatment groups. At the completion of the trial after 6 months, there was a statistically significant difference between the total WOMAC score of the glucosamine sulfate group (34% improvement) compared to placebo (22% improvement), but not between those who had received acetaminophen (30% improvement) and the placebo group. However, when the WOMAC pain subscale was assessed alone, neither glucosamine sulfate nor acetaminophen proved to be better than placebo.

The groups did not differ in the number of adverse events reported, nor were any significant abnormalities in liver function tests or serum glucose levels noted in those exposed to glucosamine. In their discussion, the authors noted that this trial importantly included an active comparator, acetaminophen, which is the medication most often recommended as first-line therapy in treatment guidelines for osteoarthritis. Interestingly, however, they found that acetaminophen fell short of its anticipated benefit, while glucosamine sulfate showed significant improvements compared to placebo in a number of outcome measures. They further noted that the improvements found were clinically significant, though with small effect sizes.[9]

One consequence of the tremendous scrutiny given to trials supporting the use of glucosamine has been the contribution critics have made to the vigorous dialog in the osteoarthritis research community regarding appropriate outcome measures in osteoarthritis. Criticism of the radiographic techniques used in the Reginster and Pavelka studies has called into question the conclusion that glucosamine has disease-modifying properties. For instance, it has been shown that the alignment of the anterior and posterior margins of the medial tibial plateau of the knee joint on knee xrays is important for being able to accurately and reproducibly measure joint space narrowing, the most widely used measurement to assess the progression of knee OA. However, in evaluating a population of patients who had X-rays performed over a 2–3 year period, investigators found that very few were routinely properly aligned. In a group of a 428 knee radiographs studied by Mazzuca and colleagues, only 14% were properly aligned. The authors concluded that poor standardization of knee positioning in serial anteroposterior radiographs has obscured the rate and variability of cartilage loss in subjects with knee OA.[10]

In addition to the controversy about the radiographic techniques used in the favorable trials, skeptics about the benefits of glucosamine point to a number of negative trials. The most recent Cochrane Collaboration meta-analysis of many of the smaller trials, published in 2005, pointed out important considerations in interpretation of the available data. Twenty randomized, controlled trials were reviewed. Overall, when compared to placebo, glucosamine showed a 28% improvement in pain and 21% improvement in function using the Lequesne Index, another osteoarthritis outcome measurement consisting of a 10-item questionnaire assessing pain, stiffness, and disability. However, WOMAC scores did not show statistical significance in outcomes. Furthermore, when the analysis was restricted to the eight higher-quality studies that utilized adequate allocation concealment, no improvement in pain or function was found. In addition, the review pointed out that the 10 trials using the Rottapharm preparation of glucosamine sulfate were more likely to have reported positive results. In those studies, glucosamine was superior for pain and function using the Lequesne Index. Rottapharm brand glucosamine was found to be superior to NSAIDs in two randomized controlled trials, and equivalent to NSAIDs in two others, and was associated with slowing radiographic progression of OA in the Reginster and Pavelka studies.[11]

Subsequently, the much-anticipated Glucosamine/chondroitin Arthritis Intervention Trial (GAIT) offered little support for the use of glucosamine in osteoarthritis, but failed to end the controversy about the efficacy of either glucosamine or chondroitin. Because many of the earlier trials had included relatively small numbers of subjects, and been sponsored by Rottapharm, many had hoped that the much larger GAIT, sponsored by the National Institutes of Health, would clarify whether or not glucosamine was a significant agent in osteoarthritis for symptom or structure modification. Unfortunately, the data on symptom relief failed to provide a definitive answer.

The 6-month-long GAIT recruited 1583 subjects and used a 5-arm intervention of either glucosamine 1500 mg daily; chondroitin 1200 mg daily; the combination of glucosamine and chondroitin; a cyclooxygenase inhibitor; and placebo. Overall, glucosamine, chondroitin and the combination of the two were no better at relieving OA symptoms than placebo measured by WOMAC, health assessment questionnaire, or patient or physician global assessments. Use of chondroitin, but not glucosamine, or the combination, was associated with a statistically significant reduction in the number of patients found to have a joint effusion or swelling on clinical examination. In subjects with moderate to severe pain, the combination of glucosamine and chondroitin—but neither of these alone, nor the cyclooxygenase inhibitor comparator—was better than placebo at relieving symptoms.[12]

These mixed results were made difficult to meaningfully interpret by the very high placebo response rate of over 60% in this trial. Presumably, the expectations of benefit from glucosamine and chondroitin were high among the participants in this trial, as the authors pointed out in their discussion. The investigators had powered the study in anticipation of a more usual 35% placebo response rate. Thus, the trial included too few subjects to ensure that the observed placebo response rate was appropriately taken into account in the statistical analysis. The investigators also noted that the outcome measures used might have been insensitive to the changes in symptoms experienced by study participants, since their symptoms were relatively mild at baseline. Other observers have noted that the use of glucosamine hydrochloride in GAIT was problematic since it precluded clear comparisons with the Rottapharm-sponsored trials that used the Dona brand glucosamine sulfate powder for oral solution.[13] It has been noted that higher plasma and synovial fluid concentrations of glucosamine might be expected with the sulfate product[14] and, therefore, the lack of efficacy documented in GAIT might, in part, be explained by the fact that the hydrochloride product could not deliver the necessary glucosamine levels needed to show a benefit.

Subsequent publication of the analysis of the radiographic data obtained during the GAIT contrasted with the earlier positive trials as well. A 572-subject subset of the original cohort underwent radiographic evaluation using a centrally standardized procedure measuring the minimum medial joint compartment joint space width. The primary longitudinal analysis compared the mean change in joint space width at two years, in each of the four intervention groups with the placebo group. The investigators found no significant difference in mean joint space narrowing between the groups. The glucosamine group had the least mean loss and the glucosamine-plus-chondroiton group had the greatest mean loss. No group differed in the likelihood of radiographic progression. Importantly, the authors noted that the loss of joint space observed in this trial was far less than they had anticipated, limiting the power of the study. In addition, the number of individuals whose films were acceptable for interpretation was fewer than expected, and the variability in joint space width measurements was greater than expected.[15]

Most glucosamine trials have limited their recruitment to subjects with knee OA. A recent publication from the Netherlands, however, focused on those with hip OA. The trial was known as the Glucosamine in Osteoarthritis: Longterm Efficacy (GOAL) study and was not industry funded. In this trial, 222 subjects with clinical and radiographic evidence of hip involvement received either glucosamine sulfate 1500 mg daily, or placebo, for 2 years. By the conclusion of the study, 13 subjects treated with glucosamine sulfate and 7 subjects treated with placebo underwent total hip arthroplasty. No clinically important differences were found between the WOMAC scores or radiographs of the treatment groups. The authors wondered if the relatively mild disease in many of the subjects, and relatively little progression seen over the 2-year study, might have made detection of a difference in effectiveness more difficult to discern.[16]

In weighing the evidence from clinical trials of glucosamine, many factors need to be taken into account. It has been noted that the heterogeneity between trials is greater than would be expected by chance. This may be attributable to the use of different glucosamine preparations (e.g., sulfate versus hydrochloride), poor study design (e.g., inadequate allocation concealment), or industry bias.[17] In addition, it is also important to keep in mind that OA is a heterogeneous disease and that currently available outcome measures may be inadequate to account for this heterogeneity.[18]

CHONDROITIN

Like glucosamine, chondroitin is an important constituent of normal joint tissue. Chondroitin contributes to the structural integrity of the joint and surrounding tissues, and chondroitin levels are altered in osteoarthritic cartilage, plasma, and synovial fluid. However, a definitive demonstration of efficacy in OA is no clearer for chondroitin than for glucosamine.

An early meta-analysis of 9 double-blind, randomized trials evaluating chondroitin use in over 750 subjects with knee OA suggested a benefit superior to that seen with glucosamine. Effect sizes were moderate to large, but the authors cautioned that the true efficacy of chondroitin might be less than expected from the meta-analysis because of methodological weaknesses in the analyzed trials. In particular, they noted that inadequate allocation concealment, and absence of intention-to-treat analysis, might affect interpretation. Nonetheless, they concluded that chondroitin was probably efficacious for OA, as well as safe and useful in the treatment of OA, and this study has been widely quoted in support of its use.[19]

A subsequent, relatively large and well-designed trial failed to show symptomatic improvement associated with the use of chondroitin in knee OA. In this randomized, double-blind, placebo-controlled trial, 300 participants received either chondroitin sulfate 800 mg of fish origin, or placebo, daily for two years. No statistically significant differences between the two groups were found in pain, stiffness or function measured by WOMAC, or in the amount of rescue medication needed for pain relief. The authors felt that this was because the initial pain level of the subjects was low, and that there was little room for improvement. However, this trial did suggest that chondroitin might have disease-modifying activity in OA, slowing the loss of cartilage. Radiographs obtained in this trial included the usual anteroposterior views of the knee in extension, as well as radiographs obtained with the knees partially flexed to about 20°. Analysis of the flexed view radiographs showed joint space narrowing in the placebo-treated group of 0.14 mm in mean joint space width. In contrast, those who received chondroitin had no progression of joint space narrowing. Adverse events did not differ between the treatment groups.[20]

A second, more recent meta-analysis of chondroitin trials involving 4056 subjects failed to substantiate the findings of the earlier meta-analysis and, as with the glucosamine trials, underscored the heterogeneity of clinical trials available for evaluation. In this meta-analysis, heterogeneity was associated with allocation concealment, intention-to-treat analysis and sample size.

Twenty trials were analyzed and all were randomized, controlled trials, comparing chondroitin to placebo or no treatment. The investigators found that higher-quality trials were less likely to show positive results, and newer publications showed smaller effects than older ones. Overall, chondroitin was associated with a large effect size for pain-related outcomes. However, effect size became considerably smaller when trials with adequate allocation concealment or intention-to-treat analysis were pooled. The authors concluded that the symptomatic benefit of chondroitin was minimal or nonexistent, and that routine clinical use of chondroitin should be discouraged. In evaluating the available radiographic evidence, the investigators found a small effect in favor of chondroitin. They noted a 0.16 mm difference in minimum joint space width and a 0.23 mm difference in mean joint space width. In their discussion, they emphasized once again the generally poor quality of many of the published studies on chondroitin and stressed the need for future studies with adherence to high methodological standards including concealed allocation, blinding of patients and outcome assessors, measures to reduce withdrawals, and intention-to-treat analysis.[21]

Vitamins

While nutritional factors are clearly important for optimal growth, development and functioning of healthy bones, joints, and connective tissues, clinical evidence in support of the use of specific vitamins in the management of arthritis has been lacking. In part, this is likely related to the heterogeneity of disease presentations and the period of time over which symptoms evolve, which can be particularly long in osteoarthritis. But it also speaks to the relatively limited number of clinical trials devoted to addressing the role of supplements in arthritis.

VITAMIN B6

Studies over many years have suggested that patients with rheumatoid arthritis have poor nutritional status. It was previously thought that this was related to the relentless systemic inflammation associated with the disease, which was not as effectively controlled by medications used to treat rheumatoid arthritis (i.e., before the advent of biologic-response-modifying drugs). However, a recent study demonstrated that lower levels of vitamin B6 and red blood cell folate can still be seen, despite the advent of these newer therapies. In a small study, 18 subjects with RA had significantly reduced levels despite similar dietary intakes of these nutrients compared to 33 controls. Interestingly, the low vitamin B6 levels were associated with high homocysteine levels that the authors hypothesized could contribute to the increased risk of cardiovascular disease observed in those with RA.[22] However, a treatment trial has failed to show that supplementing vitamin B6 improves short-term status in RA. In this study, plasma pyridoxine levels were found to be in the lowest quartile in 28 of 33 RA patients. Supplementation with pyridoxine 50 mg daily for 30 days successfully raised plasma vitamin B6 status measures, but had no effect on levels of inflammatory cytokines, plasma C-reactive protein (CRP), or the erythrocyte sedimentation rate.[23]

VITAMIN C

Laboratory studies show differing effects of vitamin C in relation to the development of arthritis depending on the animal models used—some positive and some negative. Published observational human trials have suggested a positive association between vitamin C intake and a reduced risk of arthritis, but no interventional trials have yet appeared. Early epidemiologic data from the Framingham study suggested that a high intake of antioxidant vitamins, particularly vitamin C, might reduce the risk of cartilage loss and disease progression in people with osteoarthritis. A group of 640 participants was studied, who completed food frequency questionnaires and radiographic evaluation of their knees. A threefold reduction in the risk of OA progression was noted in those with vitamin C intakes in the middle and highest tertiles. However, no preventive effect was noted.[24] A more recent survey was performed as part of the ongoing Australian epidemiologic study in Melbourne, the Melbourne Collaborative Cohort Study (MCCS). It suggested that vitamin C might have a role in affecting the incidence of OA. Members of the MCCS cohort filled out food frequency questionnaires upon entry, and a subset of 294 participants who did not have osteoarthritis were sampled 10 years later. They underwent MRI of the knee and were evaluated for the presence of a variety of radiographic abnormalities. The investigators found that vitamin C intake, as well as overall fruit intake, was inversely associated with tibial plateau bone area and the presence of bone marrow lesions, but not with the tibial cartilage volume or the presence of cartilage defects. Vegetable, vitamin E, and carotenoid intake showed no such associations. The authors hypothesized that since an increase in bone size is a potential early response to known risk factors for knee OA, and bone marrow lesions are associated with pain and progression of knee OA, their observations might provide a link between vitamin C and a reduced risk of OA.[25]

A smaller study in the United Kingdom suggested that the intake of fruits, vegetables and vitamin C could influence the development of rheumatoid arthritis as well. In a prospective, population-based, nested case-control study of 73 subjects with rheumatoid arthritis and 146 controls, 7-day food diaries were obtained and analyzed for the daily intake of nutrients of interest. The investigators found that those in the lowest tertile of vitamin C consumption had a threefold risk of RA. A less significant association was seen for combined fruit and vegetable intake, but not for either alone or for intake of vitamin E, selenium, or beta carotene.[26]

VITAMIN D

Considerable interest in vitamin D supplementation results from both its long known role in bone and cartilage health, as well as recent findings that vitamin D receptors are present on immune system cells.[27] Earlier epidemiological evidence had suggested that vitamin D intake might be linked to the incidence or progression of OA as well. Framingham data[28] suggested that the progression of OA but not the incidence of OA was related to vitamin D intake. In this study of 556 subjects, 75 had a new onset of OA and 62 had progression of known OA over an approximately 10-year period. Investigators found that the risk of progression increased threefold in those in the middle and lowest tertiles of vitamin D intake measured by serum levels of vitamin D and food frequency questionnaire. Low levels of serum vitamin D also predicted loss of cartilage as assessed by joint space narrowing and the presence of osteophytes on knee radiographs. A second epidemiologic study suggested that incident OA in the hip might, indeed, be associated with vitamin D intake.[29] In 237 subjects in the Study of Osteoporotic Fractures, investigators obtained baseline and follow-up hip radiographs an average of 8 years apart, and baseline serum vitamin D levels. The risk of incident hip OA, defined as the development of definite joint space narrowing, was increased more than threefold in subjects in the middle and lowest tertiles for 25(OH) vitamin D compared to those with the highest vitamin D levels. Because these two earlier studies were inconsistent with each other, one suggesting incidence of OA was affected, and one suggesting progression of OA was affected by vitamin D levels, a third epidemiological study was performed to clarify the potential role of vitamin D in osteoarthritis. The investigators gathered data from 715 subjects in the Framingham Osteoarthritis Study, and from 277 subjects in the Boston Osteoarthritis of the Knee Study (BOKS), and confirmed that many subjects in each study were vitamin D deficient, a well known phenomenon in northern latitudes. However, the results of this analysis were in the opposite direction of the two previous epidemiologic surveys: higher vitamin D levels were associated with worse outcomes, although the findings were not statistically significant with adjustment for other risk factors. Nonetheless, there was no confirmation of a protective effect for vitamin D, an observation with considerable public health implications. The investigators concluded that there was no relationship between vitamin D status and the risk of joint space or cartilage loss in knee OA.[30]

Conflicting results in the available epidemiologic data regarding the relationship of vitamin D levels to the risk for rheumatoid arthritis also abound. In addition to its role in calcium homeostasis, vitamin D can modulate the functioning of T cells, inhibiting cellular proliferation and decreasing the production of proinflammatory cytokines, such as interferon γ and tumor necrosis factor α. Vitamin D receptors are present on cells of the immune system, including macrophages, chondrocytes and synoviocytes, and vitamin D is produced by activated dendritic cells. These findings suggest an important role in the operation of the immune system and, thus, potentially, in the pathogenesis of RA. An observation from the Iowa Women's Health Study of 29,368 women aged 55–69 years first suggested an association. During 11 years of follow-up, 152 women in the cohort developed RA, and greater intake of vitamin D (the highest versus the lowest tertile of intake by food frequency questionnaire) was associated with a reduction in risk (RR 0.67, 95% CI 0.44–1.00, p=0.05). The authors considered this association "hypothesis generating" and noted that it could be due to chance alone.[31] A subsequent study used direct measurement of vitamin D levels from the Norfolk Arthritis Registry in the United Kingdom, a primary-care-based incidence registry of patients with inflammatory arthritis. Of the 206 subjects identified as having inflammatory arthritis, 35% met criteria for a diagnosis of RA. In those subjects who met criteria for RA, only mean levels of 1,25(OH)$_2$ vitamin D metabolites were significantly lower compared to those with other forms of inflammatory arthritis at baseline. At one-year follow up, 45% of subjects met criteria for a diagnosis of RA, and those with a lower baseline level of vitamin D were more likely to meet criteria. In all subjects with inflammatory arthritis, lower levels of vitamin D were associated with some measures of disease activity. At baseline, there was an inverse relationship between 25(OH) vitamin D levels and tender joint count, the Disease Activity Score 28-joint assessment (DAS28), and results of the Health Assessment Questionnaire (HAQ). At one-year follow-up, higher vitamin D metabolite levels were associated with lower HAQ scores. The authors postulated that vitamin D might have an immunomodulatory role in RA, but that longitudinal studies would be required to substantiate this suggestion.[32]

Most recently, however, an analysis of data from the Nurses' Health Survey found no relationship between the risk for RA and vitamin D intake.

Among 180,389 subjects followed between 1980 and 2002, 772 women developed rheumatoid arthritis. Nutrient intake was calculated from diet diaries that were collected repeatedly over the 22 years during which data was gathered. The investigators found that higher vitamin D intake was associated with other markers of healthier lifestyle, such as the absence of smoking, higher levels of physical activity, higher intake of calcium, lower intake of caffeine and a higher proportion of breastfeeding infants for a year or more. They observed no association between cumulative average vitamin D intake and the risks of RA.[33]

VITAMIN E

The appeal of using antioxidants like vitamin E derives, in part, from experimental data in which laboratory animals whose diets are supplemented develop less histologically evident changes of osteoarthritis.[34] In addition, early Framingham data suggested a weak association between vitamin E intake and a reduction in risk for osteoarthritis progression in men.[24] Subsequent data from the Johnston County Osteoarthritis Project in North Carolina suggests that α-tocopherol was not protective against radiographic knee OA. The investigators hypothesized that there was a complex relationship between vitamin E and OA, since they also found that those with the highest ratios of serum α-tocopherol to γ-tocopherol had half the odds of radiographic knee OA. This relationship was statistically significant in men and African Americans, but not for women or other ethnic groups among the 400 participants studied.[35]

This epidemiologic observation has not, however, translated into a therapeutic option for OA based upon the one prospective supplementation trial of vitamin E use for OA that has been carried out. In this study, 136 subjects were randomized to receive either vitamin E 500 IU, or placebo, for 2 years. Patients were followed with magnetic resonance imaging to measure tibial cartilage volume. There was no difference in medial or lateral tibial cartilage volume loss between those who received vitamin E supplements and those who did not. Furthermore, there was no relationship between dietary levels of antioxidants and cartilage volume loss.[36]

VITAMIN K

Vitamin K is an important regulator of bone and cartilage mineralization, and it was recently observed that low plasma levels of vitamin K1 (phylloquinone) were associated with an increased prevalence of osteoarthritis of the hand and knee. Data from 672 participants in the Framingham Offspring Study was analyzed. Plasma phylloquinone levels were measured, and bilateral hand and knee radiographs were performed, in a subset of subjects. Low plasma phylloquinone levels were strongly associated with the presence of large osteophytes on radiographs of hands and knees, a definitive sign of osteoarthritis. In addition, phylloquinone was significantly associated with joint space narrowing and osteoarthritis of the hand. The investigators noted that although phylloquinone levels were indicative of short-term dietary intake of vitamin K, they felt it was a useful measure of vitamin K status in this population study and suggested that a clinical trial was warranted to assess the potential benefit of vitamin K supplementation.[37] Results of such a trial were recently reported, but failed to support the hypothesis that vitamin K supplementation had an impact on the presence of radiographic hand OA. In a group of 378 individuals taking vitamin supplementation over 3 years, 193 received phylloquinone 500 μg, and the remainder received placebo. Hand radiographs were obtained in the last year of the study. Supplementation with vitamin K did not confer any additional benefit on radiographic hand osteoarthritis or joint-related symptoms in the healthy, community-dwelling elderly adults studied.[38]

Summary

Dietary supplements are among the most commonly used interventions chosen by arthritis patients for the options provided by complementary and alternative medicine. Considerable in vitro and animal laboratory data has suggested potential mechanisms by which dietary supplements, including vitamins, might be of benefit in slowing the progression of arthritis or treating its symptoms. Deficiencies of glucosamine, chondroitin, and vitamins are demonstrable in patients with arthritis. Yet, despite numerous clinical trials performed over the last two decades, surprisingly little data supports the routine use of supplements in arthritis treatment. In diseases that evolve over many years and involve complex genetic and environmental risk factors, it is perhaps predictable that simply adding back one of the many ingredients essential for good health would not be sufficient to reverse the course of disease. Nonetheless, the tremendous interest in seeking safer and more effective treatments for arthritis will no doubt continue to fuel future investigative work.

REFERENCES

1. Available at: http://subscribers.nutritionbusinessjournal.com/supplements/0601-supplementsbright-spot/wall.html?return=http://subscribers.nutritionbusiness journal.com/supplements/0601-supplementsbright-spot/index.html.

2. Available at: http::/www.fda.gov/RegulatoryInformation/Legislation/FederalFoodDrugandCosmeticActFDCAct/SignificantAmendmentstotheFDCAct/ucm148003.htm.
3. Available at http://www.fda.gov/OHRMS/DOCKETS/98fr/07-3039.pdf.
4. Available at: http://www.fda.gov/downloads/AboutFDA/CentersOffices/CDER/ucm102797.pdf.
5. Available at: http://www.cfsan.fda.gov/%7Edms/ds-warn.html.
6. Towheed TE, Anastassiades T. Glucosamine therapy for osteoarthritis: an update. *J Rheumatol.* 2007;34(9):1787–1790.
7. Reginster JY, Deroisy, R, Rovati LC, et al. Long-term effects of glucosamine sulphate on osteoarthritis progression: a randomized, placebo-controlled clinical tria!. *Lancet.* 2001;357(9252):251–256.
8. Pavelká K, Gatterová J, Olejarová M, Machacek S, Giacovelli G, Rovati LC. Glucosamine sulfate use and delay of progression of knee osteoarthritis: a 3-year, randomized, placebo-controlled, double-blind study. *Arch Int Med.* 2002;162(18): 2113–2123.
9. Herrero-Beaumont G, Ivorra JA, Del Carmen Trabado M, et al. Glucosamine sulfate in the treatment of knee osteoarthritis symptoms: a randomized, double-blind, placebo-controlled study using acetaminophen as a side comparator. *Arthritis Rheum.* 2007;56(2):555–567.
10. Mazzuca SA, Brandt KD, Dieppe PA, Doherty M, Katz BP, Lane KA. Effect of alignment of the medial tibial plateau and x-ray beam on apparent progression of osteoarthritis in the standing anteroposterior knee radiograph. *Arthritis Rheum.* 2001;44(8):1786–1794.
11. Towheed TE, Maxwell L, Anastassiades TP, et al. Glucosamine therapy for treating osteoarthritis. *Cochrane Database of Syst Rev.* 2005;18(2):CD002946.
12. Clegg DO, Reda DJ, Harris CL, et al. Glucosamine, chondroitin sulfate, and the two in combination for painful knee osteoarthritis. *N Engl J Med.* 2006;354(8): 795–808.
13. Hochberg MC. Nutritional supplements for knee osteoarthritis–still no resolution. *N Engl J Med.* 2006;354(8):858–860.
14. Persiani S, Rotini R, Trisolino G, et al. Synovial and plasma glucosamine concentrations in osteoarthritic patients following oral crystalline glucosamine sulphate at therapeutic dose. *Osteoarthritis Cartilage.* 2007;15(7):764–772.
15. Sawitzke AD, Shi H, Finco MF, et al. The effect of glucosamine and/or chondroitin sulfate on the progression of knee osteoarthritis: a report from the glucosamine/chondroitin arthritis intervention trial. *Arthritis Rheum.* 2008;58(10):3183–3191.
16. Rozendaal RM, Koes BW, van Osch GJ, et al. Effect of glucosamine sulfate on hip osteoarthritis: a randomized trial. *Ann Intern Med.* 2008;148(4):268–277.
17. Vlad SC, LaValley MP, McAlindon TE, Felson DT. Glucosamine for pain in osteoarthritis: why do trial results differ? *Arthritis Rheum.* 2007;56(7):2267–2277.
18. Bijlsma JW, Lafeber FP. Glucosamine sulfate in osteoarthritis: the jury is still out. *Ann Intern Med.* 2008;148(4):315–317.

19. McAlindon TE, LaValley MP, Gulin JP, Felson DT. Glucosamine and chondroitin for treatment of osteoarthritis: a systematic quality assessment and meta-analysis. *JAMA*. 2000;283(11):1469–1475.
20. Michel BA, Stucki F, Frey D, De Vathaire F, Vignon E, Bruehlmann P, Uebelhart D. Chondroitins 4 and 6 sulfate in osteoarthritis of the knee: a randomized, controlled trial. *Arthritis Rheum*. 2005;52(3):779–786.
21. Reichenbach, S, Sterchi, R, Scherer M, et al. Meta-analysis: chondroitin for osteoarthritis of the knee or hip. *Ann Intern Med*. 2007;146(8):580–590.
22. Woolf K, Manore MM. Elevated plasma homocysteine and low vitamin B-6 status in nonsupplementing older women with rheumatoid arthritis. *J Am Diet Assoc*. 2008;108(3):443–453.
23. Chiang EP, Selhub J, Bagley PJ, Dallal G, Roubenoff R. Pyridoxine supplementation corrects vitamin B6 deficiency but does not improve inflammation in patients with rheumatoid arthritis. *Arthritis Res Ther*. 2005;7(6):R1404–R1411.
24. McAlindon TE, Jacques P, Zhang Y, et al. Do antioxidant micronutrients protect against the development and progression of knee osteoarthritis? *Arthritis Rheum*. 1996;39(4):648–656.
25. Wang Y, Hodge AM, Wluka AE, et al. Effect of antioxidants on knee cartilage and bone in healthy, middle-aged subjects: a cross-sectional study. *Arthritis Res Ther*. 2007;9(4):R66.
26. Pattison DJ, Silman AJ, Goodson NJ, et al. Vitamin C and the risk of developing inflammatory polyarthritis: prospective nested case-control study. *Ann Rheum Dis*. 2004;63(7):843–847.
27. Kang J, Kolasinski SL. Vitamin D and osteoarthritis. *Alternative Med Alert*. 2008;11:85–90.
28. McAlindon TE, Felson DT, Zhang Y, et al. Relation of dietary intake and serum levels of vitamin D to progression of osteoarthritis of the knee among participants in the Framingham study. *Ann Intern Med*. 1996;125(5):353–359.
29. Lane NE, Gore LR, Cummings SR, et al. Serum vitamin D levels and incident changes of radiographic hip osteoarthritis: a longitudinal study. *Arthritis Rheum*. 1999;42(5):854–860.
30. Felson DT, Niu J, Clancy M, et al. Low levels of vitamin D and worsening of knee osteoarthritis: results of two longitudinal studies. *Arthritis Rheum*. 2007;56(1):129–136.
31. Merlino LA, Curtis J, Mikuls TR, et al. Vitamin D intake is inversely associated with rheumatoid arthritis: resuklts from the Iowa Women's Health Study. *Arthritis Rheum*. 2004;50(1):72–77.
32. Patel S, Farragher T, Berry J, Bunn D, Silman A, Symmons D. Association between serum vitamin D metabolite levels and disease activity in patients with early inflammatory polyarthritis. *Arthritis Rheum*. 2007;56(7):2143–2149.
33. Costenbader KH, Feskanich D, Holmes M, Karlson EW, Benito-Garcia E. Vitamin D intake and risks of systemic lupus erythematosus and rheumatoid arthritis in women. *Ann Rheum Dis*. 2008;67(4):530–535.

34. Kurz B, Jost B, Schünke M. Dietary vitamins and selenium diminish the development of mechanically induced osteoarthritis and increase the expression of antioxidative enzymes in the knee joint of STR/1N mice. *Osteoarthritis Cartilage.* 2002;10(2):119–126.
35. Jordan JM, De Roos AJ, Renner JB, et al. A case-control study of serum tocopherol levels and the alpha- to gamma-tocopherol ratio in radiographic knee osteoarthritis: The Johnston County Osteoarthritis Project. *Am J Epidemiol.* 2004;159(10): 968–977.
36. Wluka AE, Stuckey S, Brand C, Cicuttini FM. Supplementary vitamin E does not affect the loss of cartilage volume in knee osteoarthritis: a 2 year double blind randomized placebo controlled study. *J Rheumatol.* 2002;29(12):2585–2591.
37. Neogi T, Booth SL, Zhang YQ, et al. Low vitamin K status is associated with osteoarthritis in the hand and knee. *Arthritris Rheum.* 2006;54(4):1255–1261.
38. Neogi T, Felson DT, Sarno R, Booth SL. Vitamin K in hand osteoarthritis: results from a randomized clinical trial. *Ann Rheum Dis.* 2008;67(11):1570–1573.

7

Manual Medicine in Rheumatologic Disorders

ANASTASIA ROWLAND-SEYMOUR, MD
AND JULIA B. JERNBERG, MD

KEY CONCEPTS

- There are several different types of manual medicine; the efficacy of each can vary in different situations.
- Identification of a manual medicine practitioner who is sensible about when to apply his/her technique, and about whom you receive overwhelmingly positive feedback, may be a key step in helping to treat your patients with neck, back, and knee symptoms. We have noted that a highly skilled practitioner can have remarkable success in treating rheumatology patients, with patient improvement rates that exceed the positive data in published studies of manual manipulation, or predicted by the placebo response.
- Trigger point referral patterns can suggest myofascial patterns of pain that are amenable to easily-learned interventions (counterstrain, Travell's spray and stretch, or injections). In many cases, only a few treatments are needed to obtain long-lasting or permanent pain relief.
- Be extremely cautious if considering manipulation in patients who have ankylosing spondylitis, rheumatoid arthritis, or collagen disorders, and certainly avoid cervical manipulation in these patients altogether.

■

Case Report

A patient who had had longstanding difficulty rising from a sitting position due to anterior knee pain was seen in clinic. The treating physician was aware that anterior knee pain that can impede leg-straightening may be referred from muscular pathology in the rectus femoris muscle. Tender/trigger points were found in the proximal rectus femoris and the vastus medialis. Counterstrain, a gentle osteopathic manipulative technique, was employed to passively shorten both of these muscles and to relieve the associated tender/trigger points. By the end of the visit, the patient was able to rise from sitting without pain, and he noted with amazement that he did not need to use his cane to steady himself. He returned six months later with low back pain, but reported perfectly functioning, painless knees at that time. This case illustrates that persistent joint pain can often be relieved by treating pathologically contracted muscles, using a manual medicine technique.

Introduction

Rheumatologic conditions often present with severe pain. For centuries, manual medicine practitioners have used a vast array of techniques to ameliorate pain—some successful, others not. Manual medicine modalities remain very popular, with each technique having its own supporters. Researchers have long wondered whether there is a demonstrable, quantifiable benefit from such treatments, or whether it is all a manifestation of the placebo effect. Unfortunately, in most cases we do not have enough data to confidently attribute benefits to the manipulative interventions themselves; however, several studies do suggest that there exists a tendency for certain manipulations to benefit certain groups of patients.

If there is, indeed, a positive therapeutic effect, then other questions arise. Are some maladies particularly suited to manual manipulation interventions? If so, which techniques are most promising for specific ailments? And, what of the risks associated with manual medicine?

A Brief History of Modern Manual Medicine

To appreciate the various types of manipulation used by the different practitioners of manual medicine, it is useful to examine how the current modalities arose.

Many of our current manipulation techniques stem from the foundation of osteopathic medicine, originally conceived and taught by a 19th century American physician, Andrew Taylor Still, MD. In the mid to late 1800s, prior to the advent of antibiotics or anesthetics, conventional medicine had little in its arsenal to thwart human diseases. The state of medicine in America in the mid–late 19th century was chaotic and unregulated; often the medical remedies did more to hasten a patient's demise than did the original ailment. Professionally and personally disappointed in the medical offerings of his time (having lost three of his own children to meningitis), Still sought a different approach to medical care.[1]

Still may have derived the basis of his technique from reports of noted "bone setters" in 19th century England and America who used manual manipulation to treat all manner of ailments. Some of these bone setters attained anecdotal renown by effecting seemingly miraculous cures solely through the manipulation of the spine and musculoskeletal system.[2] According to Still's original teachings, people have a natural predisposition to be healthy, but an ailment—usually related to an abnormality in the structure of the spine—could impede the natural function of the body to attain and maintain a state of health. Since structure and function were inextricably linked, those afflicted with disease could benefit from manual manipulation of the spine or other joints. In Still's osteopathic philosophy, placement of the spine and other supporting skeletal components into the proper alignment would allow a body the freedom to achieve its optimum health. In this manner, diverse diseases could be treated with manipulation of the musculoskeletal system, including immune dysfunction and visceral disease. In 1892, Still founded an osteopathic medical school and a new branch of medicine was formed.[3]

By the early 1900s, osteopathy became such a serious contender for the minds, bodies, and dollars of the US population that the allopathic physicians and medical schools waged a multi-pronged battle against the osteopaths. Even the famed American literary humorist, Mark Twain, joined the debate (in favor of osteopathic medicine): "I don't know as I cared much about these osteopaths until I heard you were going to drive them out of the state, but since I heard that I haven't been able to sleep."[4] The friction between the two schools of medicine continued, with the allopathic schools turning away from manual therapies and embracing more pharmaceutical and surgical interventions, and the osteopaths differentiating themselves by virtue of their manipulative expertise.

Current American osteopathic medical schools (which award a DO degree to their graduates) continue to teach manual medicine, but their curriculum looks very similar to that taught in allopathic medical schools (which award an MD degree). In the 21st century in the US, many osteopaths' practices are indistinguishable from those of allopathic physicians, and many osteopaths do not practice manual medicine as part of their clinical routine.[5] It should be noted that, although both American and non-American forms of osteopathy originated from Still's 19th century osteopathic foundations, geographic separation created profound differences. In the US, osteopathic physicians complete 4 years of medical school followed by internships and residencies, typically undertaken along with allopathic physicians. The most prominent remnant of Still's teachings is the repertoire of various manipulative methods that is taught in osteopathic schools.

In the UK, Europe, and other countries, however, osteopaths are schooled in "osteopathy" and not "osteopathic medicine." Outside the US, osteopaths are non-physician manipulative clinicians, rigorously trained in osteopathic schools, but without the 4-year medical school education or the hospital-based internship and residency training that is standard in America. In the UK, there are schools for osteopathy and formal recognition by strict licensure of osteopaths by the General Osteopathic Council.

Soon after Still began promulgating osteopathy, another school of manipulative therapy developed in America. Daniel David (D.D.) Palmer, a grocer-turned-manipulator, gained his reputation by treating a deaf patient with manipulation and restoring his hearing. Similar to Still's teachings, Palmer taught that most ills were the result of abnormal alignment of the spine (subluxation), and that manipulation could aid a patient's return to health.[6]

Chiropractors study for 4–5 years in a chiropractic college, and have licensure and professional regulatory boards in each of the United States. Just as osteopathy has multiple types of techniques and practitioners, so, too, many chiropractors have diverged from Palmer's original view which taught that pathology in the integrity of the spinal structure is the main cause of disease, and that high velocity thrust techniques to realign a spine can treat most ills. The field is now divided into the "straights" who follow more closely Palmer's teachings, and the "mixers" who have incorporated many different manual and other medical techniques into their practices. Both osteopathic and chiropractic disciplines retained some of the original maneuvers and philosophies of their founders, yet grew and evolved to include numerous other techniques and approaches to patient care.

Another major category of manual medicine practitioners include physical therapists (as they are called in the US) and physiotherapists (as they are called in the UK). Physical therapists or physiotherapists have advanced masters or doctorate degrees (2 or 3 years beyond college and required clinical exposure) and also have rigorous state licensure and regulation in both countries.[7]

There are several other disciplines whose practitioners use manual techniques in order to alleviate pain and restore health. Many rheumatology patients seek relief using massage therapy or other bodywork techniques. Massage therapy practitioners vary widely, as does the regulation of the profession. In some, but not all states in the US, massage therapists are licensed and regulated, with training requirements that vary by state. In the UK, there is a movement of massage and bodyworkers attempting to regulate and license practitioners.

Patients often use other bodywork techniques such as Feldenkrais, Alexander, Structural Integration (Rolfing) and Yoga. These techniques all approach muscle dysfunction using unique and varied interventions, and may be beneficial in patients with rheumatologic conditions. Since many of these techniques are frequently used by patients with rheumatologic diseases, it is important to understand the different types of manipulation practiced today.

Types of Manual Medicine

As you might guess from the varied list of techniques employed by different manual medicine specialists, there is both considerable variability and significant overlap among the different types of manual medicine.

Manipulation techniques vary, and can include: aggressively altering joint relationships (the "high velocity thrust" so common in many chiropractic and manipulative osteopathic offices); using the patient's own counter-force to increase range of motion (muscle energy techniques used by massage therapists, -physical therapists, chiropractors and osteopaths); putting various amounts of pressure on muscles and fascia (myofascial release techniques employed by many osteopaths, chiropractors, physical therapists, and massage therapists); gently and relatively painlessly returning muscles and joints to their original, noninjured states (counterstrain technique used by osteopaths, chiropractors, physical and occupational therapists); and manipulations involving small amounts of pressure/traction to "guide" an impeded flow of central nervous system fluid (craniosacral therapies performed by many practitioners). Many other manual manipulation methods are used by therapists, in addition to those listed herein. Some practitioners consider energy healers as manual manipulators, but that area is covered elsewhere (Chapter 13).

Five common types of manipulative techniques are described below:[8]

HIGH VELOCITY/LOW AMPLITUDE THRUST

This technique represents the classic high velocity thrust applied to a joint that has pathologically restricted movement. The operator gently pushes the joint to the restricted limit of motion and then applies a quick, firm pressure on the joint in the direction of resistance, resulting in a "pop" with subsequent increased range of motion in that joint. This technique is a more direct descendent of the "bone setter" methods that may have engaged Still's attention. The application of the thrust maneuver can result in immediate increase in the range of motion. Unlike many of the other manual therapies, usually only osteopaths and chiropractors perform high velocity thrust. Not surprisingly, most of the reported risks have been associated with this technique as applied to the cervical spine.

ARTICULATION

Used for postoperative and arthritic patients, this technique uses a gentle but firm pressure against the limit of a joint's motion in order to increase the range of motion of a restricted joint. The gentle pressure is repeated as the range is pushed further—guided by the patient's pain or fatigue—each time aiming for an increase in the range of motion. This is a relatively safe form of manipulation, and is used in these more vulnerable patient populations.

MUSCLE ENERGY

This method requires active participation by the patient. The patient contracts specific muscles, with a precise configuration of the muscles/joints, and often against resistance. The position of the joints or muscles is determined by the practitioner to optimize the recruitment of the particular muscle. This technique can strengthen weakened muscles, and improve muscle health. Several different types of practitioners use this technique; osteopaths were the originators, but now chiropractors, physical therapists, and massage therapists have been trained to use muscle energy techniques with their patients.[9]

MYOFASCIAL RELEASE/SOFT TISSUE TECHNIQUES

While muscle energy requires voluntary and active muscle contraction, myofascial release usually has the patient relax while the practitioner works with the muscles and soft tissues. Various forms of direct pressure, stretching, twisting, and compressing are applied to muscles and fascia in an attempt to loosen pathologic tension, or restrictions, in the soft tissues. Tender and taut points are often used to monitor the pathology and the response to treatment. As with other soft tissue methods, this technique is practiced by many different manual clinicians.

COUNTERSTRAIN

This method was developed by an American osteopath who keenly noticed that a patient's debilitating back pain was relieved when the patient was placed on an unused exam table, in a position of comfort, while awaiting the physician. Impressed with this patient's apparent recovery while relaxing in a precisely positioned pose, Lawrence Jones, DO, spent the rest of his life developing and teaching the strain–counterstrain technique. He methodically noted hundreds of points in afflicted patients that, when treated with gentle positioning of the patient and relaxation of the target muscle (held for 90 seconds), often resulted in a symptomatic cure.[10]

Harmon Myers, DO, elaborated on Jones' findings with the notion that Jones' positions were, in fact, often shortening muscles whose tender points as mapped by Jones were very similar to Janet Travell's trigger points, which are documented in a classic text in the field.[11]

Selection of Manual Medicine Clinicians

Often, the skill of the practitioner can significantly affect (or even totally dictate) the effectiveness of the treatment. Highly talented healers can exist in any of the manual medicine realms, often with a loyal following. There are some practitioners who can effect remarkable healing with just a few sessions, with little need for follow-up. However, if a patient is required to seek manipulation regularly and frequently without any improvement in baseline symptoms, the efficacy (and, certainly, the cost-benefit ratio) of either that particular treatment, or the practitioner, should be called into question.

As desirable as it is to have evidence-based medicine guide clinical decisions, when it comes to choosing a skilled manual medicine provider, accumulated patient reports often are the best (or only) means to base a referral decision. Bear in mind, however, that even the most highly skilled healers will not be able to achieve cures in every patient; a preponderance of good reports might be all that you have to base decisions upon. If you are going to establish regular referrals to manual medicine practitioners, make sure that you obtain both positive and negative feedback from patients—often you will receive only information on the patients who are not helped, since those who achieve relief of symptoms do not return to the clinic as frequently, or their pain complaints are less.

Risks of Manual Medicine

Perhaps the most publicized and feared adverse effect of manipulation is the risk of vertebral artery dissection associated with cervical spine maneuvers. In a comparison of 150 patients with vertebral artery dissection to age/sex-matched controls without dissection, there was nearly a two-fold risk of dissection in those patients with head or neck pain versus no pain. However, there was a more than three-fold risk of dissection in those patients who had undergone cervical spine manipulation versus those who had not received manipulation.[12] Certainly, any patient with cervical instability, which is not uncommon in those with rheumatologic diseases, must use great caution if considering any manipulation of the cervical area or, to be safe, should avoid it altogether. Specifically, those patients with ankylosing spondylitis, rheumatoid arthritis[13] or collagen disorders must assiduously avoid cervical manipulation of any sort.

Dependency is a frequent concern among users of pharmaceutical analgesics, but it also can occur with manual medicine clinicians. When treatments occur frequently and regularly without significant improvement, one should be suspicious that the therapy is ineffective, or there is some dependency issue on the part of the patient (or, even a practitioner who encourages this behavior). An effective manual medicine intervention should produce noticeable relief within 5 or 6 sessions (though typically within one to three treatments). It is important that progress be regularly assessed, and if a plateau is reached, other therapies should be sought.

Application of Manual Medicine to Specific Rheumatological Conditions

The acquisition of solid, quantitative scientific data that evaluate the efficacy of manipulative medicine in different clinical situations has been difficult to achieve. The types of interventions and the skill of the manual medicine practitioners performing them can vary tremendously, even within the same clinic or institution. Anecdotal evidence suggests that the rare master manipulator can achieve near-miraculous cures of multiple ailments. However, the question of how effective a specific technique or a general type of manipulation is, in the setting of a particular pain situation, is often difficult to ascertain.

Although low back pain and neck pain (traumatic or degenerative) are the disorders most commonly treated by manual therapies, many other rheumatologic conditions, including repetitive motion injuries such as carpal tunnel syndrome, as well as ankylosing spondylitis and fibromyalgia, are commonly treated by manual medicine practitioners. We will consider these below.

LOW BACK PAIN

Spinal manipulation is often used for persistent back pain syndromes. Of all rheumatologic disorders, the use of osteopathic manipulation in low back pain has been studied most extensively. A large randomized controlled study of subacute low back pain showed that while osteopathic manipulation was comparable to standard medical care with respect to pain and functional testing, there was a dramatic and significant reduction in medication usage in the manipulation group. The use of NSAIDs was 54% for conventional care as compared to 24% for osteopathic care, while the prescription of muscle relaxants was 25% (conventional) versus 6% (osteopathic).[14] In contrast, a study that compared three interventions—chiropractic manipulation, the McKenzie method of physical therapy, and providing written information—revealed that all three interventions had similar effects and cost, with the two manual therapies providing only marginally better outcomes than the written education booklet.[15] Another study concluded that both osteopathic manipulation and sham manipulative treatment appeared to result in improvement in back pain and physical functioning, as well as greater patient satisfaction when compared to the control group.[16] Indeed, even a clinical prediction rule has been developed and validated for manipulation of back pain, to predict who might benefit from therapy.[17–19]

Given the number of studies investigating low back pain, we can utilize meta-analyses to answer this question; however, with the variation in methods and practitioners, the outcomes are difficult to interpret. A meta-analysis that reviewed 39 randomized controlled trials found that for patients with acute or chronic low back pain, there was no evidence that spinal manipulative therapy was superior to other standard treatments (sham, conventional, general practitioner care, analgesics, physical therapy, exercises, back school, or a collection of therapies).[20,21] From this meta-analysis it was unclear whether osteopathic manipulative treatment was comparable to non-osteopathic spinal manipulation performed by other practitioners. A smaller meta-analysis of

6 randomized controlled trials, specifically looking at the effect of osteopathic manipulation versus control groups, found that osteopathic manipulation significantly reduced low back pain, an effect that persisted for three months.[22] The variety of different methods of osteopathic manipulation and the varied skill levels of the different practitioners create a more difficult experimental setting relative to controlled pharmacologic studies. Case series may ultimately prove more useful in this regard.

NECK PAIN

Neck pain is often associated with significant disability in both the acute and chronic setting. In acute neck pain, a comparison between osteopathic manipulation and Ketorolac intramuscular injection found that both groups showed improvement in pain scales, with the osteopathic manipulation group having a greater decrease in pain intensity at one hour posttreatment.[23] In patients who had had neck pain for two weeks, spinal manipulation was found to be more effective and less costly than either twice-weekly physical therapy for twelve weeks or standard care by a general practitioner.[24] Manipulative therapy and a low-load exercise program were equally effective at producing sustained reductions in cervicogenic headache at 6 and 12 months in follow-up.[25] Finally, a Cochrane review of neck pain with and without headache found multiple benefits from combined programs of manipulation or mobilization with exercise therapy, but no significant advantages of either modality alone relative to controls.[26]

KNEE PAIN

Given the fact that there is a 30% coexistence rate of hip and knee arthritis,[27] it might not be surprising that hip and knee arthritic pain syndromes would be related. A clinical prediction rule has been developed to help determine which patients with knee osteoarthritis are likely to demonstrate short-term improvement in pain scales in response to hip mobilization. Five features were determined to predict the likelihood of relief of knee pain within 2 days after hip mobilization. The presence of these features are associated with increased likelihood of response to manual medicine: (1) hip or groin pain or paresthesia, (2) anterior thigh pain, (3) passive knee flexion less than 122 degrees, (4) passive hip medial (internal) rotation less than 17 degrees, and (5) pain with hip distraction. A pretest probability of success of 68% was increased to 92% if a patient had one marker present, and was increased to 97% if two markers were positive.[28] Although manipulation sounds promising in patients with osteoarthritic knee pain who meet the criteria above, manipulation does not appear to be efficacious post knee replacement.[29]

CARPAL TUNNEL SYNDROME

It has been posited that manipulation may be useful in cases of carpal tunnel syndrome from repetitive strain injuries. In cadaveric experiments, osteopathic manipulation was shown to increase the length of the transverse carpal ligament, and to increase the width of the transverse carpal arch, as demonstrated on improved measures on MRI.[30,31] In one case report, myofascial release by a physician combined with the patient's self-stretch exercises reduced pain and numbness and improved electromyographic results.[32] However, this finding was not borne out in a recent trial by Burke et al, where they found no improvement in nerve conduction studies when using chiropractic manipulation or instrument-assisted soft tissue mobilization in carpal tunnel syndrome. They did, however, note an improvement in range of motion and grip strength.[33]

Some manual medicine techniques incorporate self-stretching exercises. Yoga is a popular means of therapeutic stretching. There is one small study that details that yoga can be useful in the case of carpal tunnel syndrome.[34] Subjects in the yoga group had significant improvement in grip strength and pain reduction, but no significant difference in median nerve motor or sensory conduction.

ANKYLOSING SPONDYLITIS

Longstanding ankylosing spondylitis, characterized by fatigue, back pain, and stiffness of the sacroiliac joints and spine, can also affect the hips and shoulders. Although there is a documented case of improved quality-of-life measures and improved functional status from chiropractic manipulation in a patient with ankylosing spondylitis,[35] extreme care must be taken if one is considering manipulative therapies in this population. Consequences of ankylosing spondylitis are osteoporosis and syndesmophytosis—new vertical bone formation on the lateral spine, producing the pathognomonic "bamboo spine"—which results in a rigid and brittle spine. Rare case reports of traumatic injury after chiropractic manipulation have been noted in the literature, usually with regard to cerebrovascular accidents, myelopathy and radiculopathy.[36] A recent report detailed a cervical fracture in a patient with ankylosing spondylitis who had chiropractic spinal manipulation.[37] As one might expect, extreme caution should be used if one is considering manipulative therapy in a patient with ankylosing spondylitis, and any attempts to manipulate the spine should probably be avoided in this population.

FIBROMYALGIA

Several studies have looked at the usefulness of manipulation in fibromyalgia. The ambiguous nature of the disease itself makes for a difficult comparison between studies. Nonetheless, there are a few trials that suggest that manipulation may prove an effective adjunctive approach to managing pain in this population. A small study of 24 female patients with fibromyalgia found that osteopathic manipulation improved pain scales and functional ability over standard care alone.[38] Additionally, a small trial of chiropractic manipulation in fibromyalgia patients reported improved pain and disability scores, as well as improved cervical and lumbar range of motion with improved straight-leg-raised testing. However, the control group was without any intervention, placebo or otherwise.[39] Although data are far from conclusive or convincing, manual manipulation has been considered as a contributor to an integrative approach to fibromyalgia.[40] Unfortunately, valid studies attempting to elucidate a possible role for manipulation in fibromyalgia have been small and have had design flaws that make the resulting data difficult to interpret.

Conclusion

While it is sometimes difficult to know with certainty whether manual medicine will benefit a specific patient with a certain condition, it is reasonable to consider the use of this modality in many rheumatologic diseases. While it is important to assess risk prior to making a manual medicine referral (e.g., do not send a patient with ankylosing spondylitis, or one at risk for vertebral artery dissection, to a chiropractor for high velocity thrust to the cervical spine), the judicious use of well-trained manual medicine practitioners can help many rheumatology patients immensely. A basic knowledge of Dr. Travell's trigger points can help you determine if there is a muscular referral point that could be helped by Counterstrain or other soft tissue techniques. The ability to provide relief to a patient with pain, free from the potential adverse effects of many pharmaceuticals, is reason enough to become familiar with manual medicine practitioners in your area.

REFERENCES

1. American Osteopathic Association. Andrew Taylor Still establishes osteopathy. Available at: http://history.osteopathic.org/osteopathy.shtml. Accessed July 12, 2009.
2. Greenman PE. *Principles of Manual Medicine*. 3rd ed. Philadelphia: Lippincott, Williams & Wilkins; 2003:3–13.
3. Lane MA. *Dr. A.T. Still, Founder of Osteopathy*. Chicago: The Osteopathic Publishing Co; 1918.
4. Mark Twain, osteopath: appears at public hearing before Assembly Committee. *New York Times*. February 28, 1901:1.
5. Johnson SM, Kurtz ME. Diminished use of osteopathic manipulative treatment and its impact on the uniqueness of the osteopathic profession. *Acad Med*. 2001;76(8):821–828.
6. Palmer DD, Palmer BJ. *The Science of Chiropractic: Its Principles and Adjustments*. Davenport: The Palmer School Chiropractic; 1906.
7. Bureau of Labor Statistics. US Department of Labor, *Occupational Outlook Handbook, 2010-11 Edition, Physical Therapists*. Available at: http://www.bls.gov/oco/ocos080.htm. Accessed on: July 29, 2009.
8. The Educational Council on Osteopathic Principles (ECOP) and the American Association of Colleges of Osteopathic Medicine (AACOM). *Glossary of Osteopathic Terminology*. 2006; Available at: http://www.do-online.osteotech.org/pdf/sir_collegegloss.pdf. Accessed on: July 27, 2009.
9. Chaitow L. *Muscle Energy Techniques*. 3rd ed. New York: Elsevier Churchill-Livingstone; 2006:2–7.
10. Myers HL. *Clinical Application of Counterstrain*. Tucson: Osteopathic Press; 2006:xii–xvii.
11. McPartland JM. Travell trigger points—molecular and osteopathic perspectives. *J Am Osteopath Assoc*. 2004;104(6):244–249.
12. Smith WS, Johnston SC, Skalabrin EJ, et al. Spinal manipulative therapy is an independent risk factor for vertebral artery dissection. *Neurology*. 2003;60(9):1424–1428.
13. Neva MH, Häkkinen A, Mäkinen H, Hannonen P, Kauppi M, Sokka T. High prevalence of asymptomatic cervical spine subluxation in patients with rheumatoid arthritis waiting for orthopaedic surgery. *Ann Rheum Dis*. 2006;65(7):884–888.
14. Andersson GB, Lucente T, Davis AM, Kappler RE, Lipton JA, Leurgans S. A comparison of osteopathic spinal manipulation with standard care for patients with low back pain. *N Engl J Med*. 1999;341(19):1426–1431.
15. Cherkin DC, Deyo RA, Battié M, Street J, Barlow W. A comparison of physical therapy, chiropractic manipulation, and provision of an educational booklet for the treatment of patients with low back pain. *N Engl J Med*. 1998;339(15):1021–1029.

16. Licciardone JC, Stoll ST, Fulda KG, et al. Osteopathic manipulative treatment for chronic low back pain: a randomized controlled trial. *Spine*. 2003;28(13):1355–1362.
17. Childs JD, Fritz JM, Flynn TW, et al. A clinical prediction rule to identify patients with low back pain most likely to benefit from spinal manipulation: a validation study. *Ann Intern Med*. 2004;141(12):920–928.
18. Flynn T, Fritz J, Whitman J, et al. A clinical prediction rule for classifying patients with low back pain who demonstrate short-term improvement with spinal manipulation. *Spine*. 2002;27(24):2835–2843.
19. Fritz JM, Childs JD, Flynn TW. Pragmatic application of a clinical prediction rule in primary care to identify patients with low back pain with a good prognosis following a brief spinal manipulation intervention. *BMC Fam Pract*, 2005;6(1):29.
20. Assendelft WJ, Morton SC, Yu EI, Suttorp MJ, Shekelle PG. Spinal manipulative therapy for low back pain. A meta-analysis of effectiveness relative to other therapies. *Ann Intern Med*. 2003;138(11):871–881.
21. Assendelft WJ, Morton SC, Yu EI, Suttorp MJ, Shekelle PG. Spinal manipulative therapy for low back pain. *Cochrane Database of Syst Rev*. 2004;(1):CD000447.
22. Licciardone JC, Brimhall AK, King LN. Osteopathic manipulative treatment for low back pain: A systematic review and meta-analysis of randomized controlled trials. *BMC Musculoskeletal Disorders*, 2005;6:43.
23. McReynolds TM, Sheridan BJ. (2005). Intramuscular ketorolac versus osteopathic manipulative treatment in the management of acute neck pain in the emergency department: a randomized clinical trial. *J Am Osteopath Assoc*. 105(2):57–68.
24. Korthals-de Bos IB, Hoving JL, van Tulder MW, et al. Cost effectiveness of physiotherapy, manual therapy, and general practitioner care for neck pain: economic evaluation alongside a randomised controlled trial. *BMJ*. 2003;326(7395):911.
25. Jull G, Trott P, Potter H, et al. A randomized controlled trial of exercise and manipulative therapy for cervicogenic headache. *Spine*. 2002;27(17):1835–1843.
26. Gross AR, Hoving JL, Haines TA, et al. A Cochrane review of manipulation and mobilization for mechanical neck disorders. *Spine*. 2004;29(14):1541–1548.
27. O'Reilly SC, Muir KR, Doherty M. Occupation and knee pain: a community study. *Osteoarthritis Cartilage*, 2000;8(2):78–81.
28. Currier LL, Froehlich PJ, Carow SD, et al. Development of a clinical prediction rule to identify patients with knee pain and clinical evidence of knee osteoarthritis who demonstrate a favorable short-term response to hip mobilization. *Phys Ther*, 2007;87(9):1106–1119.
29. Licciardone JC, Stoll ST, Cardarelli KM, Gamber RG, Swift JN,Jr, Winn WB. A randomized controlled trial of osteopathic manipulative treatment following knee or hip arthroplasty. *J Am Osteopath Assoc*. 2004;104(5):193–202.
30. Sucher BM. (1993a). Myofascial manipulative release of carpal tunnel syndrome: Documentation with magnetic resonance imaging. *The Journal of the American Osteopathic Association*, *93*(12):1273–1278.
31. Sucher BM, Hinrichs RN, Welcher RL, Quiroz LD, St Laurent BF, Morrison BJ. Manipulative treatment of carpal tunnel syndrome: biomechanical and osteopathic intervention to increase the length of the transverse carpal ligament:

part 2. Effect of sex differences and manipulative "priming". *J Am Osteopath Assoc.* 2005;105(3):135–143.

32. Sucher BM. Myofascial release of carpal tunnel syndrome. *J Am Osteopath Assoc.* 1993;93(1):92–4, 100–1.
33. Burke J, Buchberger DJ, Carey-Loghmani MT, Dougherty PE, Greco DS, Dishman JD. A pilot study comparing two manual therapy interventions for carpal tunnel syndrome. *J Manipulative Physiol Ther.* 2007;30(1):50–61.
34. Garfinkel MS, Schumacher HR Jr, Husain A, Levy M, Reshetar RA. Evaluation of a yoga based regimen for treatment of osteoarthritis of the hands. *J Rheum.* 1994;21(12):2341–2343.
35. Rutherford SM, Nicolson CF, Crowther ER. Symptomatic improvement in function and disease activity in a patient with ankylosing spondylitis utilizing a course of chiropractic therapy: a prospective case study. *J Can Chiropr Assoc.* 2005;49(2):81–91.
36. Lee, KP, Carlini, WG, McCormick GF, Albers GW. Neurologic complications following chiropractic manipulation: A survey of california neurologists. *Neurology.* 1995;45(6):1213–1215.
37. Liao CC, Chen LR. Anterior and posterior fixation of a cervical fracture induced by chiropractic spinal manipulation in ankylosing spondylitis: a case report. *J Trauma.* 2007;63(4):E90–4.
38. Gamber RG, Shores JH, Russo DP, Jimenez C, Rubin BR. Osteopathic manipulative treatment in conjunction with medication relieves pain associated with fibromyalgia syndrome: results of a randomized clinical pilot project. *J Am Osteopath Assoc.* 2002;102(6):321–325.
39. Blunt KL, Rajwani MH, Guerriero RC. The effectiveness of chiropractic management of fibromyalgia patients: a pilot study. *J Manipulative Physiol Ther.* 1997;20(6):389–399.
40. Morris CR, Bowen L, Morris AJ. Integrative therapy for fibromyalgia: possible strategies for an individualized treatment program. *South Med J.* 2005;98(2): 177–184.

8

Mind-Body Medicine in Rheumatology

JOAN E. BRODERICK, PhD AND DOERTE U. JUNGHAENEL, PhD

KEY CONCEPTS

- Mind-body medicine, or behavioral medicine, is based upon the interactions among the brain, mind, body, and behavior that impact health.
- Mind-body treatments are based upon the concept that patients have the ability to influence their experience of illness through directed modification of their thoughts, emotions, and behaviors.
- The focus of mind-body medicine has been to reduce stress and physical symptoms, to enhance physical functioning and psychological wellbeing, and to curb excessive utilization of expensive and limited medical resources.
- The impact of these treatments is not only on the emotional health of the patient, but also on the physiological state, such that healthy processes are enhanced.
- Mind-body medicine is a low-risk, relatively low-cost approach that has been shown to contribute to improved status in most patients beyond what can be achieved with pharmaceutical interventions alone.
- Examples of mind-body treatments are stress management, cognitive behavioral therapies, guided imagery, relaxation training, social support interventions, and biofeedback.

■

Introduction

Mind-body medicine has an important and longstanding history in the treatment of many rheumatic conditions. Also known as *behavioral medicine* in academic settings, it is defined as a focus "on the interactions among the brain, mind, body, and behavior, and on the powerful ways in which emotional, mental, social, spiritual, and behavioral factors can directly affect health."[1] It encompasses a variety of complementary and alternative medicine (CAM) interventions that fall outside the realm of traditional biomedical treatment. These include stress management, cognitive behavioral therapies, guided imagery, relaxation training, social support interventions, and biofeedback. Over the years, numerous clinical trials have demonstrated the efficacy of mind-body interventions; however, their integration into routine medical care in the United States is still infrequent. Many medical practitioners are not familiar with these treatments and how to incorporate them into the medical regimen.

This chapter reviews the published, English-language research literature on mind-body treatments for rheumatic disease. Clinical trials often incorporate multiple mind-body components, and often do not evaluate their efficacy in isolation from one another. Most of the research in this area has involved patients with rheumatoid (RA) and osteoarthritis (OA), though some will be reported for fibromyalgia (FM), chronic fatigue syndrome (CFS), and systemic lupus erythematosus (SLE). The principles and strategies employed in mind-body interventions can be easily translated across various diagnostic groups that share similar symptomatology, such as pain and fatigue.

The Biopsychosocial Model of Chronic Disease

Mind-body medicine is focused on the complex and dynamic interplay of biological, psychological, social, and behavioral factors that are expressed as illness. The theoretical framework underlying mind-body interventions is based on the "biopsychosocial model of disease," a term coined in a seminal paper by Charles Engel in the 1970s.[2] According to this model, the experience of illness is not only determined by biological processes but also by cognitive, affective and behavioral experiences of the patient.[3] For example, cognitions and emotions can influence a patient's behavioral choices including adherence to medical treatment, exercise, nutrition, and social contact, which in turn impact on the disease process.[4,5] A given biological state (e.g., joint erosion or sedimentation rate) can be accompanied by a broad range of degrees of physical dysfunction and psychological distress.[6] Research with OA patients has found that objective evidence of disease activity, such as X-rays, explained only a small portion of patients' self-reported knee pain.[7] The dynamic and reciprocal relationship between psychosocial and biomedical factors becomes readily apparent in patients with low disease activity but significant disease burden, or, conversely, in patients with high disease activity yet minimal reduction in quality of life.

The Gate Control Theory of Pain

Another important framework of mind-body medicine in rheumatology is the gate control theory of pain.[8] This theory outlines the physiological process by which thoughts, beliefs, and emotions modulate the experience of pain. Cortical experience of pain is the culmination of both ascending nociceptive neuronal activity as well as descending inhibitory neurons; these are partially activated by affective centers in the brain.[9] The dorsal horn of the spinal cord is one of the primary locations where the gate is regulated, with either full transmission of pain signals or a reduction in afferent signals (see Figure 8.1). These findings account for "phantom pain" in amputees, the absence of pain with injury on the battlefield, neuropathic pain, and neurological differences

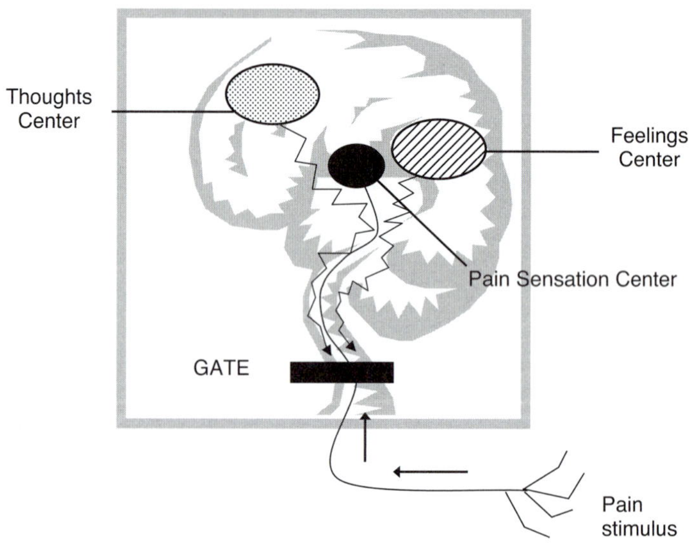

FIGURE 8.1. Gate Control Theory of Pain.

between acute and chronic pain. Psychological states, such as mood and negative cognitions (e.g., catastrophizing), have been shown to correlate with levels of pain experience. For example, among patients with RA it has been shown that feelings of helplessness are linked to higher anxiety, depression, impairment in activities of daily living,[10] and even early mortality.[11] Mind-body medicine has evolved accordingly to develop interventions designed to help patients learn how to close the pain gate and bring the body into a more relaxed affective and musculoskeletal state.

Description and History of Mind-Body Interventions for Arthritis

DISEASE EDUCATION AND SELF-MANAGEMENT TREATMENT

One of the most prominent mind-body interventions is a self-help education program for arthritis developed by Kate Lorig and her colleagues at Stanford University in the 1980s.[12,13] The Arthritis Self-Management Program is a 6-session, community-based program for patients with arthritis. Following a standardized protocol, trained peer leaders teach groups of patients the nature of the condition, the appropriate use of medication, range of motion and isometric exercises, relaxation techniques, joint protection, nutrition, interaction of patients with physicians, and evaluation of nontraditional treatments. Patients are encouraged to engage in group discussion, to keep diaries of arthritis-related content, and to self-contract for behavioral changes, such as exercise and relaxation.

COGNITIVE AND BEHAVIORAL THERAPIES (CBT)

A second important therapeutic approach is CBT, an umbrella term for a number of specific mind-body techniques:

RELAXATION EXERCISES, MEDITATION, AND IMAGERY all have the goal of teaching the patient to voluntarily reduce physiological arousal.[14] Muscle contraction and release, deep breathing, and calming imagery are among the methods used in these interventions to induce a state of relaxation. Often patients are provided with audio-recorded instructions to use in home practice.

BIOFEEDBACK is another term for external psychophysiological feedback. It entails the use of electronic or electromechanical instruments to measure and indicate ongoing somatic activities, including blood pressure, vasomotor activity, skin temperature, or electrodermal activity. Biofeedback training is typically conducted individually to guide the patient to a decreased level of physiological arousal. It can be particularly helpful for patients who have difficulty achieving a more relaxed state through other exercises.

STRESS MANAGEMENT aims to enhance patients' behavioral coping strategies to handle stress. Problem-solving of stressful situations, including homework assignments focusing on increased interpersonal assertiveness, physical exercise, sleep hygiene, and social contacts, are frequently embedded in this approach.

COGNITIVE BEHAVIORAL THERAPY is a sophisticated and comprehensive treatment delivered by a health professional, individually or in groups, with the goal of helping patients acquire disease coping skills; it incorporates a number of strategies for managing the cognitive, emotional, and behavioral experience of stressors to achieve more stability in somatic and psychological processes. Typically, this treatment is provided in 8–12 visits that are 45–90 minutes long. The concept of *self-efficacy,* first articulated by Bandura in 1977, has become an important component of CBT treatment.[15] It is defined as the extent to which a patient gains a sense of personal control over the symptoms and the disease experience. The cognitive components of CBT address illness beliefs and attitudes, such as catastrophizing and helplessness, that create negative affective states and impact on behavioral choices associated with disease management. The behavioral components target patients' activities, such as introducing management of the activity–rest cycle and reducing isolation by increasing scheduling of pleasant activities. Home practice of relaxation, scheduling activities, altering negative thinking, and other components is an essential aspect of CBT.

Treatment Outcome Studies

Mind-body treatments have been rigorously tested in clinical trials over the last 20 years and have demonstrated efficacy. Whereas disease self-management programs have demonstrated modest effect sizes,[16] CBT has yielded larger effects.[17] Nevertheless, the National Arthritis Foundation's adoption and dissemination of the Arthritis Self-Management Program has achieved a significant public health impact by virtue of its low cost (conducted by lay, peer leaders) and access throughout much of the country. Even small effects are meaningful when impacting the quality of life for millions of patients.

Research is currently being funded by the National Institute of Arthritis and Musculoskeletal and Skin Diseases (NIH) to evaluate the effectiveness of training nurse practitioners to deliver CBT in primary care offices for patients with osteoarthritis.* If treatment by nurse practitioners demonstrates efficacy, this would create the possibility of dramatically increasing the number of rheumatology patients with access to CBT.

DISEASE SELF-MANAGEMENT PROGRAMS

The first randomized controlled trial examining the efficacy of Lorig's Self-Management Program for arthritis compared 129 patients in the treatment group to 61 control patients.[12] Assessments were conducted after the 4-month treatment phase, and at 8-month and 20-month follow-ups. Patients in the treatment group reported significantly increased knowledge about arthritis, and increased frequency of exercise and relaxation exercises compared with the control group. Ratings of pain were also significantly lower for the treatment group, despite no change in the use of medications. Unaffected by the intervention were patients' ratings of disability and number of physician visits. Albeit of smaller magnitude, these effects were maintained at the 20-month follow-up assessment.

Across a number of subsequent studies, the Arthritis Self-Management Program has repeatedly demonstrated increased self-efficacy and increased knowledge about the disease.[18–20] Some studies also show reductions in pain, disability, and depression that are maintained over several years of follow-up.[21] Recently, Lorig found that programs keeping a specific focus on the disease generated better outcomes than a more generic self-management program for chronic disease.[22] The efficacy of a self-management program has also been shown in a study of 313 patients with lupus,[23] and in a randomized, controlled trial of 207 FM patients.[24] Other studies have combined physical exercise with self-management, and demonstrated efficacy in patients with FM.[25,26] However, not all self-management investigations have been as positive. Some have found very small effect sizes with fewer outcomes improved.[27,28]

COGNITIVE BEHAVIOR THERAPY

The earliest randomized, controlled studies of CBT for arthritis were conducted by Bradley and colleagues.[29,30] RA patients were assigned to CBT,

* J E. Broderick, personal communication, January 25, 2008.

supportive group therapy, or a control group. Outcomes assessed at post-treatment showed significantly greater benefit in the CBT group on pain behavior, self-reported pain, Rh factor titer, and anxiety compared with either of the other two groups. The improvement in the CBT group was maintained at the 12-month follow-up. In addition, the authors found that both disease status at baseline and compliance with the treatment moderated intervention efficacy. Patients who entered treatment with low to moderate disease status and who were highly compliant showed the best maintenance of treatment gains. In a direct comparison of CBT versus an at-home education intervention, thirty patients with arthritis were randomly assigned to the two groups. Patients in the CBT group attended five 2-hour group sessions, and patients in the education group received an arthritis education manual for study at home.[31] Patients in the CBT group reported significantly increased self-efficacy, and decreased pain, joint inflammation, and improved psychosocial functioning at post-treatment; however, the 4-month follow-up showed poor maintenance of improvement.

The success of the initial studies of CBT and educational approaches encouraged further development of the interventions. Parker and colleagues provided CBT to patients on an individual basis.[32] One-hundred-forty-one patients participated in two 10-week intervention groups: (1) a CBT group, and (2) an education group, both compared to a standard-medical-care control group. Both intervention arms were identical in the frequency of contact with patients; only the content of the individual sessions was varied. The study also incorporated an extensive maintenance phase of treatment booster sessions for both intervention arms, which were held every 3 months over a 15-month follow-up period. Consistent with previous studies, the CBT treatment produced significantly greater changes on reports of daily stressors, coping attempts, self-efficacy, helplessness, pain ratings, and extremity impairment at post-treatment. The only variable that was significantly affected by the educational intervention was experience of daily stressors. Importantly, treatment gains were maintained through the 15-month follow-up for most outcomes.

Keefe and colleagues at Duke University introduced the involvement of spouses to the treatment of chronic pain in OA and RA patients.[33] This was instigated by the increasing recognition of the role of family attitudes and reactions on the progression of arthritis disability and illness experience.[34,35] One study compared three treatment conditions with 88 OA patients with knee pain: CBT with active spouse involvement, spouse-assisted arthritis education, and traditional CBT without spouse.[36] Each treatment arm was identical in the amount of therapeutic contact. As previously shown, both CBT treatments produced superior effects over education alone. Moreover, spousal involvement in CBT yielded a significant incremental improvement on most variables over patient-only CBT. The additive effects of spousal involvement were also replicated in a brief, 4-week controlled study of 59 patients with RA.[37] Spouse-assisted treatment was found to produce improvements more rapidly than CBT alone in reducing joint pain and swelling, and in increasing physical functioning. A recent randomized controlled trial with 72 married OA patients demonstrated the salutary effects of combining spouse-assisted coping skills training with exercise training.[38]

Over the years, increasing emphasis has been placed on the importance of early treatment in RA,[39] particularly in the beginning stages of disease onset. A study by Sharpe and colleagues[40] examined the efficacy of a CBT intervention for patients with recent onset of RA (<2 years). At post-treatment, patients in the CBT groups showed significant reductions in depressive symptoms and C-reactive protein levels compared to the control participants, and improved joint involvement at the 6-month follow-up. In a similar fashion, Evers and colleagues[41] demonstrated the benefits of tailored CBT treatment in early arthritis (disease duration < 8 years).

The efficacy of CBT interventions has also been investigated in patients with FM and CFS. One-hundred-and-four patients participated in once-per-week group sessions over the span of 6 months, and were compared with 29 patients who were screened but did not participate in the program.[42] Patients in the treatment group showed significant improvement on physical function, pain, fatigue, stiffness, depression, anxiety, number of tender points, and ability to decrease and control pain compared with pretreatment levels. Nielson and colleagues applied a 3-week inpatient intervention strategy to 25 FM patients.[43] Their program consisted of a comprehensive team approach utilizing educational and cognitive-behavioral techniques. Pain and emotional distress were reduced at the end of treatment, and a sense of control over pain was increased. A 30-month follow-up found that improvement was maintained on observed pain behavior and control over pain.[44] Similar studies with CFS patients have yielded comparable outcomes.[45] Other studies find that either meditation training alone[46] or meditation-based CBT treatment yield significant benefits for FM patients.[47]

CHILDREN

In addition to clinical trials examining the efficacy of mind-body treatment in rheumatology for adults, there has been increasing recognition that pain is also a considerable burden for children with juvenile RA.[48] One 3-month study investigated the efficacy of CBT treatments for 8 children after 6 individual sessions that included involvement of mothers. Over 50% of the children experienced at least a 25% reduction in pain at post-treatment, and up to 88% of the children reported reductions in pain of at least 25% at the 6-month follow-up. Mothers' ratings of pain behavior corresponded with the children's self-reports.[49] A study of juvenile FM assigned 67 patients (age range 8 to 20 years, mean = 13.9 years) and their parents to an 8-week CBT intervention consisting of pain management, psychoeducation, relaxation and daily diaries of pain and sleep hygiene.[50] At post-treatment, children experienced significant reductions in pain, somatic and psychological symptoms, fatigue, and improvement in sleep hygiene. In addition, children had less school absenteeism and improved functional ability. Among children with chronic pain, treatment preferences among CAM interventions were found to be noninvasive treatments including biofeedback, yoga, and hypnosis.[51]

Other Developments in Mind-Body Treatment

Biofeedback is another mind-body modality increasingly being examined as a treatment for pain in rheumatology patients.[52] Flor and colleagues found that 12 sessions of EMG biofeedback yielded greater reductions in pain than either of the control groups using conventional medical care and sham biofeedback.[53] At the 2½ year follow-up, treated patients had significantly less pain-related interference and a 69% reduction in use of medical compared with the control groups.[54] A trial with lupus patients randomly assigned 92 patients to biofeedback-assisted CBT (BF/CBT), a symptom-monitoring support group, or a usual care control condition.[55] At post-treatment, patients in the BF/CBT group reported significantly greater reductions in pain and psychological dysfunction compared to the other two groups. At 9-month follow-up, improvement in psychological functioning continued to be greater in the BF/CBT group relative to the control groups.

Another remarkable development is the effect of emotionally-expressive writing on physical health. This intervention, developed by Pennebaker, has patients write essays about past traumatic events on several occasions.[56] Several studies have documented significant, positive changes in health status several months subsequent to the writing compared with a control group that writes about a neutral topic. Recently, the efficacy of the intervention has been examined in medical populations. Rheumatologists, who were blind to treatment condition, observed a 20% decrease in RA disease activity 4 months post-writing compared with a 3% decrease in the control group.[57] Another randomized controlled trial with female FM patients found significant reductions in pain and fatigue, and better psychological wellbeing, for patients in the trauma writing group at the 4-month follow-up, relative to the neutral writing and the usual care control groups. Benefits were not maintained at the 10-month follow-up.[58]

Comparison of Efficacy for NSAIDs and Mind-Body Treatment

An important factor in mind-body treatment relates to its efficacy in comparison with conventional biomedical treatment. A meta-analysis of 19 mind-body interventions (education and CBT plus medical care) and 28 nonsteroidal anti-inflammatory drug (NSAID) interventions found that mind-body treatments provided an additional 20% improvement for OA patients, and an additional 20%–40% for RA patients, over the effects of NSAIDs alone for relief from pain. For RA patients, a 40% improvement in functional ability was achieved using mind-body interventions compared to NSAIDs alone, and a 60%–80% relative decrease in tender joint count.[59] The combination of educational and cognitive behavioral components yielded the greatest benefits. In a meta-analytic review of 49 treatment outcome studies with FM patients, Rossy and colleagues[60] compared the efficacy of pharmacological and nonpharmacological treatment. The authors concluded that CBT was more effective in improving subjective symptoms and daily functioning than pharmacological treatment.

Summary

Research over the last 20 years within the new specialty of behavioral medicine, or mind-body medicine as it is colloquially known, has made significant contributions to the treatment of rheumatic disease. There has been a convergence of findings documenting the complex interplay of psychosocial and biological factors in determining patients' experience of illness. This has led to the application of educational and cognitive-behavioral intervention strategies as complementary treatment options for patients with chronic disease. These treatments are based upon the concept that patients have the ability to influence their experience of illness through directed modification of their thoughts, emotions, and behaviors. The focus of mind-body medicine has been to reduce stress and physical symptoms, to enhance physical functioning and psychological well-being, and to curb excessive utilization of expensive and limited medical resources.

This review of the scientific literature has outlined treatment outcome studies evaluating the effectiveness of mind-body interventions for several rheumatic diseases. It has been found that they provide significant, incremental symptom relief, and improvements in disability status and wellbeing, beyond that achieved through routine medical care. Issues of toxicity and side effects are virtually nonexistent. Studies find that children also experience benefit. Furthermore, there is evidence that these interventions reduce utilization of health care services, despite continuing progression of disease, a finding that has major economic implications for health policy. Mind-body researchers are currently exploring procedures that may yield improved outcome on treatment adherence, compliance, and extension of treatment effects for longer periods of time beyond the end of treatment. Finally, there is recognition that more translational and dissemination research is necessary to create effective models of treatment delivery to provide access to mind-body treatment for patients.

ACKNOWLEDGEMENTS

Preparation of this chapter was funded in part by grants AR054626 and AR052170 from the National Institute of Arthritis and Musculoskeletal and Skin Diseases.

REFERENCES

1. National Center for Complementary and Alternative Medicine. *Mind-Body Medicine: An Overview.* Available at: http://nccam.nih.gov/health/backgrounds/mindbody.htm. Accessed on December 11, 2007.
2. Engel, G. The need for a new medical model: A challenge for biomedicine. *Science.* 1977;196(4286):129–136.
3. Keefe FJ, Bonk V. Psychosocial assessment of pain in patients having rheumatic diseases. *Rheum Dis Clin North Am.* 1999;25(1):81–103.
4. DiMatteo MR, Haskard KB, Williams SL. Health beliefs, disease severity, and patient adherence: a meta-analysis. *Med Care.* 2007;45(6):521–528.
5. Halligan, PW, Aylward M, eds. The Power of Belief: Psychosocial Influence on Illness, Disability and Medicine. New York: Oxford University Press; 2006.
6. Osterweis M, Kleinman A, Mechanic D. *Pain and Disability: Clinical, Behavioral, and Public Policy Perspectives.* Washington, DC: National Academy Press; 1987.
7. Keefe F, Caldwell D, Queen K, et al. Osteoarthritic knee pain: a behavioral analysis. *Pain.* 1987;28(3):309–321.
8. Melzack R, Wall PD. Pain mechanisms: a new theory. *Science.* 1965;150(699): 971–979.
9. Kandel ER, Schwartz JH, Jessell TM. *Principles of Neural Science. 4th ed.* New York: McGraw-Hill; 2000.

10. Smith TW, Christensen AJ, Peck JR, Ward JR. Cognitive distortion, helplessness, and depressed mood in rheumatoid arthritis: a four-year longitudinal analysis. *Health Psychol.* 1994;13(3):213–217.
11. Callahan LF, Cordray DS, Wells G, Pincus T. Formal education and five-year mortality in rheumatoid arthritis: mediation by helplessness scale score. *Arthritis Care Res.* 1996;9(6):463–472.
12. Lorig K, Lubeck D, Kraines R, Seleznick M, Holman H. Outcomes of self-help education for patients with arthritis. *Arthritis Rheum.* 1985;28(6):680–685.
13. Lorig K, Seleznick M, Lubeck D, Ung E, Chastian RL, Holman H. The beneficial outcomes of the arthritis self-management course are not adequately explained by behavior change. *Arthritis Rheum.* 1989;32(1):91–95.
14. Benson H. The Relaxation response. In: Goleman D, Gurin J, eds. *Mind, Body Medicine: How to Use your Mind for Better Health.* New York: Consumers Union; 1993.
15. Bandura A. Self-efficacy: Toward a unifying theory of behavioral change. *Psychological Rev.* 1977;84(2):191–215.
16. Foster G, Taylor SJ, Eldridge SE, Ramsay J, Griffiths CJ. Self-management education programmes by lay leaders for people with chronic conditions. *Cochrane Database Syst Rev.* 2007;17(4):CD005108.
17. Morley S, Eccleston C, Williams A. Systematic review and meta-analysis of randomized controlled trials of cognitive behaviour therapy and behaviour therapy for chronic pain in adults, excluding headache. *Pain.* 1999;80(1–2):1–13.
18. Goeppinger J, Arthur MW, Baglioni AJ, Brunk SE, Brunner CM. A reexamination of the effectiveness of self-care education for persons with arthritis. *Arthritis Rheum.* 1989;32(6):706–716.
19. Lorig K, Holman H. Long term outcomes of an arthritis self-management study: effects of reinforcement efforts. *Soc Sci Med.* 1989;29(2):221–224.
20. Lorig K, & Holman H. Arthritis Self-Management studies: a twelve-year review. *Health Educ Q.* 1993;20(1):17–28.
21. Osborne RH, Wilson T, Lorig KR, McColl GJ. Does self-management lead to sustainable health benefits in people with arthritis? A 2-year transition study of 452 Australians. *J Rheumatol* 2007;34:1112–1117.
22. Lorig K, Ritter PL, Plant K. A disease-specific self-help program compared with a generalized chronic disease self-help program for arthritis patients. *Arthritis Rheum.* 2005;53(6): 950–957.
23. Braden C, McGlone K, Pennington F. Specific psychosocial and behavioral outcomes from the systemic lupus erythematosus self-help course. *Health Educ Q.* 1993;20(1):29–41.
24. Rooks DS, Gautam S., Romeling M, et al. Group exercise, education, and combination self-management in women with fibromyalgia: a randomized trial. *Arch Intern Med.* 2007;167(20):2192–2200.
25. Burckhardt CS, Mannerkorpi K, Hedenberg L, Bjelle A. A randomized, controlled clinical trial of education and physical training for women with fibromyalgia. *J Rheumatol.* 1994;21(4):714–720.

26. Cedraschi C, Desmeules J, Rapiti E, et al. Fibromyalgia: a randomised, controlled trial of a treatment programme based on self management. *Ann Rheum Dis.* 2004;63(3):290–296.
27. Buszewicz M, Rait G, Griffin M, et al. Self management of arthritis in primary care: randomised controlled trial. *BMJ.* 2006;333(7574):879.
28. Solomon DH, Warsi A, Brown-Stevenson T, et al. Does self-management education benefit all populations with arthritis? A randomized controlled trial in a primary care physician network. *J Rheumatol.* 2002;29(2):362–368.
29. Bradley LA, Young LD, Anderson KO, et al. Effects of psychological therapy on pain behavior of rheumatoid arthritis patients: Treatment outcome and six-month follow-up. *Arthritis Rheum.* 1987;30(10):1105–1114.
30. Bradley LA, Young LD, Anderson KO, et al. *Effects of cognitive-behavior therapy on rheumatoid arthritis pain behavior: One year follow-up.* In: Dubner R, Gebhart G, Bond M, eds. *Pain Research and Clinical Management. Proceedings of the 5th World Congress on Pain.* Amsterdam: Elsevier; 1988:310–314.
31. O'Leary A, Shoor S, Lorig K, Holman HR. A cognitive-behavioral treatment of rheumatoid arthritis. *Health Psychol.* 1988;7(6):527–544.
32. Parker JC, Smarr KL, Buckelew SP, et al. Effects of stress management on clinical outcomes in rheumatoid arthritis. *Arthritis Rheum.* 1995;38(12):1807–1818.
33. Keefe F, Caldwell D, Williams D, et al. Pain coping skills training in the management of osteoarthritic knee pain: A comparative study. *Behav Ther.* 1990;21: 49–62.
34. Flor H, Turk D, Rudy TE. Pain and families. II. Assessment and treatment. *Pain.* 1987;30(1):29–45.
35. Manne SL, Zautra AJ. Couples coping with chronic illness: women with rheumatoid arthritis and their healthy husbands. *J Behav Med.* 1990;13(4):327–342.
36. Keefe F, Caldwell D, Baucom D, et al. Spouse-assisted coping skills training in the management of in osteoarthritic knee pain. *Arthritis Care Res.* 1996; 9(4): 279–291.
37. Radojevic V, Nicassio P, Weisman M. Behavioral intervention with and without family support for rheumatoid arthritis. *Behav Ther.* 1992;23:13–30.
38. Keefe FJ, Blumenthal J, Baucom D, et al. Effects of spouse-assisted coping skills training and exercise training in patients with osteoarthritic knee pain: a randomized controlled study. *Pain.* 2004;110(3):539–549.
39. Parker JC, Frank RG, Beck NC, et al. Pain management in rheumatoid arthritis patients. A cognitive-behavioral approach. *Arthritis Rheum.* 1988;31(5):593–601.
40. Sharpe L, Sensky T, Timberlake N, Ryan B, Brewin CR, Allard S. A blind, randomized, controlled trial of cognitive-behavioural intervention for patients with recent onset rheumatoid arthritis: preventing psychological and physical morbidity. *Pain.* 2001;89(2–3):275–283.
41. Evers AW, Kraaimaat FW, van Riel PL, de Jong AJ. Tailored cognitive-behavioral therapy in early rheumatoid arthritis for patients at risk: a randomized controlled trial. *Pain.* 2002;100(1–2): 141–153.

42. Bennet RM, Burchkhardt CS, Clark SR, O'Reilly CA, Wiens AN, Campbell SM. Group treatment of fibromyalgia: A six-month outpatient program. *J Rheumatol.* 1996;23(3):521–528.
43. Nielson WR, Walker C, McCain GA. Cognitive behavioral treatment of fibromyalgia syndrome: preliminary findings. *J Rheumatol.* 1992;19(1):98–103.
44. White KP, Nielson WR. Cognitive behavioral treatment of fibromyalgia syndrome: a followup assessment. *J Rheumatol.* 1995;22(4):717–721.
45. Price JR, Couper J. Cognitive behaviour therapy for adults with chronic fatigue syndrome. *Cochrane Database and Syst Rev.* 2000;(2):CD001027.
46. Grossman P, Tiefenthaler-Gilmer U, Raysz A, Kesper U. Mindfulness training as an intervention for fibromyalgia: evidence of postintervention and 3-year follow-up benefits in well-being. *Psychotherapy and Psychosomatics.* 2007;76(4): 226–233.
47. Goldenberg DL, Kaplan KH, Nadeau MG, Brodeur C, Smith S, Schmid CH. A controlled study of stress-reduction, cognitive-behavioral treatment program in fibromyalgia. *Journal of Musculoskeletal Pain.* 1994;2(2):53–66.
48. Ross CK, Lavigne JV, Hayford JR, Dyer AR, Pachman LM. Validity of reported pain as a measure of clinical state in juvenile rheumatoid arthritis. *Ann Rheum Dis.* 1989;48(10):817–819.
49. Lavigne JV, Ross CK, Berry SL, Hayford JR, Pachman LM. Evaluation of a psychological treatment package for treating pain in juvenile rheumatoid arthritis. *Arthritis Care Res.* 1992;5(2):101–110.
50. Degotardi PJ, Klass ES, Rosenberg BS, Fox DG, Gallelli KA, Gottlieb BS. Development and evaluation of a cognitive-behavioral intervention for juvenile fibromyalgia. *J Pediatr Psychol.* 2006;31(7):714–723.
51. Tsao JC, Meldrum M, Kim SC, Jacob MC, Zeltzer LK. Treatment Preferences for CAM in Children with Chronic Pain. *Evid Based Complement Alternat Med.* 2007;4(3):367–374.
52. Schwartz MS, Andrasik F, eds. *Biofeedback: A practitioner's guide. 3rd ed.* New York: The Guilford Press; 2005.
53. Flor H, Haag G, Turk DC, Koehler H. Efficacy of EMG biofeedback, pseudotherapy, and conventional medical treatment for chronic rheumatic back pain. *Pain.* 1983;17(1):21–31.
54. Flor H, Haag G, Turk DC. Long-term efficacy of EMG biofeedback for chronic rheumatic back pain. *Pain.* 1986;27(2):195–202.
55. Greco CM, Rudy TE, Manzi S. Effects of a stress-reduction program on psychological function, pain, and physical function of systemic lupus erythematosus patients: a randomized controlled trial. *Arthritis Rheum.* 2004;51(4):625–634.
56. Pennebaker JW, Beall SK. Confronting a traumatic event: toward an understanding of inhibition and disease. *J Abnorm Psychol.* 1986; 95(3):274–281.
57. Smyth J, Stone A, Hurewitz A, Kaell A. Effects of writing about stressful experiences on symptom reduction in patients with asthma or rheumatoid arthritis: a randomized trial. *JAMA.* 1999;281(14):1304–1309.

58. Broderick JE, Junghaenel DU, Schwartz JE. Written emotional expression produces health benefits in fibromyalgia patients. *Psychosom Med.* 2005;67(2):326–334.
59. Superio-Cabuslay E, Ward M, Lorig K. Patient education interventions in osteoarthritis and rheumatoid arthritis: a meta-analytic comparison with nonsteroidal antiinflammatory drug treatment. *Arthritis Care Res.* 1996;9(4):92–301.
60. Rossy LA, Buckelew SP, Dorr N, et al. A meta-analysis of fibromyalgia treatment interventions. *Annals of Behavioral Medicine.* 1999;21(2):180–191.

9

Sleep Disorders in Rheumatologic Conditions: An Integrative Approach

RUBIN R. NAIMAN, PhD AND PAUL D. ABRAMSON, MD

KEY CONCEPTS

- Sleep disorders and rheumatologic conditions share many features, including underlying chronic inflammatory processes, depression, chronic pain, and functional impairment.
- Rheumatology patients should be routinely screened for sleep disturbances by primary care or specialty physicians.
- There is a growing body of data supporting an integrative, whole-person approach to treating sleep disorders that includes mind-body, nutritional and botanical medicine interventions.
- The integrative treatment of sleep disorders in rheumatology patients must be personalized and comprehensive. It often requires an ongoing, systematic program rather than a single intervention, and may require a team approach.
- Our clinical model for treating insomnia, the Noise Reduction Model, helps patients conceptualize and manage complex factors influencing their sleep.
- Cognitive behavioral therapies (CBT) are among the most effective strategies available to manage insomnia.

■

Introduction

The past two decades have witnessed significant advances in the understanding of sleep disorders, as well as their role in the pathogenesis of a broad range of medical and psychological illnesses. Although sleep disturbance is frequently mentioned in discussions of rheumatologic conditions, conventional treatment considerations often overlook the critical role that poor sleep may play in the disease process. Once identified, sleep disorders may be readily treated with an integrative approach, relieving many of the symptoms that overlap with rheumatologic conditions and perhaps even ameliorating the underlying inflammatory pathophysiology. Complicating the situation is the possibility that the inflammatory processes and pain associated with rheumatologic conditions may themselves disrupt sleep, creating a runaway feedback loop.

Rheumatologic conditions are strongly correlated with poor sleep. The National Sleep Foundation's 2003 *Sleep in America* poll[1] reported that among the 46% of older adults with arthritis, 15% reported sleeping less than 6 hours per night, 29% rate their sleep quality as poor, 18% have a diagnosed sleep disorder, 18% report daytime sleepiness, 34% report waking unrefreshed, and 56% report a symptom of insomnia,[2] found that among arthritis patients over the age of 65, approximately one-third of survey respondents reported disrupted sleep, which was associated with increased use of medical, complementary, and self-care strategies.

Sleep disorders and rheumatologic conditions share many features, including underlying chronic inflammatory processes, depression, chronic pain, and functional impairment. Intertwined with these are sleep symptoms, such as insomnia, sleep fragmentation with increased arousals, impaired sleep quality, and excessive daytime sleepiness and fatigue. Both sleep disorders and rheumatologic conditions are also complicated by iatrogenic effects of conventional treatments, especially medications.

This will emphasize two points: first, care of patients with rheumatologic conditions should include screening and evaluation for sleep disorders, with treatment as indicated. Second, there is a growing body of data supporting an integrative, whole-person approach to treating sleep disorders, and broadening conventional medical treatment to emphasize modalities such as mind-body techniques, nutritional interventions, dietary supplements, and botanical medicines.

Overview of Sleep Disorders

Physicians frequently encounter complaints of disturbed sleep. The 2008 Sleep in America Poll found that 65% of adults report at least one sleep problem a few nights a week or more, with 44% reporting problems every night or almost every night and 28% reporting that sleepiness interferes with daily activities at least a few days a month.

Sleep problems may also contribute to medical and psychiatric disorders. Historically, many sleep complaints have been empirically treated with hypnotic medications, but in recent decades a systematic approach to classifying disorders of sleep and arousal disorders has allowed for a more nuanced approach to treatment.

Insomnia is the most common sleep symptom, characterized by difficulty falling asleep (onset insomnia), staying asleep (maintenance insomnia), or not feeling refreshed upon waking (nonrestorative sleep). Insomnia may be associated with a number of underlying medical conditions including obstructive sleep apnea (OSA), narcolepsy, restless legs syndrome (RLS), periodic limb movements in sleep (PLMS), parasomnias, alpha intrusion, and reduced REM latencies. Other conditions associated with insomnia include anxiety, depression, adjustment disorders, pain, and hormonal changes associated with menstruation and menopause. Substance use, including caffeine, alcohol, and pharmaceuticals can also contribute to insomnia.

Excessive daytime sleepiness and fatigue are symptoms common to rheumatologic conditions and sleep disorders, and are frequently dismissed as inevitable features of rheumatologic problems. In fact, they may be associated with an insufficient amount of sleep or compromised sleep quality that remains unexamined by physicians, or denied and masked by patients.

Sleepiness is essentially the propensity to fall asleep, while **fatigue** is a subjective sense of physical exhaustion but with an active mind and a propensity to rest that is independent of sleepiness. When fatigue occurs independently of sleepiness, patients commonly report insomnia associated with physical exhaustion and a frustratingly active mind. Patients reporting fatigue may or may not have a concomitant sleep disorder.

Excessive daytime sleepiness (EDS) is the most immediate symptom of disordered sleep, though it is commonly masked by physiological or psychological states such as hyperarousal[3] as well as the use of "counterfeit energies" such as caffeine and high-glycemic-index foods. Patients with primary insomnia have an elevated metabolic rate across the 24-hour circadian cycle[4] and elevated nocturnal catecholamine levels.[5] As a group, primary insomniacs appear to be less sleepy during the day by objective measures than normal sleepers, possibly because the primary underlying condition is hyperarousal that is secondarily disrupting their sleep.[3] Excessive daytime sleepiness warrants an evaluation for an underlying sleep disorder, as well as causes of overstimulation and hyperarousal.

Fatigue, on the other hand, is often part of a complex of symptoms and may have multifactorial origins, including direct effects of elevated cytokine levels in inflammatory disorders.[6,7] Physical correlates of fatigue may include generalized weakness, heaviness of limbs and postexertional malaise lasting several hours. Psychological features may include difficulty with concentration or attention, diminished motivation, short-term memory loss, and a tendency to struggle against inactivity. These symptoms may be associated with significant impairment in social and occupational functioning. Fatigue is also considered a core symptom of major depression, and is often the main residual symptom persisting after treatment interventions.[8]

Approximately 40%–80% of outpatients with rheumatoid arthritis (RA) report struggling with significant levels of fatigue.[9–12] Pollard et al[13] found that fatigue in RA was more strongly associated with pain and depression than the severity of disease.[9–11,14,15] Other factors in fatigue include subjective perception of illness, general health beliefs, and inadequate social support.[14,16]

In a large-scale study of the prevalence and meaning of fatigue in rheumatic disease, Wolfe, et al[11] concluded:

> "Fatigue is common across all rheumatic diseases, associates with all measures of distress, and is a predictor of work dysfunction and overall health status. The correlates of fatigue are generally similar across RA, OA and FM. Fatigue assessment adds much to understanding and management of patients and diseases."

Sleep Disorders, Inflammation, and Immune Function

The relationship between sleep disruption and inflammation is likely bidirectional. Insufficient sleep appears to promote inflammation, while inflammatory disorders disrupt sleep.

Impaired sleep is independently linked to the risk of chronic medical conditions associated with inflammation, such as insulin resistance,[17] type II diabetes,[18-21] and atherosclerosis.[22,23] In particular, patients with obstructive sleep apnea (OSA) who have associated cardiovascular disease have elevated levels of C-reactive protein (CRP) compared with patients with OSA but without cardiovascular disease.[24]

A number of studies have looked at the effects of sleep deprivation on markers and mediators of inflammation and immunity.[25] Experimental sleep deprivation of as little as one night's sleep has been found to alter cellular immune responses in humans[25,26] and also to increase serum levels of inflammatory markers such as the cytokines[7] tumor necrosis factor alpha (TNF-alpha), TNF-R p55,[27] and the acute phase reactant C-reactive protein (CRP).[6,28–31]

Conversely, inflammatory conditions with elevated cytokine levels may in turn disrupt sleep via several mechanisms including increased pain, depression, and anxiety, and possibly by a direct sleep-modulating effect of inflammatory cytokines such as IL-6[32] and TNF-alpha.[33] It appears reasonable to hypothesize that proper treatment of sleep symptoms could break such a cycle and allow more effective treatment of the inflammatory condition.

Sleep Disorders Associated with Rheumatologic Conditions

The association between various rheumatologic conditions and particular sleep disorders is well documented in a recent review by Abad et al.[34] Fibromyalgia syndrome (FMS) is the best studied rheumatologic conditions with respect to sleep disorders. FMS is associated with symptoms of excessive daytime sleepiness, fatigue, and insomnia, as well as obstructive sleep apnea (OSA), restless legs syndrome (RLS) and periodic limb movements in sleep (PLMS).[34] Intrusion of alpha waves into delta (deep) sleep, known as alpha-intrusion or alpha-delta sleep, is a common feature in FMS and RA.[35] Alpha-delta sleep, particularly a variant known as "phasic alpha activity," is associated with pain, decreased total sleep time, lower sleep efficiency, and less slow-wave sleep.[36]

Rheumatoid arthritis is associated with symptoms of excessive daytime sleepiness and fatigue. Specific to rheumatoid arthritis is worsening of OSA by destruction of the temporomandibular joint, acquired retrognathia and micrognathia. Vertical luxation of the odontoid process may also compress the brainstem, leading to central sleep apnea. RA has also been associated with sleep state misperception, OSA, RLS, and PLMD.[34] There is also evidence that patients with insomnia can improve their rheumatoid arthritis symptoms by improving their sleep.[37]

The experimental disruption of slow-wave (delta) sleep by noise[38] or painful stimuli[39] in healthy persons induces alpha-delta sleep and fibromyalgia-like symptoms of musculoskeletal pain and negative mood changes. A return to normal sleep leads to the alleviation of symptoms.[38] Another study of experimentally-induced slow-wave sleep disruption in healthy middle-aged subjects found increased musculoskeletal pain, decreased pain threshold and fatigue after three nights, although the alpha-delta anomaly was not observed.[40] Thus, sleep disruption may contribute to fibromyalgia symptoms, perhaps via upregulation of inflammatory mediators or another mechanism yet to be elucidated.

Screening and Evaluating Sleep Concerns in Rheumatology

Rheumatology patients should be routinely screened for sleep disturbances by primary care or specialty physicians. Effective sleep screening and evaluation must be sensitive to subjective factors including possible anxiety about evaluation procedures and treatment options, possible patient bias, and other patient emotional needs. We feel that an integrative evaluation should include serious consideration of both standardized objective data as well as relevant subjective experience of patients. Unfortunately, formal sleep evaluations can be impersonal and offer little if any regard for important subjective and psychological aspects of sleep. Many sleep patients are routed through polysomnography studies without ever meeting their sleep specialist or having a meaningful discussion about sleep with their personal physician.

Ultimately, sleep screening and evaluation represents an important part the treatment process and should also be therapeutic; that is, informative and encouraging. An integrative approach to sleep screening and evaluation is comprehensive, accounting for biomedical, psychological (including psychosocial) and environmental factors.

SLEEP DISORDERS SCREENING

The Epworth Sleepiness Scale (ESS) is a widely used standardized sleepiness scale that provides a quick and valid subjective measure of sleepiness. Although it does not offer good discriminatory sensitivity among sleep disorders, it is an excellent sleep-screening device. A score of 10 or greater suggests a need for further evaluation.

Epworth Sleepiness Scale

In contrast to just feeling tired, how likely are you to doze off or fall asleep in the following situations? (Even if you have not done some of these things

Table 9.1.

0 = Would never doze 1 = Slight chance of dozing 2 = Moderate chance of dozing
3 = High chance of dozing

Situation	*Chance of Dozing*
a. Sitting & Reading	a. ______
b. Watching TV	b. ______
c. Sitting inactive in a public place (i.e. theater)	c. ______
d. As a car passenger for an hour without a break	d. ______
e. Lying down to rest in the afternoon	e. ______
f. Sitting & talking to someone	f. ______
g. Sitting quietly after lunch without alcohol	g. ______
h. In a car, while stopping for a few minutes in traffic	h. ______
Total Score	________

recently, try to work out how they would have affected you.) Use the following scale to choose the most appropriate number for each situation:

Although they often coexist, sleepiness and fatigue are discrete symptoms suggestive of different problems that may call for different treatments. Patients frequently fail to make adequate discriminations among different kinds of low-energy states. The term "tired," for example, is commonly used to refer to sleepiness, fatigue, and even depression. It is useful to help patients better discriminate among these different experiences with further questioning. Discriminating between sleepiness and fatigue is of particular importance with regard to rheumatologic conditions such as FMS that may be associated less with daytime sleepiness and more with fatigue. In a systematic review of 23 scales used to measure fatigue in rheumatoid arthritis, Hewlett et al[41] found reasonable evidence of validation in only six scales, concluding that caution should be exercised in selecting such scales.

Evaluating Insomnia

Insomnia is evaluated through clinical interview and history, and does not usually require polysomnography (PSG) unless it is intractable or there is suspicion of secondary concerns (such as PLMS, OSA, or alpha intrusion) that need to be evaluated. Because patients may be poor historians, the use of a sleep diary to collect data over a number of days may be helpful.

The etiology of insomnia is commonly understood in terms of predisposing, precipitating, and perpetuating factors. Factors that can predispose one to insomnia include the use of drugs, medications, alcohol, caffeine or nicotine; nocturnal pain or discomfort; primary sleep disorders such as OSA, RLS/PLMS or GERD; sleep phase or rhythm disorders, shift-work, chronic jet lag, and psychological factors such as depression, anxiety, PTSD, OCD or being Type A. Precipitating factors include stressful medical, social, vocational or other events that compromise one's coping capacity. Perpetuating factors refer to failed attempts to remedy, manage, adapt or cope with insomnia. These include excessive time in bed, an irregular sleep/wake schedule, daytime napping and dozing, compensatory caffeine, alcohol, and drug use, anxiety about daytime consequences, attempts to control sleep, hypnotic use and rebound effects, and possible secondary gain.

Biomedical evaluation involves assessment of general nutrition, exercise habits, substance use, medical conditions, and sleep side effects of medications. Our clinical experience suggests a common tendency to underestimate both caffeine consumption and its potential for disrupting sleep. It may be helpful to remind patients that a cup is only 8 oz. Failure to report nighttime wakefulness may result from its masking with evening alcohol, marijuana, or hypnotics and other sedating medications.

Psychological factors in insomnia include psychiatric symptoms (particularly depression and anxiety) stress, conditioned insomnia (resulting from prolonged association of the bed and bedroom with wakefulness), and engaging in stimulating activity in the evening. More specifically, sleep efficiency (SE) is a useful measure of the extent to which insomnia may result from a conditioned association of the bed with wakefulness.

Cognitive factors—including faulty beliefs about sleep, and thought patterns that generate anxiety—figure prominently in insomnia as well as depression and anxiety disorders, and will be addressed in greater detail in the discussion of treatment.

Evaluation of environmental factors in insomnia involves determining the quality of the patient's physical, circadian (or temporal), and social sleep environment. Questions are directed at determining if the patient's bedroom is sufficiently cool, dark, quiet, and otherwise comfortable. Is sleep disrupted by children, pets, a spouse's snoring? It is also essential to determine if a patient feels psychologically safe in his or her bedroom. Psychological safety may be compromised by current threat, or a history of trauma or abuse in the bedroom. The sleep environment is also defined in terms of timing, or circadian factors. This refers to questions about sleep schedule, its regularity or disruption by shift work, or frequent jet lag.

"A Good Sleeper?" Normal sleep onset latency ranges from approximately 5 to 20 or more minutes. Although frequently touted as a sign of being a good sleeper, a consistently rapid sleep onset is frequently a sign of an accruing sleep debt and may actually be symptomatic of an underlying sleep disorder.

Evaluating Sleep in Fibromyalgia Syndrome Patients

As suggested earlier, fibromyalgia patients commonly struggle with both OSA and insomnia. Insomnia in FMS is characterized by alpha intrusion, the presence of alpha EEG activity in sleep or dream (REM) states. Associated with a drowsy state of wakefulness, alpha activity signals a relaxed but waking state that can compromise both sleep and dream quality. There is little research on the intrusion of alpha into REM, but significant data confirming alpha intrusion into deep or delta sleep among FMS patients, as well as others with chronic fatigue and RA.36 Alpha intrusions may be due to surges of nocturnal pain that do not necessarily result in frank awakenings. Possibly due to the presence of delta waves, FMS patients may be receiving some degree of restorative sleep. Patients with alpha-delta intrusion may complain less of sleepiness and more of fatigue. 8,9 In addition to alpha intrusion, FMS patients have a high incidence of RLS and PLMS. Evaluation of alpha intrusion and the probable comorbitity of OSA and RLS/PLMS requires polysomnography.

Integrative Approaches to Treating Sleep Disorders

OVERVIEW

Because the treatment of sleep concerns is typically complex, challenging, and potentially emotionally-charged, a one-size-fits-all approach (e.g., treating the ICD-9 code) may limit both effectiveness and patient adherence. The integrative treatment of sleep disorders in rheumatology patients must be personalized and comprehensive.

More often than not, patients are called upon to make challenging lifestyle changes to improve their sleep. Turk and Meichenbaum found adherence to treatment recommendations depended strongly on the face validity.[42] The *Noise Reduction Model* described below offers a face-valid rationale and framework for planning and implementing treatment. Ultimately, the lifestyle changes required to improve sleep will likely contribute significantly to overall health and wellbeing.

In contrast to the common primary care practices of simply offering sleep hygiene tips or conventional hypnotics, an integrative approach is comprehensive, and especially sensitive to mind and environmental factors, addressing the entire scope of biomedical, psychological, environmental and even spiritual factors that impact sleep. The treatment of sleep disorders is often an ongoing, systematic program rather than a single intervention, and may require a team approach. In an ideal situation, practitioners will have skills in or access to associates with special skills in counseling and psychotherapy, medical hypnosis, clinical nutrition, and other effective specialty modalities. Although too complex to address here, other total systems of healing such as traditional Chinese medicine, homeopathy, and Ayurveda may be helpful for some patients (see appropriate chapters in this text).

The "Noise Reduction" Approach to Treating Insomnia

Our clinical model for treating insomnia is called the *Noise Reduction Model.* It helps patients to better conceptualize and manage complex factors influencing their sleep.

Sleep involves a reduction, diversion, and dissipation of energy. Factors that interfere with sleep and promote nighttime wakefulness can be thought of as excessive energy or "noise." Noise can occur in biological (body), psychological (mind), and environmental (bed) arenas. Examples of "body noise" include excessive caffeine intake, pain or discomfort, inadequate exercise, and the side effects of certain medications. Examples of "mind noise" include anxiety, stress, troublesome emotions, and obsessive thoughts. Examples of "bed noise" include exposure to too much light at night, an uncomfortable mattress, a warm or noisy bedroom, and not feeling calm and safe in one's bedroom.

"Noise" from various sources is additive, both over the course of a day and over longer periods of time. "Sleepiness" is also cumulative. Periods of poor sleep can drive sleepiness up, resulting in a temporarily increased resistance to noise. Sleeping well is, in large part, about reducing noise and simultaneously maintaining normal levels of nighttime sleepiness. This perspective lends itself to a noise-reduction approach that is readily understood and accepted by patients.

Patients with insomnia frequently report a subjective sense of not feeling sufficiently sleepy during the night. In actuality, it may be that they are simply too "noisy." Commonly used sleep-promoting substances, including alcohol and sedative-hypnotics, do not effectively diminish noise but essentially override it by increasing sleepiness. This is largely a symptom-suppressive strategy that can backfire with habituation, dependence, and other sleep-disruptive side effects. Nonetheless, this "taking something to sleep" approach is not mutually exclusive with the noise reduction, or "letting go of something to sleep" approach.

Reducing Body, Mind and Bed Noise

BODY NOISE REDUCTION

Techniques to reduce "body noise" and thereby improve sleep include nutrition, exercise, dietary supplements, medication management, weight management, and pain management.

Nutrition

Obesity is strongly linked to poor sleep, clearly in obstructive sleep apnea but also via an inflammatory mechanism, or because of the effects of overweight on gastroesophageal reflux, nighttime pain and discomfort, and other medical conditions that interfere with sleep. Thus, a program of weight optimization is an important part of a sleep treatment plan in patients who are overweight.

Nutrition can also play a direct role in reducing inflammation both by limiting elevations in blood glucose and by direct anti-inflammatory effects

Table 9.2. Treatment modalities.

1. BODY a - Clinical nutrition, including dietary supplements b - Sleep medication management: hypnotics and medications with sleep-disruptive side effects c - Botanical medicine: orally-administered herbal preparations and aromatherapy d - Special Concerns: nocturnal pain and discomfort, obstructive sleep apnea (OSA)
2. MIND a - Psychological strategies: counseling, psychotherapy, journaling, spiritual b - Behavioral interventions: stimulus control, bedtime rituals c - Rest practices: hypnotherapy, guided imagery breathing exercises, meditation, tai chi, yoga
3. BED a - Sleep environment management b - Circadian rhythms: light and dark therapies c - Social sleep issues

of an increased ratio of dietary omega-3 to omega-6 fats. A high-glycemic-load diet has been linked to elevated plasma CRP concentrations.[43] The mechanism by which elevated glucose levels increase inflammation is likely mediated by several mechanisms, including the inflammatory consequences of elevated insulin levels, and, possibly, increased production of TNF-alpha.[42]

Heavy meals near bedtime should be avoided, instead using a small nighttime snack to decrease the chances of waking later due to hunger. A recent study indicated that a high-glycemic-index meal eaten one hour prior to bedtime was associated with a significantly longer sleep onset than the same meal eaten 4 hours prior to sleep.[43]

Limiting caffeine, alcohol, nicotine, and other stimulant drug use is often helpful for patients with insomnia and other sleep disorders.

Dietary triggers of gastroesophageal reflux, such as fatty foods, alcohol, caffeine, and peppermint, should be avoided in patients with GERD.

In patients with restless legs syndrome (RLS), a serum ferritin should be checked and iron deficiency with or without anemia corrected, since low iron levels (evidenced by a ferritin less than 50 ng/mL) can worsen symptoms.[45] Although little information is available on the effects of lifestyle on RLS, limiting caffeine, tobacco, and alcohol is often recommended.

Exercise

Improved sleep is among the many benefits of adequate exercise.[46] Exercise can raise core body temperature, which needs to drop to support sleep. Therefore, strenuous exercise should be avoided within 3-6 hours of sleep onset.

A small trial showed improvements in RLS symptoms with an exercise regimen consisting of resistance training and aerobic conditioning.[47]

We generally recommend regular resistance, aerobic, and stretching exercise to all patients with sleep disorders. However, vigorous exercise should be avoided in the several hours prior to bedtime to avoid overstimulation.

Substance Management

Most sleep hygiene recommendations do not adequately address caffeine and alcohol. Simply advising a patient to discontinue using a substance that is detrimental, but otherwise functional in their lives, is unlikely effect behavior change. It is important to be sensitive to the fact that patients taking sedating medications such as analgesics may rely on stimulants like caffeine and nicotine to help them manage the diminished energy side effects of these drugs.

It is helpful to convey that the treatment goal is to restore normal energy levels without the use of these substances.

Caffeine has a half-life that can range from 4 to over 36 hours depending on age and liver detoxification systems. Thus, even coffee in the morning can cause substantial serum caffeine levels at bedtime and disrupt sleep in some people. Dosages of caffeine in many products is much higher than one might think. One popular chain's large-sized drip coffee has over 400 mg of caffeine.

Nicotine is also very stimulating. Data from the 2005 National Sleep Foundation Poll showed that daily smokers were significantly more likely to report RLS symptoms.[48]

Alcohol is the most common ingested substance used as a sleep aid, according to the 2005 Sleep in America Poll.[49] Alcohol may seem to help with reducing sleep onset, but actually suppresses deep sleep and increases awakenings after the brief hypnotic effects wear off. We recommend avoiding alcohol within 4 hours of sleep onset.

Sleep Medication Management

SEDATIVE-HYPNOTIC MEDICATIONS Two-thirds of patients prescribed pharmaceutical sleep medications will use them long-term. This has a profound implication for sleep health, since many of these medications have significant side effects, while not promoting high-quality sleep. Many medications also frequently induce physical and/or psychological dependency, particularly in the benzodiazepine class. Sleep architecture is often disrupted, and despite feeling "knocked out" the patient is often getting inadequate stage III and IV sleep. Excessive morning sedation is common, and even in the absence of overt sedation many of these medications cause significant cognitive dysfunction persisting into the next day. Newer non-benzodiazepine hypnotics such as zolpidem are also known to produce anterograde amnesia and a variety of parasomnias such as nighttime binge eating. Medications prescribed to improve sleep also have not been demonstrated to provide lasting benefit for pain in fibromyalgia patients. Furthermore, sleep EEG studies suggested that neither cyclobenzaprine nor amitryptiline reduces the alpha-delta sleep disorder common in fibromyalgia and RA.[50]

CONVENTIONAL MEDICATIONS WITH SLEEP-RELATED SIDE EFFECTS Medications, including steroids, benzodiazepines, antihypertensives, antidepressants and analgesics, which are commonly prescribed to patients with rheumatologic conditions, may also disrupt sleep.[51–53]

Table 9.3. Effects of Common Medications on Sleep Architecture.

Benzodiazepines	Suppress REM sleep
Classic antiepileptic agents	Suppress REM sleep
SSRI Antidepressants	Stimulating, suppress REM sleep; cause RLS and PLMD
TCA Antidepressants	Some stimulating, suppress REM sleep; cause RLS and PLMD
Opioid Analgesics	Increase wake time, reduce slow wave and REM sleep
NSAID Analgesics	Increase wake time, possibly by inhibiting prostaglandin synthesis
Corticosteroids	Suppress REM sleep
CNS Stimulants, including caffeine	Suppress stage 3-4 and REM sleep
Beta Blockers (lipophilic) e.g. propranolol, pindolol, metoprolol. (effects not seen with hydrophilic agents like atenolol and sotalol)	Increase number of awakenings and wake time, suppress REM sleep, increases daytime sleepiness, may cause nightmares
Alpha Agonist (Clonidine)	Increases wake time, suppresses REM sleep, increases daytime sleepiness
Cigarettes (current use)	Increase sleep latency, decreases total sleep time, decreases slow wave sleep
Caffeine and other methylxanthines	Cause RLS and PLMD
Infliximab	Can worsen OSA(Zamarrón et al. 2004)

Given the sleep-related side effects of common antidepressant medications, we recommend consideration of alternative treatment regimens for depression. James Lake, MD, provides a comprehensive review of such complementary and alternative treatments from an evidence-based perspective.[54]

Botanical Medicine and Dietary Supplements

Botanical remedies and dietary supplements mentioned here are essentially different from hypnotic medications, in that no evidence of habituation or tolerance has been documented. Subjectively, they offer less of a "knockout" and more of a gentle assist.

There are dozens of botanical substances that have been used, some for many centuries, to support sleep and even to directly encourage dreaming. Only some of these products have been tested in clinical trials, and the quality of data is often marginal. Nonetheless, their adverse effect profile is generally quite benign compared to pharmaceutical alternatives.

CAM Sleep Aids

1. Melatonin
2. Valerian
3. Hops
4. 5-hydroxytryptophan (5-HTP)
5. Lemon Balm
6. Lavender

MELATONIN Melatonin is a naturally-occurring substance in most animals, and some other living organisms such as algae. Secreted in humans by the pineal gland, retina, lens, gastrointestinal tract, bone marrow cells,[55] lymphocytes, and epithelial cells, melatonin is synthesized from the amino acid tryptophan via synthesis of serotonin by the enzyme 5-hydroxyindole-O-methyltransferase. Melatonin is also synthesized by certain plants, including rice, and melatonin consumed in plant form has been shown to be orally active in mammals.[56]

Melatonin secretion by the pineal gland is regulated by information about the daily pattern of light and dark received from the retina via the suprachiasmatic nucleus of the hypothalamus, exhibiting a circadian rhythm with nocturnal melatonin plasma concentrations several times higher than daytime concentrations.[57] Production in the gastrointestinal tract and elsewhere may not be regulated by external lighting conditions.

As well as playing a role in initiating and maintaining sleep, higher nighttime melatonin concentrations may have a wide variety of other effects on bodily tissues, including an anti-inflammatory effect, immune-modulating effects, free-radical scavenging effects, and influences on bone growth and osteoporosis. These effects may take place via receptor-mediated and non-receptor-mediated pathways.[58]

The significance of suppressed nocturnal melatonin levels may be significant. Factors contributing to melatonin suppression include exposure to light at night (LAN),[59–61] advancing age,[62] and common medications (e.g. beta blockers,[63] caffeine, alcohol, 8-methoxypsoralen).

Some literature in recent years has suggested a possible proinflammatory effect of high-dose melatonin administered to patients with rheumatoid arthritis, possibly related to its immune-modulating effects.[64,65] These preliminary findings warrant caution when administering supplemental melatonin to patients with RA.

Effects of Drugs on Melatonin Levels. Caffeine, nicotine, alcohol, beta blockers, diuretics, calcium channel blockers, and over-the-counter analgesics suppress endogenous melatonin levels. Tetrahydrocannibinol (THC) has been shown to markedly increase melatonin secretion in humans, but by such a marked amount (more than 400-fold) that it may not be clinically useful.[66]

Melatonin for Insomnia. A recent study suggested that prolonged-release melatonin administered to patients aged 55-80 with insomnia was significantly more effective than placebo in improving sleep latency, sleep quality, and quality of life, similar to that seen with pharmaceutical sleep medications. The medication was administered for 3 weeks at a dosage of 2 mg.[67]

Preparations: Melatonin can be taken in oral or sublingual form (tablet or liquid). Sustained-release preparations are also available as a sublingual spray and tablet. Sublingual forms bypass first-pass liver metabolism, which may result in more reliable serum levels. Sustained-release forms may more accurately simulate the normal physiologic peak of melatonin levels midway through the night.

Dosage: We usually recommend lower bedtime doses of melatonin of approximately 0.25-0.5 mg in adults, based on research showing a more physiologic response at these dosages, without extending elevated melatonin levels into waking hours.[68]

Adverse Effects: Adverse effects including autoimmune hepatitis, confusion, seizures, and headache have been reported, but case reports are few and

Pro-Inflammatory Effect of Melatonin in Rheumatoid Arthritis?

Questions have been raised about a potential proinflammatory effect of melatonin in patients with rheumatoid arthritis. These concerns are based on animal studies, a population study in Northern Europe, and small human studies[64]. The one human study that showed increases of certain inflammatory markers (but not cytokines or symptoms) administered a high dose of melatonin (10mg) nightly for 6 months.[65] So far, no study has demonstrated worsening of disease endpoints or symptoms in humans with melatonin therapy, but some concern is warranted and further study will be important.

dosages were often extremely high. One study involved a literature search for reports of adverse effects over a 35-year time period, finding that adverse effects were uncommon and occurred only with high-dose melatonin regimens (1 to 36 mg).[69] Long-term effects have been not studied, although melatonin has been in widespread use for decades.

VALERIAN ROOT (*VALERIANA OFFICINALIS*) Valerian is a nonaddictive and safe botanical with mild anxiolytic and hypnotic properties, thought to be due to actions on the gamma aminobutyric acid (GABA) system, but, unlike pharmaceutical alternatives, valerian does not impair psychomotor or cognitive performance.[70,71] A recent systematic review concluded that valerian was safe, but did not have significant effects on sleep.[72] However, we have found valerian to be useful in many patients when a standardized extract is used in sufficient dosage, in combination with other botanicals and behavioral measures.

Unlike prescription hypnotic agents, valerian does not have addictive potential, and there is no withdrawal syndrome upon discontinuation. Valerian often does not have immediate effects, and it may take 2-4 weeks of nightly use to see a significant effect.[73] Valerian may thus be more helpful for chronic sleep maintenance insomnia and less helpful for jet lag and short-term treatment of sleep-onset insomnia.

Preparation: Aqueous or ethanolic extract standardized to 0.8% valerenate. High-quality products will have an unpleasant "dirty socks" smell, confirming potency.

Dosage: 800-1200 mg, 30-60 minutes prior to bedtime. Use nightly for 2-4 weeks to assess effectiveness in a patient.

Precautions: Do not use during pregnancy.

HOPS (*HUMULUS LUPULUS*) Hops refers to the clusters of flowers of female plants of species *Humulus lupulus*. More commonly used in the production of beer, extracts of hops have also been traditionally used by practitioners of herbal medicine in Europe and North America for treatment of insomnia, mania, anxiety, toothache, and nerve pain. Menstrual disturbances among female hops-pickers also suggest possible endocrine effects of constituents of the hops plant, such as 8-prenylnaringenin which shows potent in vitro estrogen agonist activity. The German Commission E Monographs list hops as approved for anxiety and sleep disturbance.[74] The sedative effects of hops may have their basis in a sedative volatile alcohol, dimethylvinyl carbinol, which comprises up to 0.15% of the dried leaves.[75]

Small, methodologically limited studies have looked at the combination of valerian and hops for insomnia and suggested helpful effects.[76–78]

Preparation: Ethanolic 5:1 extract

Dosage: ½ to 1 dropper full, 30–60 minutes prior to bedtime

Precautions: Reported cases of dermatitis in hops workers, but no evidence of toxicity in medicinal dosages. Avoid driving or operating machinery when using hops.

5-HYDROXYTRYPTOPHAN (5-HTP) 5-hydroxytryptophan is a precursor in serotonin synthesis, with vitamin B6 as a cofactor. Synthesis occurs in the brain and liver, and 5-HTP crosses the blood-brain barrier. Theoretically, administration of 5-HTP may increase serotonin production and release.

Common uses include as an antidepressant, sleep aid, and in the treatment of chronic pain including fibromyalgia.[79,80]

Preparation: Powder in capsules, or tablets

Dosage: For depression and anxiety, 50-100 mg, one to three times per day. For sleep, 50-100 mg, 30-60 min prior to bedtime.

Precautions: Serotonin syndrome in combination with SSRI medication is a theoretical concern, but studies using 5-HTP to augment traditional antidepressant therapy have not observed any interactions. High doses (over 300 mg per day) may cause nausea.

LEMON BALM (*MELISSA OFFICINALIS*) Lemon balm is a plant native to southern Europe and the Mediterranean which now grows in North America, and is frequently used in cosmetics, furniture polish, and as a flavoring in ice cream and teas. Medicinally, it has been used traditionally as a "calming herb," a mosquito repellant, digestive, and an antiviral (including herpes) and antibacterial agent. Components include eugenol and tannins, as well as terpenes.

In modern herbal medicine, it is often combined with other calming herbs such as valerian, chamomile, and hops to obtain an additive effect, and several small studies have found that these combinations reduce anxiety and promote sleep. A recent double-blind, placebo-controlled study of 18 healthy subjects found that a standardized lemon balm extract in a dose of 600mg increased calmness and alertness more than placebo.[81]

Preparation: Available as dried leaf, tea, and in capsules, extracts, tinctures, and essential oil fractions.

Dosage: In adults, choose from tea (¼-1 teaspoonful of dried leaves in hot water up to 4 times a day); tincture ([1:5], 2-3 mL [40-90 drops] 3 times a day); or capsules (300-600mg dried lemon balm, 3 times a day or as needed).

Precautions: No side effects have been reported. Contraindicated in pregnant or breastfeeding women.

LAVENDER (*LAVANDULA AUGUSTIFOLIA*) Lavender essential oil has been used traditionally by the olfactory route as a mild anxiolytic and sedative. One small study suggested benefit, but had methodological limitations.[82]

Nocturnal Pain

Botanicals with muscle-relaxing properties, such as hops, may be helpful in patients with pain associated with muscular tension.

MANAGING MIND NOISE

Psychological Therapy

CBT FOR INSOMNIA Cognitive behavioral therapies (CBT) are among the most effective strategies available to manage insomnia. Through identifying specific patterns of dysfunctional thoughts and faulty beliefs that are associated with arousal, anxiety, and sleep-inhibiting behaviors, patients not only learn effective strategies, but also have their sense of self-efficacy around sleep restored.

Insomnia patients frequently have unrealistic expectations about sleep. These include the belief that sleep onset should be rapid, that virtually any nocturnal awakening is problematic, and that even a single night of poor sleep will have dire consequences.

Normal sleep onset latency can range from about 5 to 20 minutes. A pattern of rapid sleep onset, e.g., "going out like a light when one's head hits the pillow," is not a sign of being a good sleeper. It is more likely an indication of the presence of an excessive sleep load at bedtime, and possibly suggestive of a sleep disorder.

Nocturnal awakenings are not necessarily symptomatic of sleep concerns. Healthy sleepers can experience momentary awakenings between sleep cycles and to use the restroom. Recent historical evidence suggests that an extended period of middle-of-the-night awakening was common prior to the industrial revolution. The belief that any wakefulness during sleep is problematic can trigger anxiety-provoking judgments that, in turn, extend that wakefulness and result in a vicious cycle. Aware of the potentially dire health consequences of chronically poor sleep, many insomniacs will worry excessively about the effects of a single bad night, dialing up their anxiety and further compromising their sleep.

Another common belief held by insomniacs is that they must somehow control sleep. Although we can control our approach to sleep, we have no control over sleep itself. Any attempt to impose control over what is not controllable will inevitably increase anxiety.

Faulty beliefs about sleep damage sleep with anxiety. CBT approaches, which require specialized training, teach patients to identify and manage faulty beliefs and associated dysfunctional thoughts, thereby diminishing anxiety and allowing sleep to come. We believe that CBT approaches provide a foundation for understanding what many might view as a spiritual component of sleep.

The common notion of "going to sleep" implies a sense of intention, activity and even control. There is a delicate balance necessary between intention and effort, on the one hand, and receptivity and surrender on the other. Allowing for the latter is related to the spiritual component of sleep. It calls for a letting-go, or a psychological posture of surrender. What makes this spiritual is that such a practice presupposes some kind of faith in something beyond the sense of self that is being "let go of." It is not surprising to find a preponderance of prayer and ritual centered around night and sleep in world spiritual traditions.

Behavioral Interventions

SLEEP HYGIENE Sleep hygiene recommendations are designed break the association of the bed and bedtime with wakefulness, and strengthen their association with drowsiness and sleep. These include:

Table 9.4. Stimulus Control Measures.

1. Go to bed only when feeling sleepy.
2. Use the bed only for sleep and sexual activity.
3. If can't sleep, get out of bed and do relaxing activity until drowsy, then return to bed.
4. Repeat Step 3 as often as is necessary.
5. Get up at same time every day even if haven't slept well.
6. Don't nap during day until nighttime sleep improves.

Adapted from *No More Sleepless Nights, Hauri, P. & Linde, S., 1996*

Bedtime Rituals and Rest Practices Bedtime rituals refer to a set of personalized behaviors that can decrease sleep-related anxiety and promote rest, relaxation, and the natural onset of sleepiness at bedtime. In lieu of common evening activities that can result in overarousal, bedtime rituals might include a warm bath, a rest practice (described below), self-caring behaviors, and journaling. Journaling may be particularly helpful in processing unresolved emotions prior to getting into bed.

Actively engaging in pre-sleep practices that produce a relaxation response has been shown to help promote sleep onset and sleep maintenance.[37] We use the term *rest practices* to refer to psychological and behavioral exercises that help reduce mind noise, and probably body and bed noise as well.

Rest practices can readily bring one into an alpha EEG state that is similar to Stage 1, or transitional, sleep. Such practice sensitizes one to that experience, essentially teaching the coordinates of that psychological place. This state of rest is an essential bridge to sleep

Examples of rest practices include hypnotherapy, guided imagery, meditation, neurofeedback, muscular relaxation, heart rate variability techniques, Tai Chi, and gentle yoga or breathing exercises. Patients should be encouraged to explore these and choose a practice that suits them.

Because breathing exercises are easy to learn and portable, they lend themselves well to inclusion in bedtime rituals. Reversing the usual pattern of respiration to a mode where the exhalation is longer than the inhalation, the practice described below (4-7-8 Breathing Technique) reduces sympathetic "fight or flight" signals and increases parasympathetic "rest and digest" signals. Activation of the parasympathetic nervous system via stimulation of the vagus nerve has been shown to reduce inflammation and prevent the release of TNF-alpha and IL-6 in vitro, and TNF-alpha in vivo, in response to endotoxin exposure.[83] This result suggests one possible mechanism by which vagal-stimulating breathing techniques might reduce inflammation. These safe and

4-7-8 Breathing Technique

- **Count to four (1, 2, 3, 4) as you inhale deeply through your nose, with closed mouth.**
- **Hold your breath to the count of seven (1, 2, 3, 4, 5, 6, 7)**
- **Then exhale slowly through pursed lips to the count of eight (1, 2, 3, 4, 5, 6, 7, 8) with an audible "whoosh" sound, feeling your ribs contract inward at the end.**
- **Repeat this exercise 4 times, twice daily. You can also use it when you are feeling stressed or worried.**

inexpensive breathing techniques may offer an attractive addition or alternative to more costly and toxic immune-suppressant medications.

REDUCING BED NOISE: THE SLEEP ENVIRONMENT

The need to minimize body and mind noise as well as support the psychological surrender into sleep requires an optimal sleep environment. If lifestyle is a key factor in sleep, then the sleep environment is the structure that both supports and reveals sleep lifestyle. In years past, when physicians routinely made house calls and treated patients in their bedrooms, they had direct, invaluable insight into the sleep environment.

The physical sleep environment should be cool, quiet, comfortable, and otherwise conducive to sleep. Data suggests that a temperature of about 68 degrees may be ideal because it supports a normal drop in body temperature through the night. A source of white noise can be effective in drowning out audible noise that can be a problem in urban areas. Beyond obvious considerations, a comfortable sleep surface or mattress is a matter of personal taste. Patients should be advised to position their clocks so that they cannot readily check the time if sleepless.

The circadian sleep environment refers to the internal pacemaker, which is considered disrupted when subjective time becomes desynchronized with objective time. The timing and intensity of first morning light exposure essentially signals the brain that it is a new day. Rising at about the same time every day to significant light exposure can help regulate circadian rhythms. Likewise, as suggested earlier, exposure to evening dim light triggers the production and release of melatonin, which in turn supports sleep. Dusk simulation refers to a nightly practice of considerably dimming home lighting for one to three hours prior to bed. Exposure to excessive light at night (LAN) not only delays melatonin onset, but also encourages excessive activity. For this reason, bedtime rituals are best experienced with dusk simulation.

The social sleep environment, or "sleeping together" needs to be liberated from its limited sexual connotations. Beyond the obvious bed partnership associated with primary relationships, people may sleep together as families, roommates, in dormitories or barracks, in hostels and on airplanes. The social sleep environment may be a source of "noise" if there is a history or a current concern about psychological or physical safety. Childhood trauma around excessive punishment, neglect, and abuse is frequently associated with the sleep environment. Twenty-four percent of US couples reportedly sleep apart for reasons ranging from loud snoring to marital discord. Social sleep-environment noise may also be associated with current relationship difficulties, the loss of a loved

To Nap or Not To Nap? Or "When to sleep"

Napping less than 30 minutes during the day may improve wakefulness and promote cognitive performance. However, frequent or long naps may be associated with increased morbidity and mortality, especially in the elderly.[84] Further research is needed to determine causality.

one, and conflicting or desynchronized sleep-wake schedules. Sensitizing patients to the role of social factors in sleep may help them identify and correct problems in this arena.

Summary

The proper quantity and quality of sleep is essential for proper physical, psychological, and cognitive function. In addition, there is strong evidence that sleep is essential for proper immune function. In many rheumatological conditions, sleep is disrupted due to pain or anxiety. Addressing these concerns with conventional pharmacotherapy can produce unwanted adverse effects, including dependence, disrupted REM sleep, or even daytime somnolence. Therapeutic approaches to sleep restoration is critical in the care of the patient with a rheumatological condition, and must address obstacles—both physical and psychological.

REFERENCES

1. National Sleep Foundation. (2000) *Omnibus Sleep in America Poll.* Washington, DC: National Sleep Foundation; 2000.
2. Jordan JM, Bernard SL, Callahan LF, Kincade JE, Konrad TR, DeFriese GH. Self-reported arthritis-related disruptions in sleep and daily life and the use of medical, complementary, and self-care strategies for arthritis: the National Survey of Self-care and Aging. *Arch Fam Med.* 2000;9(2):143–149.
3. Bonnet MH, Arand DL. Hyperarousal and insomnia. *Sleep Med Rev.* 1997;1(2): 97–108.
4. Bonnet MH, Arand DL. 24-Hour metabolic rate in insomniacs and matched normal sleepers. *Sleep.* 1995;18(7):581–588.
5. Irwin M, Clark C, Kennedy B, Christian Gillin J, Ziegler M. Nocturnal catecholamines and immune function in insomniacs, depressed patients, and control subjects. *Brain Behav Immun.* 2003;17(5):365–372.

6. Vgontzas AN, Papanicolaou DA, Bixler EO, Lotsikas A, Zachman K, Kales A, Prolo P, Wong ML, Licinio J, Gold PW, Hermida RC, Mastorakos G, Chrousos GP. Circadian interleukin-6 secretion and quantity and depth of sleep. *The Journal of clinical endocrinology and metabolism*. 1999;84(8):2603-7.
7. Vgontzas AN, Zoumakis E, Bixler EO, et al. Adverse effects of modest sleep restriction on sleepiness, performance, and inflammatory cytokines. *J Clin Endocrinol Metab*. 2004;89:2119–26.
8. Ferentinos PP, Kontaxakis VP, Havaki-Kontaxaki BJ, Paplos KG, Soldatos CR. The measurement of fatigue in depression. *Psychopathology*. 2007;40(2):133–134.
9. Belza BL. Comparison of self-reported fatigue in rheumatoid arthritis and controls. *J Rheumatol*. 1995;22(4):639–643.
10. Belza BL, Henke CJ, Yelin EH, Epstein WV, Gilliss CL. Correlates of fatigue in older adults with rheumatoid arthritis. *Nurs Res*. 1993;42(2):93–99.
11. Wolfe F, Hawley DJ, Wilson K. The prevalence and meaning of fatigue in rheumatic disease. *J Rheumatol*. 1996;23(8):1407–1417.
12. Hewlett S, Cockshott Z, Byron M, et. al. Patients' perceptions of fatigue in rheumatoid arthritis: overwhelming, uncontrollable, ignored. *Arthritis Rheum*. 2005;53(5):697–702.
13. Pollard LC, Choy EH, Gonzalez J, Khoshaba B, Scott DL. Fatigue in rheumatoid arthritis reflects pain, not disease activity. *Rheumatology*. 2006;45(7):885–889.
14. Huyser BA, Parker JC, Thoreson R, Smarr KL, Johnson JC, Hoffman R. Predictors of subjective fatigue among individuals with rheumatoid arthritis. *Arthritis Rheum*. 1998;41(12):2230–2237.
15. Jump RL, Fifield J, Tennen H, Reisine S, Giuliano AJ. History of affective disorder and the experience of fatigue in rheumatoid arthritis. *Arthritis Rheum*. 2004;51(2):239–245.
16. Riemsma RP, Rasker JJ, Taal E, Griep EN, Wouters JM, Wiegman O. Fatigue in rheumatoid arthritis: the role of self-efficacy and problematic social support. *Br J Rheumatol*. 1998;37(10):1042–1046.
17. Gonzalez-Ortiz M, Martinez-Abundis E. Impact of sleep deprivation on insulin secretion, insulin sensitivity, and other hormonal regulations. *Metab Syndr Relat Disord*. 2005;3(1):3–7.
18. Knutson KL, Van Cauter E. Associations between sleep loss and increased risk of obesity and diabetes. *Ann N Y Acad Sci*. 2008;1129:287–304.
19. Nakajima H, Kaneita Y, Yokoyama E, et al. Association between sleep duration and hemoglobin A1c level. *Sleep Med*. 2008;9(7):745–752.
20. Chaput JP, Despres JP, Bouchard C, Tremblay A. Association of sleep duration with type 2 diabetes and impaired glucose tolerance. *Diabetologia*. 2007;50(11): 2298–2304.
21. Gottlieb DJ, Punjabi NM, Newman AB, et al. Association of sleep time with diabetes mellitus and impaired glucose tolerance. *Arch Intern Med*. 2005;165(8):863–867.
22. Appels A, Bär FW, Bär J, Bruggeman C, de Baets M. Inflammation, depressive symptomtology, and coronary artery disease. *Psychosom Med*. 2000;62(5):601–605.

23. Eaker ED, Pinsky J, Castelli WP. Myocardial infarction and coronary death among women: psychosocial predictors from a 20-year follow-up of women in the Framingham Study. *Am J Epidemiol.* 1992;135(8):854–864.
24. Kokturk O, Ciftci TU, Mollarecep E, Ciftci B. Elevated C-reactive protein levels and increased cardiovascular risk in patients with obstructive sleep apnea syndrome. *Int Heart J.* 2005;46(5):801–809.
25. Irwin MR, Wang M, Campomayor CO, Collado-Hidalgo A, Cole S. Sleep deprivation and activation of morning levels of cellular and genomic markers of inflammation. *Arch Intern Med.* 2006;166(16):1756–1762.
26. Born J, Lange T, Hansen K, Molle M, Fehm HL. Effects of sleep and circadian rhythm on human circulating immune cells. *J Immunol.* 1997;158(9):4454–4464.
27. Shearer WT. Consequences of contamination of the spacecraft environment: immunologic consequences. *Gravit Space Biol Bull.* 2001 Jun;14(2):7-14.
28. Kapsimalis F, Basta M, Varouchakis G, Gourgoulianis K, Vgontzas A, Kryger M. Cytokines and pathological sleep. *Sleep Med.* 2008;9(6):603–614.
29. Opp MR. Cytokines and sleep. *Sleep Med Rev.* 2005;9(5):355–364.
30. Burgos I, Richter L, Klein T, et al. Increased nocturnal interleukin-6 excretion in patients with primary insomnia: a pilot study. *Brain Behav Immun.* 2006;20(3): 246–253.
31. Meier-Ewert HK, Ridker PM, Rifai N, Regan MM, Price NJ, Dinges DF, Mullington JM. Effect of sleep loss on C-reactive protein, an inflammatory marker of cardiovascular risk. *J Am Coll Cardiol.* 2004 Feb 18;43(4):678-83.
32. Hogan D, Morrow JD, Smith EM, Opp MR. Interleukin-6 alters sleep of rats. *J Neuroimmunol.* 2003;137(1-2):59–66.
33. Zamarrón C, Maceiras F, Mera A, Gómez-Reino JJ. Effect of the first infliximab infusion on sleep and alertness in patients with active rheumatoid arthritis. *Ann Rheum Dis.* 2004;63(1):88–90.
34. Abad VC, Sarinas PS, Guilleminault C. Sleep and rheumatologic disorders. *Sleep Med Rev.* 2008;12(3):211–228.
35. Harding SM. Sleep in fibromyalgia patients: subjective and objective findings. *Am J Med Sci.* 1998;315(6):367–376.
36. Roizenblatt S, Moldofsky H, Benedito-Silva AA, Tufik S. Alpha sleep characteristics in fibromyalgia. *Arthritis Rheum.* 2001;44(1):222–230.
37. Morin AK, Jarvis CI, Lynch AM. Therapeutic options for sleep-maintenance and sleep-onset insomnia. *Pharmacotherapy.* 2007;27(1):89–110.
38. Moldofsky H, Scarisbrick P. Induction of neurasthenic musculoskeletal pain syndrome by selective sleep stage deprivation. *Psychosom Med.* 1976;38(1):35–44.
39. Drewes AM, Nielsen KD, Arendt-Nielsen L, Birket-Smith L, Hansen LM. The effect of cutaneous and deep pain on the electroencephalogram during sleep–an experimental study. *Sleep.* 1997;20(8):632–640.
40. Lentz MJ, Landis CA, Rothermel J, Shaver JL. Effects of selective slow wave sleep disruption on musculoskeletal pain and fatigue in middle aged women. *J Rheumatol.* 1999;26(7):1586–1592.

41. Hewlett S, M. Hehir M, Kirwan JR. Measuring fatigue in rheumatoid arthritis: A systematic review of scales in use. *Arthritis Rheum.* 2007;57(3):429–439.
42. Turk DC, Meichenbaum, D, Genest, M. (1983). Pain and behavioral medicine: A cognitive-behavioral perspective. New York: Guilford Press.
43. Liu S, Manson JE, Buring JE, Stampfer MJ, Willett WC, Ridker PM. Relation between a diet with a high glycemic load and plasma concentrations of high-sensitivity C-reactive protein in middle-aged women. *Am J Clin Nutr.* 2002 Mar;75(3):492–8.
44. Afaghi A, O'Connor H, Chow CM. High-glycemic-index carbohydrate meals shorten sleep onset. *Am J Clin Nutr.* 2007;85(2):426–430.
45. Moldofsky H. Management of sleep disorders in fibromyalgia. *Rheum Dis Clin North Am.* 2002;28(2):353–365.
46. King AC, Pruitt LA, Woo S, et al. Effects of moderate-intensity exercise on polysomnographic and subjective sleep quality in older adults with mild to moderate sleep complaints. *J Gerontol A Biol Sci Med Sci.* 2008;63(9):997–1004.
47. Aukerman MM, Aukerman D, Bayard M, Tudiver F, Thorp L, Bailey B. Exercise and restless legs syndrome: a randomized controlled trial. *J Am Board Fam Med.* 2006;19(5):487–493.
48. Phillips B, Hening W, Britz P, Mannino D. Prevalence and correlates of restless legs syndrome: results from the 2005 National Sleep Foundation Poll. *Chest.* 2006;129(1):76–80.
49. National Sleep Foundation. Sleep in America Poll 2005. Washington, DC: National Sleep Foundation; 2005. http://www.sleepfoundation.org/article/sleep-america-polls/2005-adult-sleep-habits-and-styles. Accessed on 10/10/09
50. Carette S, Oakson G, Guimont C, Steriade M. Sleep electroencephalography and the clinical response to amitriptyline in patients with fibromyalgia. Arthritis Rheum. 1995 Sep;38(9):1211–7.
51. Schweitzer, PK. Drugs that disturb sleep and wakefulness. In Principles and practice of sleep medicine. 4th edition. Edited by: Kryger MH, Roth T, Dement WC. New York: Elesevier Saunders; 2005:499–518.
52. Dimsdale JE, Norman D, DeJardin D, Wallace MS. The effect of opioids on sleep architecture. *J Clin Sleep Med.* 2007 Feb 15;3(1):33–6.
53. Gillin JC, Jacobs LS, Fram DH, Snyder F. Acute effect of a glucocorticoid on normal human sleep. *Nature.* 1972 Jun 16;237(5355):398–9.
54. Lake J. Textbook of Integrative Mental Health Care.1st edition. Thieme; 2006.
55. Conti A, Conconi S, Hertens E, Skwarlo-Sonta K, Markowska M, Maestroni JM. Evidence for melatonin synthesis in mouse and human bone marrow cells. *J Pineal Res.* 2000;28(4):193–202.
56. Hattori A, Migitaka H, Iigo M, et al. Identification of melatonin in plants and its effects on plasma melatonin levels and binding to melatonin receptors in vertebrates. *Biochem mol boil Int.* 1995;35(3):627–634.
57. Lynch HJ, Wurtman RJ, Moskowitz MA, Archer MC, Ho MH. Daily rhythm in human urinary melatonin. *Science.* 1975;187(4172):169–171.
58. Reiter RJ, Tan DX, Manchester LC, Pilar Terron M, Flores LJ, Koppisepi S. Medical implications of melatonin: receptor-mediated and receptor-independent actions. *Adv Med Sci.* 2007;52:11–28.

59. Reiter RJ, Gultekin F, Manchester LC, Tan DX. Light pollution, melatonin suppression and cancer growth. *J Pineal Res.* 2006;40(4):357–358.
60. Evans JA, Elliott JA, Gorman MR. Circadian effects of light no brighter than moonlight. *J Biol Rhythms.* 2007;22(4):356–367.
61. Blask DE, Dauchy RT, Sauer LA, Krause JA, Brainard GC. Light during darkness, melatonin suppression and cancer progression. *Neuro Endocrinol Lett.* 2002; 23(suppl 2):52–6.
62. Mahlberg R, Tilmann A, Salewski L, Kunz D. Normative data on the daily profile of urinary 6-sulfatoxymelatonin in healthy subjects between the ages of 20 and 84. *Psychoneuroendocrinology.* 2006;31(5):634–641.
63. Brismar K, Hylander B, Eliasson K, Rossner S, Wetterberg L. Melatonin secretion related to side-effects of beta-blockers from the central nervous system. *Acta Med Scand.* 1988;223(6):525–530.
64. Cutolo M, Maestroni GJM. The melatonin-cytokine connection in rheumatoid arthritis. *Ann Rheum Dis.* 2005;64(8):1109–1111.
65. Forrest CM, Mackay GM, Stoy N, Stone TW, Darlington LG. Inflammatory status and kynurenine metabolism in rheumatoid arthritis treated with melatonin. *Br J Clin Pharm.* 2007;64(4):517–526.
66. Lissoni, P., Resentini, M., and Fraschini, F. “Effects of Tetrahydrocannabinol on Melatonin Secretion in Man.” Hormone and Metabolic Research 1986; 77–78.
67. Wade AG, Ford I, Crawford G, et al. Efficacy of prolonged release melatonin in insomnia patients aged 55-80 years: quality of sleep and next-day alertness outcomes. *Curr Med Res Opin.* 2007;23(10):2597–2605.
68. Zhdanova IV, Wurtman RJ, Regan MM, Taylor JA, Shi JP, Leclair OU. Melatonin treatment for age-related insomnia. *J Clin Endocrinol Metab.* 2001 Oct;86(10): 4727–30.
69. Morera AL, Henry M, de La Varga M. Safety in melatonin use Actas Esp Psiquiatr. 2001 Sep-Oct;29(5):334–7.
70. Gutierrez S, Ang-Lee MK, Walker DJ, Zacny JP. Assessing subjective and psychomotor effects of the herbal medication valerian in healthy volunteers. *Pharmacol Biochem Behav.* 2004;78(1):57–64.
71. Hallam KT, Olver JS, McGrath C, Norman TR. Comparative cognitive and psychomotor effects of single doses of Valeriana officianalis and triazolam in healthy volunteers. *Hum Psychopharmacol.* 2003;18(8):619–625.
72. Taibi DM, Landis CA, Petry H, Vitiello MV. A systematic review of valerian as a sleep aid: safe but not effective. *Sleep Med Rev.* 2007;11(3):209–230.
73. Wheatley D. Medicinal plants for insomnia: a review of their pharmacology, efficacy and tolerability. *J Psychopharmacol.* 2005;19(4):414–421.
74. The Complete German Commission E Monographs, Therapeutic Guide to Herbal Medicines, 1st ed. 1998, Integrative Medicine Communications, pub; Bk&CD-Rom edition, 1999.
75. Small E, Catling PM. Canadian Medicinal Crops. National Research Council of Canada Monograph Publishing Program, NRC Research Press; 1999:74–80.
76. Koetter U, Schrader E, Käufeler R, Brattström A. A randomized, double blind, placebo-controlled, prospective clinical study to demonstrate clinical efficacy of

a fixed valerian hops extract combination (Ze 91019) in patients suffering from non-organic sleep disorder. *Phytother Res*. 2007;21(9):847–851.

77. Morin CM, Koetter U, Bastien C, Ware JC, Wooten V. Valerian-hops combination and diphenhydramine for treating insomnia: a randomized placebo-controlled clinical trial. *Sleep*. 2005;28(11):1465–1471.
78. Fussel A, Wolf A, Brattstrom A. Effect of a fixed valerian-Hop extract combination (Ze 91019) on sleep polygraphy in patients with non-organic insomnia: a pilot study. *Eur J Med Res*. 2000;5(9):385–390.
79. 516 Bruni, O. 2004.
80. 517 Sarzi Puttini, P. 1992.
81. Kennedy DO, Little W, Scholey AB. Attenuation of laboratory-induced stress in humans after acute administration of Melissa officinalis (Lemon Balm). *Psychosom Med*. 2004 Jul-Aug;66(4):607–13.
82. Lewith GT, Godfrey AD, Prescott P. A single-blinded, randomized pilot study evaluating the aroma of Lavandula augustifolia as a treatment for mild insomnia. *J Altern Complement Med*. 2005 Aug;11(4):631–7.
83. Borovikova LV, Ivanova S, Zhang M, Yang H, Botchkina GI, Watkins LR, Wang H, Abumrad N, Eaton JW, Tracey KJ. Vagus nerve stimulation attenuates the systemic inflammatory response to endotoxin. *Nature*. 2000 May 25;405(6785):458–62.
84. Dhand R, Sohal H. 2006, Good sleep, bad sleep! The role of daytime naps in healthy adults. *Curr Opin Pulm Med*. 2006;12(6):379–382.

10

Acupuncture and Traditional Chinese Medicine (TCM) in Arthritis

PETER WHITE, PhD, BSc, MCSP AND
GEORGE LEWITH, MD, FRCP, MRCGP

KEY CONCEPTS

- Acupuncture is increasing in popularity and is becoming much more "mainstream" in terms of its acceptability.
- When compared to many other interventions such as pharmacology, acupuncture is considered to be an extremely safe treatment for pain.
- Traditional Chinese theory underpinning acupuncture centers around the flow of energy in the body. Western scientific theory suggests that acupuncture works through neural mechanisms.
- There is an increasing body of evidence which suggests that acupuncture has efficacy for the treatment of painful conditions.

■

Introduction

Over the past 15 years, there has been a huge increase in the popularity and use of Complementary and Alternative Medicine (CAM).[1,2] Ernst and White[3] estimated that £1.6 billion is spent on CAM annually within the UK. It may, however, be used as a last resort by many patients,[4] either as a result of dissatisfaction with routine care (i.e., the failure of conventional medicine to deliver a satisfactory outcome for many patients with chronic conditions), or because of the many adverse effects associated with conventional medicines.[5,6]

Acupuncture is one of the most popular and widely used CAM interventions for pain—especially for patients suffering from osteoarthritis (OA).[3,7] It has been reported that 71% of visits to CAM practitioners in the UK are due to musculoskeletal problems.[8] More than 600,000 adults in the UK, and 1 million people in the US use acupuncture annually for the relief of pain.[9]

Traditional Chinese Medicine (TCM)

The TCM theories that underpin acupuncture revolve around the concepts of balance and the flow of energy within the body. It is thought that illness is the result of an imbalance in qi (pronounced *chee*) or "vital energy."[10] By placing needles into specific points, and influencing the body's energy, the acupuncturist can balance the qi, thus creating equilibrium and enabling the body to heal itself.

Chinese medicine in its traditional form is more than simply a method to treat illness; it is a philosophy in itself, and is concerned with the balance not only of the forces within man, but of man within nature. It has its own well-developed system of anatomy and physiology. Illnesses and symptoms are simply outward manifestations of imbalance. Great emphasis is therefore placed upon tracing and treating the cause of the imbalance, rather than the symptoms, in order to maintain health.

By 200 BC, some 1700 years before the West adopted this view, the Chinese had hypothesized the circulation of the blood through two types of vessels, arteries and veins, as well as qi. It is thought that qi is in fact the "life force" and that the presence of qi is what differentiates living beings from inanimate objects.

> "It is the cohesion of our mind, body and spirit and is integrated into the myriad aspects of every being."[11]

The qi in the body is thought to circulate through discrete pathways called meridians. These meridians have superficial "access points" on the body where the practitioner can modulate qi. These access points are known as acupuncture points, and are well defined on the body.[12] Stimulation of the points by pressure, heat, or wounding can have an influence on the meridian, as well as on the qi circulating within it. This could then affect the injured part of the body.[13]

There are many external factors that may influence qi. Various organs of the body play an important role in modulating qi. These include the liver, gall bladder, and spleen. In addition, emotional states may impact the distribution and intensity of qi. Finally, the climate, time of year, time of day, the phases of the moon, and the presence and balance of various elements (the 5-element theory) all have a role to play in maintaining equilibrium.[14,13]

Diagnosis using TCM is holistic and includes a combination of observation of the various physical characteristics of the patient and their demeanor.[13] Some aspects of TCM diagnosis include: the shape, color, moisture, and coating of the tongue; the patient's manner and tone of voice;[10] an evaluation of various bodily functions; and the quality and intensity of the radial pulse, which is thought to yield a great deal of information about the organs and meridians within the body.

The common TCM syndromes that relate to arthritis are called "bi" syndromes. These may be related to many different TCM "pathogens," particularly "damp" and "cold." Within a TCM approach there are particular acupuncture points that dispel damp, and specific techniques designed to treat cold, such as moxibustion (heat) and cupping (vacuum).[15]

Western Acupuncture

The introduction of acupuncture to the Western world has led to the development of the field of medical acupuncture, which is widely taught in the US. The Western practitioner aims to integrate a knowledge of anatomy, physiology, and pathology with a more basic understanding of acupuncture, to arrive at a more prescriptive "scientific" point prescription. The actual points used for a particular painful condition may be the same as those used within TCM, but the route to choosing them is entirely different. The distinction between TCM and "Westernized" acupuncture is important, however, as Western acupuncture tends to be much more formulaic.[16] Those using a Westernized form of acupuncture may still have many options to treating one condition. These may be points on meridians that pass over or near the painful area, as well as associated points further along the meridian. Added to this are the options of using trigger, or *Ah shi,* points (points that are painful on palpation), which may not coincide with a recognized acupuncture point.

Typical Treatment

Treatment of conditions with acupuncture must be viewed as a fluid modality—that is, responsive to the changing condition of the patient. Acupuncture points used for treatment may vary from session to session depending on the response of the patient. This is because there may be several possible point prescriptions for the same condition. This explains the substantial variability and flexibility for the treatment options, all of which can be individualized. Should a treatment fail to resolve the problem, the combination of points may therefore be changed.

In a Westernized treatment for pain, typically anything between three to ten needles may be used, although evidence would suggest that 6 would be the minimum.[17] Some of these would be placed in close proximity to the painful area, and others might be on associated meridians distal to the problem. Reactions of patients during acupuncture treatment can vary. The needle is inserted fairly quickly into the chosen point, and this may or may not cause mild discomfort as the needle pierces the skin. Depth of penetration will vary according to the anatomical area being needled (amount of soft tissue and size of patient), as well as the specific location of the point itself—not all points are "needled" at the same depth.

Point location is most commonly determined via palpation and a good working knowledge of surface anatomy. Once the needle has been inserted, the patient should feel some sensation. This is most typically described as a deep ache, although feelings of warmth, heaviness, tingling or even numbness have been described. This sensation is called *deqi* (pronounced *der-chee*) and it is thought to be important in the treatment of pain.[18,19] The intensity of this sensation can also vary from person to person, with some feeling little more than mild sensation and others describing intense and sometimes quite uncomfortable feelings. The needles are typically left in place for 10-20 minutes, although some practitioners may simply insert and immediately withdraw the needle.[20]

Efficacy

While there is little doubt that for many painful conditions, acupuncture is an effective and safe treatment (see below), the question of efficacy remains debatable. The reason for this is multifaceted, but might in part be due to the poor quality of early trials that have thus far made up the evidence base for acupuncture effectiveness.

Patel et al[21] conducted a meta-analysis for several chronic pain conditions, but divided this into subsections for different sites (e.g., head and neck). When results were pooled, it appeared as though the only subgroups that obtained significance were the trials for head and neck pain, although Patel commented that the blinding was poor in all of these trials. Patel noted that patients who received strict "formula type" acupuncture tended to do less well than those who were treated with a more flexible approach. This could, of course, be a reflection of the need to maintain therapeutic flexibility and adequate treatment when using acupuncture. It was also noted that the more rigorous the blinding was in a trial, the less significant the difference between real treatment and control, an observation also suggested by ter Riet[22] and Ernst.[23] Patel concluded that on the whole, "results favorable to acupuncture were obtained significantly more than chance alone would allow."

Another meta-analysis, by ter Riet et al,[22] also examined acupuncture and chronic pain. Two of the main criticisms that the authors state are the very low case numbers used in the trials, and the poor quality of all the trials reviewed. It was, therefore, felt that no definitive conclusions as to effectiveness could be drawn, but that efficacy remained doubtful. Ter Riet et al, however, failed to differentiate between different sites of pain, despite the fact that pain from several areas had been included in the analysis. This implied that all pain reacts to acupuncture in the same way, regardless of location; this may not be the case. Also, no account was taken of the adequacy of the treatment given in the reviewed trials.[23] Interestingly, Kjellman et al[24] reviewed the literature for all randomized trials of neck pain, covering a wide range of interventions including acupuncture and conventional therapies. They found that again, quality was generally very low for all trials. This suggests that many trials are poorly executed, not just those evaluating acupuncture. They also noted that the more recent trials tended to be of better quality than the older ones, and perhaps this marks a change for the better in the rigor of clinical trials.

In a systematic review of acupuncture for the treatment of OA, 13 appropriate studies were found.[7] The overall conclusion of this was that there was no uniform picture as to the efficacy of acupuncture. In view of the high number of methodological flaws displayed in these early trials, however, it is not surprising that a systematic review would fail to provide conclusive answers.

Smith et al[25] also carried out a systematic review, drawing on studies that used acupuncture for the treatment of back and neck pain. They included randomized trials that used acupuncture needling or laser stimulation, and an inert control. They did not exclude trials that were not blinded. Both chronic and acute conditions were included, and 13 trials met their inclusion criteria. The authors concluded that acupuncture was no more effective than placebo, and that there was an inverse relationship between the quality of the trial and its findings; i.e., better-quality trials were more likely to produce a negative result for acupuncture. Once again, however, homogeneity was not maintained in this systematic review, either in terms of the condition being examined or the type of control used. Nor was there any consideration for the type or adequacy of treatment being used; e.g., laser vs. needling, formulaic vs. flexible treatment, multiple vs. single sessions.

Ezzo et al[17] conducted a systematic review to examine the effectiveness of acupuncture for various painful conditions. Studies were included if they were randomized, had a control group, used needles, had a measurement of pain relief, and dealt with chronic pain. The authors also examined specific aspects of acupuncture treatment (i.e., the number of treatment sessions and the number of needles needed to be used in order to provide an adequate treatment). To aid homogeneity, they divided the studies depending on the type of control that was used. After reviewing the 51 appropriate trials, they found that results were inconsistent, and that no firm conclusions could be drawn as to the efficacy of acupuncture. This was largely attributed to the poor quality of the trials. They did, however, conclude that treatments consisting of at least six sessions and using at least six needles per session were consistently associated with a positive result. They suggested that this might be due to a cumulative effect of treatment.

A systematic review of knee pain trials evaluated by the same researcher (7 trials, 393 patients) concluded that acupuncture was more effective than "sham" acupuncture in terms of pain relief, although all of the included trials were small.[26]

A Cochrane review of the literature evaluating the effectiveness of acupuncture in the treatment of tennis elbow[27] identified only 4 trials that met their criteria, all of which were underpowered and of poor rigor. It was concluded that acupuncture might have a short-term benefit when treating this condition, but owing to the small number of trials included, firm conclusions could not be made.

Three systematic reviews of acupuncture for low back pain were conducted by Ernst and White, Furlan, et al, and Manheimer, et al.[28–30] These involved 12, 35 and 33 randomized controlled trials, respectively. Ernst concluded that the results suggested that acupuncture was an effective treatment for back pain, but because of the large variation in trial methodology, firm conclusions were difficult. Furlan et al concluded that for chronic back pain, acupuncture is more effective for pain relief and functional improvement than either no treatment or sham treatment. Average reductions in pain were on the order of 32% for acupuncture and 23% for sham interventions. They concluded that it would be a useful adjunct to other conventional treatments, but also pointed out that the quality of trials included in the review was very low, and so, as with the Ernst review, clear recommendations could not be made. The conclusions by Manheimer et al were similar, insomuch as they felt that acupuncture was effective at reducing chronic back pain, but that it was not more effective than other therapies. They also stated that there was great heterogeneity between trials.

Thus, many early trials were underpowered, nonrandomized, unblinded, employed a substandard treatment regime, and used controls of unknown physiological effect. Furthermore, these poor trials were included in systematic reviews, thus making conclusions difficult.[31] More recently, however, the quality of research has changed and researchers are much more cognizant of the methodological issues involved. This has recently led to more rigorous and reliable data, although the problem remains that the absence of a standardized placebo control for acupuncture makes interpretation of efficacy trials difficult to perform.

A large trial of acupuncture therapy for the treatment of chronic OA of the neck was recently performed involving 135 patients and a course of 8 treatments (average of 6 needles per treatment) over 4 weeks.[32] Patients were randomly allocated to either real treatment or a placebo group that received mock electrical stimulation of acupuncture points. This trial demonstrated nearly a 60% fall in pain from baseline in the acupuncture group, compared to a 42% fall in the placebo group (the primary study outcome). Secondary outcomes (SF36, Neck Disability Index, and range of movement) similarly improved. Furthermore, this study also included a long-term follow-up that found that patients continued to show a significant improvement at one year post-treatment. This improvement in pain was *statistically* significant compared to the control group. However, the authors felt that this difference was not *clinically* significant, although the difference from baseline clearly was. The trial, although rigorous, can be criticized because it did not include a non-treatment arm; therefore, the effect of regression to the mean could not be assessed. Also, this was effectively a single-practitioner study, and therefore it is not known if these results are generalizable to other practitioners.

Two other large and recent studies by Berman et al[33] and by Witt et al[34] examined the effectiveness of acupuncture for OA of the knee. Berman enrolled 570 patients and randomized them to one of 3 groups: real acupuncture, an "education" control group (in which patients received advice only), and an acupuncture sham control. The acupuncture control consisted of a combination of inserting needles at non-classic acupuncture points, as well as tapping a plastic needle against the real points. Patients were screened so that they could not view the procedure. This study found a significant improvement in Western Ontario and McMaster Universities Osteoarthritis Index (WOMAC) pain and function scores for the acupuncture group over the other interventions. They concluded that due to the lack of any side effects, and because the improvement was over and above those achieved with conventional therapy, that acupuncture has an important role to play as an adjunctive therapy in osteoarthritis. This study was also rigorous, and therefore produced valid results—but, could be criticised for the excessively long treatment regime, which spanned 26 weeks with varying intensity. It could be said that this would render such treatments financially unviable. There was also a very high drop-out rate: 25% in the acupuncture groups, and 43% in the advice group.

A trial by Witt et al,[35] enrolled 294 patients with chronic knee OA, who were randomly assigned to 8 weeks of acupuncture, minimal acupuncture (superficial needling at non-acupuncture points) or a waitlist control. This trial also used the WOMAC score as the primary outcome measure. Immediately post-treatment, the baseline adjusted scores showed an improvement for the acupuncture group of 8.8 points over the minimal acupuncture, and 22.7 points over the waitlist control. These differences were highly statistically and clinically significant, thus concluding that efficacy was demonstrated. The authors point out, however, that at the long-term follow-up (one year) this statistical difference had disappeared.

These result are summarized in Table 10.1.

Table 10.1. Trials of Acupuncture in Pain & Arthritis.

Study	*Type*	*Site/ Condition*	*Intervention*	*Result*	*Conclusion*
Patel (1989)	SR	Pain various	-	-	In favour of AP
Ter Riet (1990)	SR	Pain various	-	-	Doubtful efficacy for AP
Ernst (1997)	SR	Neck Pain	-	-	Inconclusive
Smith (2000)	SR	Back Pain	-	-	AP no better than placebo
Ezzo (2000)	SR	Pain various	-	-	Inconclusive
Ezzo (2001)	SR	Knee	-	-	AP better than sham
Green (2002)	SR	Tennis elbow	-	-	Some short term benefit/inconclusive
Ernst (1998)	SR	Back pain	-	-	Efficacy shown
Furlan (2005)	SR	Back pain	-	-	Efficacy shown
Manheimer (2005)	SR	Back pain	-	-	Efficacy shown

Table 10.1. (Continued)

Study	*Type*	*Site/ Condition*	*Intervention*	*Result*	*Conclusion*
White (2004)	RCT	Neck pain	AP vs mock electrical stimulation	58% improvement for AP, 42% improvement for placebo	Large effect, but not clinically better than placebo
Berman (2005)	RCT	Knee pain	AP vs Advice vs Sham intervention	Pain improved by -0.87 & function by -2.5 (WOMAC) over sham	AP demonstrates greater improvement in pain than sham
Witt (2005)	RCT	Knee pain	AP vs superficial needling vs Wait list	8.8 points improvement over control acupuncture (WOMAC)	AP demonstrates greater improvement than control AP

Key: SR=Systematic review; RCT=Randomised controlled trial; AP=Acupuncture

Safety

Acupuncture is not completely free of risk, but the risks are very low. It has been estimated that major complications of acupuncture occur with an incidence of between 1:10 000 and 1:100 000.[36] MacPherson[37] surveyed 574 practitioners (34,407 treatments) and found no serious adverse events. Minor events, the most common being nausea or fainting, were noted in 1.3 per 1000 treatments. Another survey[38] found 14 "significant" (e.g. fainting, nausea, drowsiness, anxiety, lost needle, etc.) events per 10,000 treatments, although they also reported 671 "minor" adverse events (including bleeding and discomfort) per 10,000. Norheim and Fonnebo,[39] in Norway, suggested that there were 0.21 incidents of any nature, serious or otherwise, per year of acupuncture practice. The low risk is particularly illustrated when considered within the context of conventional medicine. For example, side effects from NSAIDs are generally dose-related and increase with increasing age. It has been suggested that on average, 1 in 1200 patients will die from complications as a result of taking NSAIDs for at least two months (i.e., approximately 2000 deaths each year in the UK).[40] MacPherson[41] points out that in New York State, 3%–7% of all hospital admissions were due to adverse drug reactions, and that 1% of all patients admitted to the hospital were seriously harmed by conventional treatment. Compared to this number, acupuncture seems very safe.[42] Ernst and White[43] observed that if one takes into account the vast number of acupuncturists practicing worldwide, and the many millions of treatment sessions performed each year, then the incidence of serious complication is very low. It should be pointed out, however, that acupuncture should be used with caution where pregnancy is suspected, as it is thought that certain points may induce labor, or when patients are using anticoagulants.

Summary

Acupuncture is an ancient yet rapidly expanding modality that is becoming increasingly popular for musculoskeletal problems, including arthritis. It is safe and relatively free of adverse effects. The evidence base for acupuncture is steadily growing as more rigorous trials are completed, and this is tending to show that acupuncture does have a place in treating chronic painful musculoskeletal conditions.

REFERENCES

1. Anderson E, Anderson, P. General practitioners and alternative medicine. *J R Coll Gen Pract*. 1987;37(295):52–55.
2. Wharton R, Lewith G. Complementary medicine and the general practitioner. *Br Med J. (Clin Res Ed)*. 1986;292(6534):1498–1500.
3. Ernst E, White A. The BBC survey of complementary medicine use in the UK. *Complement Ther Med*. 2000;8(1):32–36.
4. Finnigan M. The Centre for the Study of Complementary Medicine: an attempt to understand its popularity through psychological, demographic and operational criteria. *Complement Med Res*. 1991;5(2):83–87.
5. Berman BM, Swyers JP. Establishing a research agenda for investigating alternative medical interventions for chronic pain. *Prim Care*. 1997;24(4):743–758.
6. Ernst E. The role of complementary and alternative medicine. *BMJ*. 2000;321(7269): 1133–1135.
7. Ernst E. Acupuncture as a symptomatic treatment of osteoarthritis. A systematic review. *Scand J Rheumatol*. 1997;26(6):444–447.
8. Thomas KJ, Nicholl JP, Coleman P. Use and expenditure on complementary medicine in England: a population based survey. *Complement Ther Med*. 2001;9(1):2–11.
9. Paramore LC. Use of alternative therapies: estimates from the 1994 Robert Wood Johnson Foundation National Access to Care Survey. *J Pain Symptom Manage*. 1997;13(2):83–89.

10. Ellis N. *Acupuncture in Clinical Practice*. London: Chapman and Hall; 1994.
11. Salzberg C, Miller A, Johnson LK. Acupuncture: history, clinical uses, and proposed physiology. *Phys Med Rehabil Clin N Am*. 1995;6(4):905–916.
12. Lynn J. Using complementary therapies: acupuncture. *Prof Nurse*. 1996;11(11): 722–724.
13. Wu JN. A short history of acupuncture. *J Altern Complement Med*. 1996;2(1):19–21.
14. Stux G, Pomeranz B. *Basics of acupuncture*. New York: Springer Verlag; 1995: 309.
15. Lewith GT, Lewith NR. *Modern Chinese Acupuncture. 2nd ed*. London: Thorsons Publishers; 1983.
16. Ryan D. The logic of acupuncture. *Pacific Journal of Oriental Medicine*. 1996;(8): 24–27.
17. Ezzo J, Berman B, Hadhazy VA, Jadad AR, Lao L, Singh BB. Is acupuncture effective for the treatment of chronic pain? A systematic review. *Pain*. 2000;86(3):217–225.
18. Hobbs B. The application of electricity to acupuncture needles: a review of the current literature and research with a brief outline of the principles involved. *Complement Ther Med*. 1994;2(1):36–40.
19. Pomeranz, B. Bruce Pomeranz, PHD. Acupuncture and the raison d'être for alternative medicine. Interview by Bonnie Horrigan. *Altern Ther Health Med*. 1996;2(6):85–91.
20. Ceniceros S, Brown GR. Acupuncture: A review of its history, theories, and indications. *South Med J*. 1998;91(12):1121–1125.
21. Patel M, Gutzwiller F, Paccaud F, Marazzi A. A meta-analysis of acupuncture for chronic pain. *Int J Epidemiol*. 1989;18(4):900–906.
22. ter Riet G, Kleijnen J, Knipschild P. Acupuncture and chronic pain: a criteria-based meta-analysis. *J Clin Epidemiol*. 1990;43(11):1191–1199.
23. Ernst E. Is acupuncture effective for pain control? [letter], *J Pain Symptom.Manage*. 1994;9(2):72–74.
24. Birch, S. 1997, Issues to consider in determining an adequate treatment in a clinical trial of acupuncture. *Complementary Therapies in Medicine*. 5(1):8–12.
25. Kjellman GV, Skargren EI, Oberg BE. A critical analysis of randomised clinical trials on neck pain and treatment efficacy. A review of the literature. *Scand J Rehab Med*. 1999;31(3):139–152.
26. Smith LA, Oldman AD, McQuay HJ, Moore RA. Teasing apart quality and validity in systematic reviews: an example from acupuncture trials in chronic neck and back pain. *Pain*. 2000;86(1-2):119–132.
27. Ezzo J, Hadhazy V, Birch S, et al. Acupuncture for Osteoarthritis of the knee: a systematic review. *Arthritis Rheum*. 2001;44(4):819–825.
28. Green S, Buchbinder R, Barnsley L, et al. Acupuncture for lateral elbow pain. *Cochrane Database Syst Rev*. 2002;(1):CD003527.
29. Ernst E, White AR. Acupuncture for back pain: a meta-analysis of randomized controlled trials. *Arch Intern Med*. 1998;158(20):2235–2241.
30. Furlan AD, van Tulder M, Cherkin D, et al. Acupuncture and dry-needling for low back pain: an updated systematic review within the framework of the cochrane collaboration. *Spine*. 2005; 30(8):944–963.

31. Manheimer E, White A, Berman B, Forys K, Ernst E. Meta-analysis: acupuncture for low back pain. *Ann Intern Med.* 2005;142(8):651–663.
32. White P, Lewith G, Berman B, Birch S. Reviews of acupuncture for chronic neck pain: pitfalls in conducting systematic reviews. *Rheumatology.* 2002;41(11):1224–1231.
33. White P, Lewith G, Prescott P, Conway J. Acupuncture versus placebo for the treatment of chronic mechanical neck pain: a randomized, controlled trial. *Ann Intern Med.* 2004;141(12):911–919.
34. Berman BM, Lao L, Langenberg P, Lee W, Gilpin A, Hochberg MC. Effectiveness of acupuncture as adjunctive therapy in osteoarthritis of the knee: a randomized controlled trial. *Ann Intern Med.* 2004;141(12):901–911.
35. Witt C, Brinkhaus B, Jena S, et al. Acupuncture in patients with osteoarthritis of the knee: a randomised trial. *Lancet.* 2005;366(9480):136–143.
36. White A, Hayhoe S, Ernst E. Survey of Adverse Events Following Acupuncture. *Acupunct Med.* 1997;15(2):80–83.
37. MacPherson H, Lewith G. Reporting adverse events following acupuncture. *Physiotherapy.* 2001;87(1):21–23.
38. White A, Hayhoe S, Hart A, Ernst E. Adverse events following acupuncture: Prospective survey of 32 000 consultations with doctors and physiotherapists. *BMJ.* 2001;323(7311):485–486.
39. Norheim AJ, Fønnebø V. Acupuncture adverse effects are more than occasional case reports: results from questionnaires among 1135 randomly selected doctors, and 197 acupuncturists. *Complement Ther Med.* 1996;4(1):8–13.
40. Tramèr MR, Moore RA, Reynolds DJ, McQuay HJ. Quantitative estimation of rare adverse events which follow a biological progression: a new model applied to chronic NSAID use. *Pain.* 2000;85(1-2):169–182.
41. MacPherson H. Fatal and adverse events from acupuncture: allegation, evidence. and the implications. *J Altern Complement Med.* 1999;5(1):47–56.
42. MacPherson H, Thomas K, Walters S, Fitter M. The York acupuncture safety study: prospective survey of 34 000 treatments by traditional acupuncturists. *BMJ.* 2001;323(7311):486–487.
43. Ernst E, White A. Life-threatening adverse reactions after acupuncture? A systematic review. *Pain.* 1997;71(2):123–126.

11

Energy Medicine and Rheumatologic Disorders

ANN MARIE CHIASSON, MD, MPH

KEY CONCEPTS

- Energy medicine is defined as any modality in medicine, or complementary and alternative medicine, that works with the body's underlying electromagnetic field.
- Rheumatologic patients with more severe symptoms are more likely to seek an energy medicine modality.
- Early research weakly supports using energy medicine in rheumatologic disease for pain control and symptom relief.
- A multidisciplinary approach to fibromyalgia is effective; this approach can include energy medicine (EM) techniques if the patient's belief system is aligned with EM techniques.

■

What is Energy Medicine?

The term *energy medicine* has many, varied definitions. In the broadest sense, the field of energy medicine (EM) can be explained in the context of the whole person: "…in addition to a system of physical and chemical processes, the human being is made up of a complex system of energy."[1] In this view, energy is described as being within (or underlying) the physical body, depending upon the healing tradition. The composite of all energy in the body is often referred to as the energy body, the biofield, or the subtle body. A recent, formal definition of energy medicine is delineated in Table 11.1.

Table 11.1. Definition of Energy Medicine from ISSSEEM, the International Society for the Study of Subtle Energies and Energy Medicine.

"Energy Medicine includes all energetic and informational interactions resulting from self-regulation or brought about through other energy linkages to mind and body. In addition to various therapeutic energies which we may use, there are also energy pulses from the environment which influence humans and animals in a variety of ways. For instance, low-level changes in magnetic, electric, electromagnetic, acoustic, and gravitational fields often have profound effects on both biology and psychology. In addition to energies originating in the environment, it has been documented that humans are capable of generating and controlling subtle, not-yet-measurable energies that seem to influence both physiological and physical mechanisms." ~ISSSEEM (International Society for the Study of Subtle Energies and Energy Medicine)

Reprinted from the ISSSEEM website, www.issseem.org.

The National Center for Complementary and Alternative Medicine (NCCAM), further delineates two types of energy fields: veritable and putative. They consider veritable energy as that which can be measured, and putative energy as that which has yet to be measured (using our current technology).[2] Veritable energies may include light, with measurable wavelengths and frequencies, or sound, which employs mechanical vibrations. Electromagnetic forces, including magnetism, monochromatic radiation (such as laser beams), and rays from other parts of the electromagnetic spectrum are also examples of veritable energy.[2] There are many conventional medical interventions that employ veritable energy, including electromagnetic fields used in magnetic resonance imaging, cardiac pacemakers, radiation therapy, ultraviolet light for psoriasis, and laser keratoplasty.[2]

Putative fields, according to NCCAM "have defied measurement to date by reproducible methods."[2] The bulk of energy medicine as currently practiced in the United States uses modalities that modify the putative field, or biofield. With regard to the biofield or subtle body, NCCAM recognizes that the concept that human beings are infused with a subtle form of energy has persisted for 2000 years, and has many names, "such as *Qi* in traditional Chinese medicine (TCM), *ki* in the Japanese Kampo system, *doshas* in Ayurvedic medicine, and elsewhere as *prana*, etheric energy, *fohat*, orgone, odic force, *mana*, and homeopathic resonance."[2] Further, "therapists claim that they can work with

> It is interesting that once the positive effects of a CAM therapy are measurable and reproducible, it often permeates conventional medicine, and is not longer considered CAM.

this subtle energy, see it with their own eyes, and use it to effect changes in the physical body and influence health."[2]

The authenticity of the "subtle body" is a central dilemma for energy medicine practitioners, and has proved to be an impediment with respect to acceptance by conventional medical practitioners and researchers. While 94 cultures have been documented to have a concept which describes this underlying energy of the body, they lack a unified set of characteristics. Thus, the characterization of energy medicine as spiritual healing, energy healing, or aspects of traditional Chinese medicine (TCM) and mind-body medicine is ambiguous. These confusions will likely continue until a method is devised to accurately measure the body's subtle field. Work in this area is continuing, and the technology of gas discharge visualization (GDV) for the measurement of biophoton emission, superconducting quantum interference device (SQUID), and low-frequency pulsed electromagnetic field (PEMF) are being developed to demonstrate the electromagnetic field of the body, although with difficulty.[3] Despite the uncertainty of verification or definition, EM modalities are frequently being used in the United States. The 2000 NHIS study on CAM revealed that at least 1% of people in the US seek Reiki or another form of energy medicine, and this number is growing.[4] This percentage is much greater in persons suffering from chronic pain and chronic illness. As of 2002, more than 50 hospitals and clinics in the US provided energy medicine as an adjunct.[3]

The scope of energy medicine (i.e., which modalities are considered energy medicine and which are not) is not well defined. Since many EM practitioners postulate that everything is energy, one can place much of CAM within the EM paradigm, including TCM and homeopathy (Table 11.2).[5] For the purpose of this chapter, we will discuss EM with regard to modalities that directly address the biofield or subtle body. These include: therapeutic touch, healing touch, Reiki, Johrei, sound healing, Zero Balancing, Barbara Brennan's work, and Rosalyn Bruyere's healing. For many, EM also includes spiritual healing, natural healing, and shamanic healing—paradigms that do not have well-delineated training and certification programs, and thus have variable structure.

Anatomy of the Energy Field

The anatomical composition of the energy field varies according to the belief system in each healing tradition. An overview of how these anatomical components interact can be described as "layers." Different energy medicine techniques are based on different layers of the biofield. A simple map of such

Table 11.2. A List of Common Energy Medicine Techniques.

Technique	*Theory*
Acupuncture	Involves using needles to stimulate energy flow at meridian points on the body. Part of Traditional Chinese Medicine.
Healing Touch	Energy transfer by laying of hands onto the body, based in the chakra system.
Homeopathy	Considered a vibrational remedy. Remedies use high diluted elements of substances that would cause symptoms in undiluted quantities. At high dilution they stimulate the body's innate ability to heal.
Joh Rei	A technique for detoxification of the energy body through sending universal energy to the patient from the healers hands from a short distance.
Polarity Therapy	A touch therapy based on balancing positive and negative energy flows in the body.
Prayer	Uses pure energy and intention from a universal healing source to heal a patient through distance healing.
Qi-Gong	A self healing practice using movement and laying of hands to cultivate balanced energy flow through the body.
Reiki	Of Japanese origin, a technique that channels universal energy into the patient's body through the hands of the healer.
Sound and Light Therapies	Uses vibration through sound or light to heal or shift the energetic body of the patient. Can be done on or off the body.
Tai Chi	A series of movements postures and exercises to stimulate energy flow and increased energy in the body.
Therapeutic Touch	Energy transfer by placing hands into the patients' auric field of the body.
Yoga	Philosophy, poses and breathing techniques to promote energy flow and balanced energy in the body.
Zero Balancing	A touch therapy that balances energy at the zero-point field of the body. Uses slight movement and touch.

Adapted from Baggott A: The Encyclopedia of Energy Healing. New York, Sterling Publishing, 1999.

Table 11.3. A Summary of Energy Anatomy.

Energy Fields These are energetic and encompass the body. This model was developed in India and is the most inclusive model.
Seven Chakras This model is also from India and other cultures as well. These are the main energetic centers of the body responsible for metabolizing and storing specific types of energy.
Twelve Meridians (**or Twelve Energetic Pathways**) This model was developed in China. These specialized maps provide us with information about how energy circulates throughout the body.
The energy bodies: the **most interior body** represented by a small blue light, is in the chest. On top of that we place the **causal body**, or dan-tien, the small red ball, a few inches in diameter and a few inches below the navel. Over this is the **subtle body**, which contains the seven chakras and the energy field extending to arm's length. Over this is the **physical body** containing the 12 meridians of energy.

Adapted from the University of Arizona, Program in Integrative Medicine Fellowship, 2007.

layers is presented in Table 11.3.[6] For example, the technique of Zero Balancing is targeted at the deepest layer; healing touch works at the chakra layer, while TCM works with the meridians at the most superficial layer of the energy field.

Energy Medicine and the Basis of Illness

Pathology, or illness, as viewed from an energy medicine perspective, first develops when there is a problem in the subtle body or biofield. In the natural history of the disease, the energetic field becomes unbalanced, then pathology develops, and finally, clinical symptoms appear. Major cellular pathology typically appears weeks to years after a block in the natural flow of energy has occurred. Pain, a symptom that represents blocked energy, can occur right away. Infection is thought to occur from a weakness in the energy field that causes immunosupression.

Factors that contribute to or cause energy blocks include external insults, genetic or hereditary causes, and physical or emotional trauma. Treatment is based upon energy transfer in order to remove blocks, and to ultimately restore normal energy flow. Keeping the energy field as clear as possible, and the energy flowing, promotes health and healing.[6]

HOW THE ENERGY BODY IS ALTERED

Energy medicine therapies rely upon methods to shift or change the underlying energy field of the body. The most common technique involves the laying of the hands on the patient's body, or over the body. However, different techniques employ vibration, light, sound, movement, magnets, or direct current.

Energy Medicine and the Autonomic Nervous System

In the 1970's, Dr Herbert Benson's work demonstrated the effects of relaxation on the body to improve blood pressure and heart rate, and to enhance immune function, gastrointestinal peristalsis, kidney function, and brain wave activity.[7] Energy medicine modalities are thought to function in a similar fashion to relaxation—shifting autonomic nervous system function to improve health and reduce inflammation. Research on Reiki has demonstrated physiological changes after treatment. Wetzel demonstrated a significant increase in hemoglobin and hematocrit levels in healthy persons learning Reiki.[8] Wardell, et al reported decreased blood pressure (BP), increased IgA levels, changes in skin response, and no shift in cortisol with 30 minutes of Reiki.[8] With respect to chronic illness and pain, Olson, et al demonstrated a reduction in pain, and improved sleep and mood, although this study was only of fair quality.[8]

Placebo effect, relaxation, and the effects of human touch and healer/patient relationship may be most important in the physiological and psychological aspects of the EM treatments. These aspects of EM sessions (which are usually an hour long) can be quite helpful with patient perception and coping ability with their illness.

Research on EM

While there are few high-quality EM studies in the literature, some provocative findings may be gleaned. In 2003, NCCAM concluded that the research on veritable EM to date includes some uses of magnet therapy, millimeter wave therapy, sound energy therapy, and light therapy.[2] With respect to putative energy field work, NCCAM concludes that the data is scant and of poor quality. This chapter will discuss a few positive studies of good quality. In addition, three systematic reviews have been published since 2000. Most studies to date have focused upon therapeutic touch (TT), developed by Delores Krieger in the 70's, and Reiki, a Japanese form of healing that originated in Japan in the early twentieth century. Most EM practitioners claim that the biggest benefits of EM work include decreases in pain, anxiety, and healing times.

Multiple studies using therapeutic touch have been published with positive findings. Movaffaghi et al showed that therapeutic touch was able to elevate hemoglobin and hematocrit levels in healthy students.[9] Experienced therapueutic touch practitioners can alleviate anxiety, with the experience of the practitioner positively correlated with the amount of benefit.[10] Stress reduction was also demonstrated using therapeutic touch following a natural disaster (Hurricane Hugo).[11] Meehan, et al published three studies that demonstrated significant effects of therapeutic touch on pain reduction after surgery, with decreasing frequency in patient requests for prn analgesic medication.[12–14]

A few systematic reviews have also been done on EM in various setting and outcomes. Approximately half of the studies examined showed benefit, but the quality of the studies varies greatly. Jonas et al looked at 19 randomized controlled trials most using therapeutic touch, and found that 11 of 19 showed statistically significant treatment effects, with a mean effect size of 0.60. They conclude that the evidence for EM modalities to relieve pain and anxiety was poor to fair (evidence level B).[15] Astin et al performed a systematic review of 11 TT studies and reported a mean effect of 0.63 with respect to symptom reduction. Seven of the 11 studies showed a positive effect on at least one outcome. When all healing trials (including prayer and distant healing) were reviewed, the mean effect size was 0.40. The mean effect score for distant healing, which included Reiki, was 0.38.[16] Finally, Abbot et al reviewed 22 trials of EM healing. This review concluded that 10 trials had a significant positive outcome for healing, 11 had no significant outcome, and 1 study was indeterminate due to poor study design. They then examined the trials based upon Jadad score, a measure of study quality. Five of 8 studies with a Jadad score of 5 showed significant differences between the EM treatment group and the control group. Yet, due to the variation of quality of studies, they conclude that firm conclusions cannot be drawn about the efficacy or inefficacy of EM.[17]

CAM AND RHEUMATOLOGIC DISEASE

Research on EM in rheumatological conditions is even more limited. There are data describing prevalence of CAM use and EM modalities in rheumatology patients, and there are data to correlate increased pain and chronic illness with increased CAM use. There have been few studies that describe the prevalence of referrals of rheumatology patients to CAM by health care providers.

Hagen et al, in 2003, published a cross-sectional descriptive survey from a Toronto pediatric rheumatology clinic. Sixty-four percent of respondents used one form of CAM, with half of these using more than one form of CAM. While energy medicine was not specifically named, 22% used relaxation techniques, and 17% used "other CAM practitioner." Duration of illness was positively associated with use of CAM.[18] Rao et al used a representative sample of rheumatology patients, representing a range of socioeconomic levels, to examine CAM use and related variables. Sixty-three percent of patients reported using at least one type of CAM; most patients used 2.6 types of CAM. Among those that used CAM, 75% reported that spiritual healers were useful. Many spiritual healers use forms of EM, and this is the first published data describing such a high of use of EM. The most common reason to use CAM was for pain control and to help treat the underlying condition. Education and having osteoarthritis were both associated with CAM use. Rao[19] reported that most patients use CAM for symptom relief, rather than cure. His group completed a one-year longitudinal study of CAM use and its impact with a cohort of rheumatology patients. They reported no difference in outcomes for objective symptoms and severity of illness. Fifty-six percent used CAM at the time of the survey, and 24% used three or more modalities of CAM. Patients most commonly reported that it reduced pain. Increased use of CAM modalities was associated with more severe pain and higher education.[20]

The confusion in defining EM, and the multiple names of EM modalities, make it very difficult to research prevalence of use. Some studies specifically ask about EM, healing, spiritual healing, or by specific modality name. Most studies have not asked questions thoroughly enough to capture the range of EM modalities. Therefore, estimates of patient use are quite poor, and vary from 1% of the population to up to 45% of patients with chronic illness or pain.

Berman et al surveyed all physician members of the American College of Rheumatology for physician self-reported knowledge, perceptions of legitimacy, referral patterns, and use (in practice) of 22 different CAM therapies. Eleven percent stated that they had enough knowledge of CAM to discuss it with patients, and 5% referred patients to CAM practitioners.[21] Osborn et al surveyed rheumatology nurses in the UK, and reported that CAM therapies were provided by 8.3% of the nurses, with 51.6% of the nurses providing advice about CAM to patients. The nurses believed that adjunctive CAM therapies were used mostly by RA patients. Eighty three percent of the nurses believed that CAM would relieve symptoms in patients with rheumatologic disease.[22]

EM AND RHEUMATOLOGIC DISEASES

Recently, there has been a series of reviews in the literature looking at CAM and rheumatologic diseases. Most conclude that there is promising early evidence for adjuvant use of CAM modalities for pain relief and quality of life. Most did not specifically investigate EM in their reviews, as very few studies on EM alone have been done. The majority of the studies published to date explore the use of CAM as adjuvant therapy for fibromyalgia. Most conclude there is good evidence for exercise, cognitive behavior therapy (CBT), education, and social support. A recent Cochrane review concluded that multidisciplinary rehabilitation is an effective approach for fibromyalgia.[23] A recent study looked at 5 patients with chronic illness, (MS, lupus, fibromyalgia, and goiter) who were given 11 Reiki treatments.[24] This study found decreased skin resistance over acupuncture meridians, with patients reporting decreased pain and anxiety. This was a very small study and was not controlled, or blinded.

Ernst[25] reviewed the evidence for CAM and fibromyalgia—primarily acupuncture, herbal medicine, homeopathy, magnet therapy, and dietary supplements—as treatments for OA, RA, and fibromyalgia. They reported that magnet therapy, as measured by PEMF (low-frequency pulsed electromagnetic field), was tested on patients in a randomized double-blind placebo controlled with 75 patients with knee OA. While there was no difference overall between the experimental and the control group, magnet therapy showed increase in quality of life secondary measures in the intervention group when analyzed by paired analysis. Significant differences were seen in WOMAC (Western Ontario and McMaster University Osteoarthritis index) global score, WOMAC pain score and WOMAC disability score when compared to baseline.[25]

A systematic review of 25 randomized controlled trials on no pharmacological interventions for fibromyalgia concluded that exercise and education were effective, along with a multidisciplinary team approach.[26] Denison et al did a small study on therapeutic touch for persons with fibromyalgia, in which they examined the effectiveness of 6 TT treatments on patients. Dependent variables included experience of pain, QOL, and cutaneous skin temperature measured by electronic infrared ski thermography (EIT). The study confirmed that the most beneficial treatment of fibromyalgia is exercise and restoration of normal sleep cycle. However, they found TT reduced the experience of pain in the study participants. In addition, there was significant decrease in EIT on "hot spots" from pre-TT treatment to post-TT treatment.[27] This study, too, points out that conventional treatment often fails to help patients with fibromyalgia, necessitating the use of adjunctive therapies.

NEGATIVE EFFECTS OF ENERGY MEDICINE

Properly used, there are negligible adverse effects of energy medicine modalities. The most common is an occasional increase in the symptom of pain following the first few treatments. Skilled practitioners feel that this represents the beginning of a release of blocked energy, and it typically diminishes and dissipates with subsequent treatments.

Rheumatologic Disease and Fibromyalgia by Healing Modality

Most EM paradigms do not diagnose conditions using conventional medical terminology. Thus, it is difficult to directly translate the medical diagnoses to allow easy comparison between energy modalities. However, when asked, energy healers will give an impression of what each disease may represent. For example, heat may be considered excess energy to be drained or removed, while cold spots are a decrease or block in energy that energy can be added to.

Energy medicine therapies often consider the mind and body as one entity, with the illness expressing something that the mind cannot. In terms of the common symptoms of rheumatologic disease, the body is attacking itself. The underlying issues might be self-rejection, feeling unloved, or resentment and rigidity in the patient's world view. These are seen as the metaphors that the body is expressing.[28] Table 11.4 summarizes a few interpretations of fibromyalgia by healers from different modalities.[6]

Referral and Certification

When considering referral to an EM practitioner, it is important to match the patients' belief system to modalities considered for referral. Patients who are seeking adjunctive therapies for their pain or related symptoms with a belief, openness, or cultural alignment to EM, may be appropriate for referral to EM. It can be a useful addition to their medical management, with few side effects. Patients with longer duration of illness and more severe pain are good candidates. If a patient does not experience positive physical or mental effects within a few visits, discuss this with the patient; it may be more appropriate for the patient to use their resources on another adjunct CAM modality.

Most EM modalities have websites with certification guidelines and lists of certified practitioners. These include: Reiki, Healing Touch International,

Table 11.4. Healer views of Fibromylagia, by modality.

Illness and Consciousness The patient has a deep unconscious meaningful relationship to pain and conflict as it is suffering that engages them in life. Resistance to the pain makes the pain more pronounced. The patient carries the bulk of their conflict somatically, more than emotionally, mentally, or spiritually. The way it is carried is not volitional and will not shift without deep physical and psychodynamic work. The concept that they are in relationship to pain is too difficult at first. Begin by working with how the illness serves (what is right about it?), moving very small amounts of energy, and having them practice carrying the tension or pain in different ways. This approach is appropriate for many chronic pain patients, not just fibromyalgia.
Joh Rei Joh Rei can be highly effective for rheumatism. With Joh Rei, joints may swell, fever and pain would increase, and then symptoms may gradually disappear through increased urination. Fibromyalgia includes joint pain as well as muscle pain and mental and sleep disturbances. This is caused by the accumulation of medicines in the central nervous system, which irritate the nerves as they slowly dissolve as a deeper form of rheumatism.
Reiki Often so much of the body is in chaos and in pain that the feeling can be on pins and needles or actually painful to the healer's hands. This is a case where distant healing can be done first to provide some relief to the patient. Anything that helps the patient relax will assist and many are helped by giving daily self treatments. This is disease where it is likely to be a complex of energetic situations, such as cords to unhealthy relationships, charkas that need clearing, past lives of poor judgment, depression from the disease process, unresolved cords, etc.
Healing Touch Fibromyalgia may stem from a variety of issues. On a physical level, whiplash may create fibromyalgia, with congestion around the neck and shoulders and a disturbance in the throat chakra. The Healing Touch neck and back techniques are very effective in releasing this pain and tension.There is often a strong emotional component. The client is energetically and physically clenched, the chakras may be blocked/closed. The energy field assessment shows a condensed field, cold areas around the hips, low back, mid back at the base of the trapesius muscles and up into the neck and shoulders. As a pattern, the clients tend to hold the breath, breathe in a shallow manner and have very inflated chests which are held extremely tightly. Often hip muscles and low back are clenched while abdominal muscles are loose and slack. As part of the emotional/mental pattern, clients with this diagnosis tend have control issues, hold tightly, stuffs emotions - especially anger and rage, and care for everyone to the exclusion of the self. Chakras related to these issues must be addressed as well. Clenching in the pelvic girdle can become so tight that it may radiate to the thighs. The same may occur in the shoulder girdle and the through at the throat chakra. Back and neck techniques are effective. Exploring the pent up emotions while working energetically allows them to release, clearing the energy field and body, decreasing pain and increasing energy flow to support the healing process.

(*continued*)

Table 11.4. (Continued)

Healing Touch
More than one session is needed when working with this diagnosis so that self care teaching can be put in place to break old coping patterns and new methods of self care can be slowly put in place with the support of the practitioner. Self care teaching includes learning to breathe and let go, move with the breath, stretch, relax rather than clench, write in a journal, release pent up anger. Counseling may be warranted to assist with the emotional component.

Adapted from University of Arizona, Program in Integrative Medicine, Energy Medicine Module, 2007.

Therapeutic Touch, Polarity Therapy, Johrei, Zero Balancing, Jin Shin Jytsu, Barbara Brennan Healing, and Rosalyn Bruyere's work. Since EM skills involve both expertise and sensitivity, counsel patients to consider choosing a practitioner with multiple years of experience.

Conclusion

While EM may be helpful in many conditions, there is a lack of convincing data to support efficacy of EM as a treatment for specific rheumatologic disease. However, rheumatology patients seek CAM modalities for adjunctive treatment in 64% of cases, and CAM use is positively correlated with severity of disease and severity of pain. As rheumatologic diseases, especially fibromyalgia, respond better to a multidisciplinary approach, it may be appropriate to refer patients to EM if they have an interest or belief system that includes an EM modality. Further, the comorbid symptoms of pain and anxiety often respond to the use of EM modalities, as seen in several studies. The relaxing benefits of EM may be helpful to patients.

REFERENCES

1. Hurwitz W. Energy Medicine. In: Micozzi MS, ed. *Fundamentals of Complementary and Alternative Medicine*. New York: Churchill Livingstone; 2001:238–256.
2. National Center for Complementary and Alternative Medicine (NCCAM). Energy Medicine: An Overview. *Backgrounder*. National Institute for Health; 2003.
3. Di Nucci EM. Energy healing: a complementary treatment for orthopaedic and other conditions. *Orthop Nurs*. 2005;24(4):259–269.
4. Barnes PM. Powell-Griner E, McFann K, Nahin RL. Complementary and alternative medicine use among adults: United State, 2002. U.S. Department of Health

and Human Services, Centers for Disease Control and Prevention, National Center for Health Statistics. CDC Advance Data 2004;343.

5. D'Aprile J. Energy Medicine. In: Kohatsu MD, Wendy ed. *Complementary and Alternative Medicine Secrets.* Philadelphia: Hanley & Belfus, Inc.; 2002: 153–162.
6. University of Arizona Fellowship Curriculum. Program in Integrative Medicine, Energy Medicine Module. University of Arizona Board of Regents, 2007.
7. Benson H. *The Relaxation Response.* New York: HarperCollins; 1976.
8. Miles P, True G. Reiki—review of biofeild therapy, history, theory, practice, and research. *Altern Ther Health Med.* 2003;9(2):62–72.
9. Movaffaghi Z, Hasanpoor M, Farsi M, Hooshmand P, Abrishami F. Effects of therapeutic touch on blood hemoglobin and hematocrit level. *J Holist Nurs.* 2006;24(1):41–48.
10. Ferguson CK. Subjective experience of therapeutic touch (SETTS): Psychometric examination of an instrument. [Unpublished Ph. dissertation]. Austin: University of Texas at Austin; 1986.
11. Olson M, Sneed N, Bonadonna R, Ratliff J, Dias J. Therapeutic touch and post-Hurricane Hugo stress. *J Holist Nurs.* 1992;10(2):120–136.
12. Meehan TC. An abstract of the effect of therapeutic touch on the experience of acute pain in post-operative patients [dissertation]. New York: New York University; 1985.
13. Meehan TC, Mersmann CA, Wiseman M, Wolff, BB, Malgady R. The effect of therapeutic touch on postoperative pain. *Pain.* 1990;(Suppl):149.
14. Meehan TC. Therapeutic touch and postoperative pain: a Rogerian research study. *Nurs Sci Q.* 1993;6(2):69–78.
15. Jonas WB, Crawford CC. Science and spiritual healing: a critical review of spiritual healing, "energy" medicine, and intentionality. *Altern Ther Health Med.* 2003;9(2):56–61.
16. Astin J, Harkness E, Ernst E. The efficacy of "distant healing": a systematic review of randomized trials. *Ann Intern Med.* 2000;132(11):903–910.
17. Abbot N. Healing as a therapy for human disease: a systematic review. *J Altern Complement Med.* 2000;6(2):159–169.
18. Hagen LE, Schneider R, Stephens D, Modrusan D, Feldman BM. Use of complementary and alternative medicine by pediatric rheumatology patients. *Arthritis Rheum.* 2003;49(1):3–6.
19. Rao JK, Mihaliak K, Kroenke K, Bradley J, Tierney WM, Weinberger M. Use of complementary therapies for arthritis among patients of rheumatologists. *Ann Intern Med.* 1999;131(6):409–416.
20. Rao JK, Kroenke K, Mihaliak KA, Grambow SC, Weinberger M. Rheumatology patients' use of complementary therapies: results from a one-year longitudinal study. *Arthritis Rheum.* 2003;49(5):619–625.
21. Berman BM. Bausell RB, Lee WL. Use and referral patterns for 22 complementary and alternative medical therapies by members of the American college of Rheumatology: results of a national survey. *Arch Intern Med.* 2002;162(7):766–770.

22. Osborn C, Baxter GD, Barlas P, Barlow J. Complementary and alternative medicine and rheumatology nurses: A survey of current use and perceptions. *NT Res.* 2004;9(2):110–119.
23. Karjalainen K, Malmivaara A, van Tulder M, et al. Multidisciplinary rehabilitation for fibromyalgia and musculoskeletal pain in working age adults. *Cochrane Database of Syst Rev.* 2000;(2):CD001984.
24. Brewitt B, Hartwell B, Vittetoe T. The efficacy of Reiki: Improvements in spleen and nervous system function as qualified by electro-dermal screening. *Alter Ther.* 1997;3:89–97.
25. Ernst E. Complementary and alternative medicine in rheumatology. *Baillieres Best Pract Res Clin Rheumatol.* 2000;14(4):731–749.
26. Sim J, Adams N. Systematic review of randomized controlled trials of nonpharmacological interventions for fibromyalgia. *Clin J Pain.* 2002;18(5):324–336.
27. Denison B. Touch the pain away: new research on therapeutic touch and persons with fibromyalgia syndrome. *Holist Nurs Pract.* 2004;18(3):142–151.
28. Hay LL. *Heal Your Body.* Santa Monica: Hay House Inc.; 1984:60.

12

Ayurveda and Rheumatologic Disorders

MALYNN UTZINGER, MA, MD

KEY CONCEPTS

- Ayurveda is a system of medicine originating up to five thousand years ago in India, where early sages noted that patterns in nature are reflected in the human body through circadian rhythms and changes throughout the life cycle.
- The goal of Ayurveda is to clear the mind and harmonize bodily functions. Each patient is said to have a unique combination of the five elements, (space, air, fire, water, and earth), linked to anatomic and physiologic functions now described in more modern, scientific terms. As life challenges our bodily systems and creates imbalances, Ayurveda seeks to reestablish the original or healthiest constitutional blend of elements, thus allowing full and healthy expression of a person's body and mind. The metaphorical language of Ayurveda can be appreciated as a poetic reminder to tune in to and creatively explore healing experiences found in nature itself.
- Specific recommendations in Ayurvedic medicine include reestablishing daily and seasonal routines involving habits of sleep, reflection/meditation, meals, exercise, and even, in some instances, specific colors, textures, sounds, aromas, and tastes. In Ayurveda, activating the senses allows people to take in information about the environment and reeducates the body and mind to restore balance.
- In Ayurveda, foods and herbs are categorized according to the degree to which they express one or more of the "six tastes": sweet, salty, sour, pungent, bitter, and astringent, each one necessary in the proper proportion. Certain foods and herbal

remedies are prescribed to help a person build up deficient qualities and reduce unwanted excesses.

- Studies reveal that several of the herbal remedies and common ingredients in Ayurvedic cooking, such as ginger and turmeric, for example, have healing properties based on their anti-inflammatory actions and immunomodulating capacities.
- Finally, Ayurvedic medicine includes an elaborate system of cleansing called *panchakarma*. Such cleanses may last from a few days to, more often, several weeks and are best supervised by an Ayurvedic physician.

■

Background

Ayurveda, a Sanskrit word meaning the "science of life," emerged in India over 5000 years ago and today is practiced around the world. In all of its forms, Ayurveda is as much a philosophy as an elegant medical system involving treatment with foods, herbs, meditation, yoga, cleansing routines, and specialized massages.

The overarching goal of Ayurveda is to harmonize our human rhythms of appetite, digestion, elimination, sleep, and thinking with the cycles of nature. A passage in the *Chakara Samhita*, an Ayurvedic text from the third century BC, translates loosely to, "a quack is a doctor who treats symptoms only and does not address the underlying cause of disease." Ayurveda therefore emphasizes nourishing the body and cultivating a clear mind through meditation and yoga. In fact, the Sanskrit word for health, *swastha*, translates to "established in the self," or grounded in healthy self-awareness.[1,2]

Scope of Ayurvedic Applications

Research has shown that Ayurvedic protocols may be valuable in the treatment of chronic diseases, such as diabetes,[3–6] cardiovascular disease,[7–9] neurological conditions,[10,11] and cancer.[2,12,13] Costs and unwanted side effects are low with administration of Ayurvedic herbs,[14–17] and studies suggest that Ayurvedic cleansing can remove toxins from the body.[14,15] Specific anti-rheumatic properties are discussed under herbal preparations below.

An Ayurvedic Understanding of the Body

The early Ayurvedic scholars observed five *great elements*—space, air, fire, water, and earth—in nature and in humans. These elements pair up to form three *constitutional types,* or *doshas,* describing body type, personality, and behavioral tendencies. The first dosha is called *vata* (space and air). The second is *pitta* (fire and water), and the third is *kapha* (water and earth).

The doshic blend we express at birth is known as *prakruti,* or "basic nature." Subsequently the stresses of life and environmental conditions lead to different disruptions in health called *vikruti,* or "current imbalance."

Doshas are more than mere metaphor. New research suggests genomic differences between the doshas. For example, a *kapha*-dominant (water and earth) person, classically described as vulnerable to diabetes and heart disease, appears to express genes that may be in part responsible for this correlation.[18] This study indicates that number of other significant differences may exist between people of different doshic phenotypes: liver function, hemoglobin levels, regulation of cyclin-dependent protein kinase, immune responses, regulation of blood coagulation, and even expression of disease-related hub and housekeeping genes. Future study may strengthen links between Ayurvedic phenotypes and metabolic, immunological, infectious, cardiovascular, and neuropsychiatric disease, and certain cancers.[18]

The Doshas

Vata dosha (space and air) governs movement in the body and is cold, quick, vast, changeable, rough, dry, subtle and light. People dominant in these qualities are generally thin with fine bones, small muscles, and fast metabolism. Their skin tends to be dry and rough, and their eyes are small and lively. By nature, vatas are prone to irritable bowel syndrome, constipation and nervous system issues: tight muscles, spasms, tremors, unexplained pains, or other "tics" that are bothersome and may defy medical diagnosis.

Vata-dominant people are spontaneous, changeable, and tend to think and speak quickly. The vata mind is expansive, tending to look at the big picture and potential ideas over operational details. Vata prefers to initiate a new project than finish an old one. Finally, vata-dominant people tend to be articulate communicators.

The primary functions of vata are related to movement, breath, circulation, speech, memory, and elimination—especially those aspects of each that are controlled by the nervous system.

When a vata person is in balance, he or she is trim, full of energy and enthusiasm, flexible, expressive, and an initiator of change. Classically, vata people are said to have a highly lucid or illuminated mind.

In poor balance, vata qualities are exaggerated. A lively mind turns to racing thoughts, anxiety, and insomnia. Flexibility and spontaneity become ungroundedness and unpredictability in work or relationships. A love of new projects becomes an inability to follow through. An effervescent nature becomes excessive chatter and difficulty listening. Most importantly, vata may strenuously resist routine of all kinds. Yet, restoring routine is the primary prescription for balancing vata.

It is possible that rheumatologic problems may be generated in vata through a vulnerability in the gut, such as IBS or leaky gut syndrome, as irritability in digestion is part of this dosha's tendency when imbalance occurs. Furthermore, vata's anxious nature and difficulty sleeping can erode wellbeing and worsen symptoms.[1]

Pitta dosha (fire and water) governs metabolism and is hot, intense, steamy, acidic, aggressive, and action-oriented. Good digestive fire is responsible for chemical and enzymatic *transformation* throughout the body, but especially in the stomach and small intestine. The pitta-dominant person tends to have a moderate-sized frame and the ability to gain or lose weight easily. He or she is often a versatile athlete with loose joints. The skin of a pitta person appears moist, glowing, and freckled with a reddish or ruddy tone. Hair is red or warm-colored with a tendency for early graying or balding. The person with a predominance of pitta has a strong appetite and may exhibit a fondness for hot foods, but excessive acid potentially leads to heartburn, reflux, diarrhea and gas.

The pitta-dominant person uses keen vision to set and achieve goals. His or her warmth, charisma, and joie de vivre attract and inspire others. Pittas' work ethic and abundant energy make for natural leaders whose uncompromising vision, love of beauty, and demand for perfection in herself or himself and others result in excellent work, albeit with a sometimes-critical nature. Still, pitta doesn't dwell on past problems, but rather expresses emotion/anger and moves on. Pitta expects and appreciates this same honesty from others.

When pitta is out of balance, good qualities can go sour. Keen vision can turn into unhealthy perfectionism and rage over perceived mistakes. Similarly, a strong work ethic may lead to burnout. If the pitta is ill, he or she may feel angry with the body for interrupting work or play. According to Ayurvedic physicians, when a pitta person does not leave time for proper rest and digestion, toxins*

* NB: The accumulation of toxins is referred to in Ayurveda as *ama*, which Western practitioners know as gallstones, LDL cholesterol, inflammation, and other forms of excess. Ama may aggravate any dosha and even "spill over" into other doshas, causing widespread imbalance.

build up and create inflammation, which may become chronic. The prescription for pitta is appreciation of beauty, life, and people. Music, nature, or art can all have a tremendously healing affect on pitta.

In the pitta person, rheumatologic dysfunction is hypothesized to be generated through inflammation. Failing to manage stress may be a key contributor, as demonstrated in a host of studies over the years.[17,19]

Kapha dosha (water and earth) creates structure in the body and is responsible for lubrication of joints and mucosal membranes. It is cool, cohesive, smooth, slow, solid, stable, and enduring. People expressing kapha tend to have a large, muscular build, with solid bones, stable joints, and broad shoulders and chest. Their vulnerability is in the chest (or sinuses) where they are more prone than others to develop respiratory congestion, asthma, or sinusitis.

Kapha is led by the taste buds, and loves sweet and sumptuous tastes and smells. However, kapha people do not digest quickly and report feeling full longer than their vata and pitta counterparts. Kapha generally needs more strenuous exercise than the other types to keep excess weight off.

In their interactions, kapha people tend to be reserved, preferring to listen and carefully choose words than to chat casually. Their voices are smooth, deep, and sonorous. They are gentle, trustworthy, loyal and even-keeled. Methodical by nature, they generally dislike having to change routines abruptly.

Key physiologic functions of kapha are protection of the tissues and bodily cavities (chest, pelvis, brain) through strong bones and solid muscle mass. Kapha also lubricates and cushions through saliva and mucous membranes, cerebrospinal fluid (CSF) and synovial fluid.

A balanced kapha has a strong body and unusually good health, compounded by high tolerance for discomfort. (Contrast this with the vata, who has a "twitchier" nervous system and worries about unusual sensations, and the pitta, who may have pain but chooses to "work through it.") Kapha in balance has excellent endurance, sound sleep, smooth digestion and elimination, and relaxed enjoyment of sensual pleasures.

In contrast, the unbalanced kapha may have developed a sedentary lifestyle, which can lead to exhaustion and sluggishness. When stressed, the kaphic person seeks sweet foods, leading to weight gain or edema. Classically, kapha tends to form cysts, tumors, and enclosed pockets of disease, all reflecting kapha's inward tendencies. All of these processes worsen rheumatologic conditions or help to usher in comorbid conditions.

Emotionally, an out-of-balance kapha person can become rigid, sullen, withdrawn. In relationships, a kapha's gentle, loyal ways may turn to jealousy or clinginess. At work, a reliable kapha may become resistant to any change. When it comes to disease management, the kapha's tendency to withdraw or feel guilty may bring on isolation, which has been shown to worsen outcomes in a number of diseases.[19–21]

How to Determine the Dosha or Doshas of Your Patients

According to Ayurvedic wisdom, all of us contain all three doshas, although most people are thought to have one or two dominant doshas. Approximately 5% of all people are *tridoshic*, with a relatively equal balance of all three.[1] A person is said to be in balance when he or she is expressing his or her particular doshic constitution (prakruti) in a healthy manner. Excellent self-guided questionnaires are available to determine prakruti, basic nature, and vikruti, the imbalances to be corrected. (See resource list at the end of the chapter.)

Ayurvedic Diagnosis and Treatment

The Ayurvedic practitioner takes a detailed history, focusing on current symptoms, sleep, appetite, diet, digestion, elimination, allergies, menstrual cycles, relationships, sexuality, and engagement in life. The exam includes a careful Ayurvedic analysis of the pulses, tongue, fingernails, and eyes as well as standard elements of the Western exam.

Diseases are seen as being uniquely expressed in people according to their prakruti and vikruti. While rheumatoid arthritis has primarily pitta and kapha components (inflammation and edema), autoimmune diseases in general can be described by an overly vigilant (vata) immune system inappropriately attacking (pitta) or protecting (kapha) the self from self. Once disease is advanced, it is likely that all doshas are affected.

When every dosha is out of balance, vata-calming therapies can be a wise place to start. Vata is considered the leader of all the doshas; when vata is healthy, the rest of the doshas are pulled toward health. Therapies that calm the mind, relax tense muscles, and create good sympathetic-parasympathetic balance and tone will tend to have beneficial effects throughout the body-mind.

Universal Ayurvedic Guidelines

No matter what the condition, Ayurveda recommends an ideal daily routine to help reset the system. Following even one or two of these steps may provide some physical relief and a sense of pride in achieving a goal.

AYURVEDA AND THE IDEAL DAILY AND SEASONAL ROUTINES

Ideally, early morning, from 2–6am, is quiet, fresh, undisturbed, and full of potential, just like the qualities of the *healthy* vata mind. Ayurvedic texts recommend early-morning meditation, before or near sunrise, when the mind has stirred out of deep sleep into dreaming (REM) and liminal states.

Kapha time (6 am to 10 am) is a heavier period for the body and mind. Indeed, oversleeping well into these kapha hours sometimes makes it harder, not easier, to arise. For those people who experience midmorning sluggishness, morning exercise or a stretch break may help.

From 10 am to 2 pm is pitta time, the hottest time of day when the body's digestive fires are said to be strongest. In Ayurveda, it is suggested to eat the biggest meal between 10 am and 2 pm and then to allow for a brief period of stillness followed by a gentle walk to aid digestion.

From 2 pm to 6 pm is again vata time. Although ideally a time of mental clarity, many experience fatigue, possibly driven by poor nutrition, post-caffeine crash, or an overfull schedule. To remedy this, Ayurveda suggests a brief period of meditation in the late afternoon, just before dinner.

From 6 pm to 10 pm is kapha time, when daily rhythms slow down. A light dinner is recommended and, whenever possible, it is suggested to make one's last media intake or conversations light, humorous, or inspiring. Journaling before bed can help address the mind's concerns and cultivate deep sleep.

From 10 pm to 2 am is pitta time, when, according to Ayurveda, the body wants to be in deep sleep in order to complete its digestive functions, which culminate in separating out and removing wastes.

It is important to note that life simply does not allow perfect adherence to these "rules" all of the time. However, even small shifts toward healthy routines may be worthwhile. It is up to our patients to do the experiments and decide which changes are helpful.

There are also seasonal recommendations for each dosha, but a detailed listing is beyond the scope of this chapter. A simple summary is to pay attention to temperature and seek appropriate clothing and food for the day. On cold, dry, windy days, seek warm clothing, humidified air, and warm soups or teas. On cool, soggy days, sitting in a warm, dry sauna, taking a dessert vacation, or eating warm, astringent (drying) foods may help alleviate symptoms. As simple as these remedies are, they are profound in their ability to increase quality of life through regular attention to the body's signals.

Exercise and Ayurveda

Exercise guidelines must be flexibly applied due individual patients' conditioning or injuries. In general, vata people have quick bursts of energy and are prone to tiring with exertion. Thus, gentle exercise, such as Hatha yoga, light walking, or tai chi may be best, especially in conditions such as fibromyalgia, in which strenuous exercise can be depleting and painful. As a practitioner I have found, however, it is best not to try, for example, to talk a runner out of running if he or she feels enriched by it. Far better to be doing something regularly and joyfully than to stop completely or overanalyze. At most, encourage the substitution of a day a week of yoga and let your patient evaluate the difference.

The pitta person is often a versatile, competitive athlete who needs no more than a reminder to modify intensity. Pittas who do not exercise may respond to a direct statement that lack of exercise will quite possibly harm their capacity to perform in other ways. If overuse injuries occur, moderately intense yoga or cross-training may help. For the pitta, the best recommendation may be simply to *remember to enjoy* the activity, and not participate solely to beat the competition.

Kapha, with its potential build-up of weight, fluid, and *ama*, needs to sweat, burn calories, and release toxins through vigorous exercise, unless badly deconditioned. Once cleared for exercise, the most important thing for kapha is to be invigorated and in touch, once again, with inner vitality that trumps sluggishness.

Healing Foods and Aromas

In Ayurveda, there are no "low carb" or "high protein" diets. Rather, there are six "tastes" that should be included at every meal.

- **Sweet**—most carbohydrates, breads, grains, oils and fats, unprepared meats, and sugar/sweeteners. Most of our calories are derived from "sweet" foods, as they are energy-rich and necessary for life. Seek complex carbohydrates when possible, and minimize simple, refined sugars. High-quality oils are best, such as first-cold-pressed extra virgin olive oil or flaxseed oil with lignans. These should always be taken over artificially hydrogenated oils and trans-fats.
- **Salty**—salt and salty fish, soy sauce, seaweed.

- **Sour**—lemons, citrus fruits, cheese, chutney, yogurt, relish, pickles.
- **Pungent**—hot foods and spices, such as cayenne peppers. Most herbs and spices have some element of pungent flavor: e.g. cinnamon, cloves, oregano, thyme, and parsley.
- **Bitter**—dark, leafy greens such as chard, kale, arugula.
- **Astringent**—tannic tastes that make your mouth feel dry, such as Granny Smith apples, pomegranates, some teas, or foods that soak up water when cooking, such as lentils and other beans.

When weight loss is desired, it is best to emphasize the pungent, bitter, and astringent foods, which are higher in nutrients and lower in calories. Still, all diets must include "sweet" as a source of energy.

The goal is for meals to contain all 6 of these in the proper proportion. Some foods have multiple tastes—such as oranges, which are sweet and sour, or dark chocolate, which is sweet, bitter, and astringent. For detailed instructions on doshic balance, it is helpful to consult a trained Ayurvedic practitioner. Basic guidelines follow.

- Vata people are best balanced by sweet, salty, and sour tastes, which are heavier, warming, lubricating, and grounding. In situations of extreme vata imbalance, vegetables are better eaten sautéed/cooked, as raw vegetables are poorly digested.
- Pitta people are balanced by sweet, bitter, and astringent, and aggravated by salty, sour, and pungent foods eaten in excess.
- Kapha people are balanced by pungent, bitter, and astringent foods, and should lower proportions of sweet, salty, and sour or gravitate to their lighter forms.

Lists of foods and their primary and secondary (and even tertiary qualities) in Ayurveda are vast. The goal of this chapter is not to provide a complete list, but rather an initial sense of direction. As always, high-quality, fresh foods, as free as possible from pesticides and other synthetic chemicals, are desired. Raw foods in general are minimized in Ayurveda, especially for vata, but when cooking vegetables, a light steaming or sautéing is fine. You want to leave life in the food. Raw fruits are fine, especially in season and in keeping with the body's preferences; e.g., a pitta person might pass by the sour grapefruit in favor of the sweeter mango or peach. With intuition, common sense, and these short guidelines, one can make good food choices without turning shopping and eating into a stressful event, which would be counterproductive.

Panchakarma and Herbal Remedies

Thus far, recommendations in this chapter have been designed to be used readily by the reader/practitioner without special training. *Panchakarma*, on the other hand, is a specialized system of cleansing that requires specific Ayurvedic training. Inpatient and outpatient programs exist, lasting from days to months. The purpose is a profound, yet gentle cleansing of metabolic wastes and habits that are not nourishing. Controlled studies are rare, but simple pre-/post-design studies suggest improvements in multiple chronic conditions.[14] Key steps are as follows:

- Oleation (*snehana*)—ingestion of sesame seeds and clarified butter (*ghee*) to quiet the digestive fires, soften wastes, and prepare for deeper cleansing.
- Laxative (*virechana*) to clear the lower digestive track. (May be eliminated for some patients.)
- Oil Massage (*abhyanga*) with dosha-specific oils in patterns that direct wastes to the body's organs of elimination. An oil massage in which warm oil is dripped on the forehead (*shirodhara*) may be added to balance vata.
- Sweat treatments (*swedana*) is used to promote release of toxins through the skin.
- Enemas (*basti*) with medical herbs are administered to those without health contraindications to help clear the intestines and nourish mucosa.
- Neti Pot/medicated nasal lavage is used to clear sinus passages of excess kaphic mucus. This is followed by an oil infused with aromatic herbs to protect and open the nasal passageways.
- *Vamana* (emesis) is used to clear excess phlegm and toxins from the upper GI system. It is prescribed rarely in the West, where there is a disturbingly high incidence of eating disorders.

Although these practices stretch our modern understanding, patients often express renewed energy by the end of the procedure, not to mention significantly less pain and physical limitation. One study suggests panchakarma results in overall reduction in toxicity load, specifically 46% less dichlorodiphenyldichloroethylene (DDE) and 58% less polychlorinated biphenyls (PCBs), both of which appear to contribute to hormone disruption, immune dysregulation, reproductive disorders, several types of cancer and other diseases.[14]

Ayurvedic Herbal Remedies

The last section of this chapter covers Ayurvedic herbs, several of which have been covered in the chapter on Herbal Remedies (Chapter 5). While there are literally hundreds of herbs used in Ayurveda, made even harder to study given their often combined nature, a few single herbs stand out as being commonly used and more frequently studied in a modern, Western lab or clinic.

KEY INGREDIENTS IN AYURVEDIC REMEDIES FOR RHEUMATIC CONDITIONS

Turmeric (*Curcumin longa*) appears to modulate inflammation via down-regulation of NF-κB and subsequent suppression of the expression of COX-2, 5-LOX, TNF-α, IL-1β, IL-6, IL-8, MMPs (matrix metalloproteinases) and AM (adhesion molecules).[22] In a small study, curcumin compared favorably to ibuprofen and phenylbutazone for morning stiffness, joint swelling, and walking distance, but was not rated higher in terms of overall effectiveness.[23] Animal studies show curcumin administered before injury can reduce inflammation.[24] Finally, a crossover RTC showed curcumin combined with ashwagandha, boswellia, and zinc to effect significant reduction in pain and disability.[25] The lack of negative side effects, especially gastric distress, make it attractive as a therapeutic choice.[15,22]

Ginger (*Zingebar officinalis*) contains 6-shogaol, which appears to be one of the multiple chemicals responsible for its anti-inflammatory effect.[26] Ginger has also demonstrated reduction in pain and improvement in mobility in humans, likely through the inhibition of the formation of cytokines. In a small study of patients with RA, cooked, fresh, and powdered forms led to pain relief, better joint mobility, and decreased swelling and morning stiffness.[27] In a follow-up observational study, 75% of patients with OA/RA had improvement in pain or swelling while taking ginger, up to 4000 mg.[28] A recent review found moderate evidence for the anti-inflammatory properties of ginger in OA and low back pain.[29] For practical uses, one gram powdered root is equivalent to approximately 10 grams or 1/3 oz fresh ginger root (1 1/3 to 1 1/2-inch slice). Ayurvedic remedies use ginger in teas, soups, sauces, and topical poultices.

Guggul (*Commiphora mukul*) use correlates with significant reduction of pain, stiffness, and improved function without side effects, in subjective and objective measures for older people with osteoarthritis.[30] Guggul is used alone and in Ayurvedic formulations for pain and cleansing, but does not have common culinary uses. The main side effect is reduced platelet stickiness.

Ashwagandha (*Withania somnifera*) is known in classical Ayurveda as a powerful rejuvenative to slow aging and treat a broad range of conditions from cancer to depression.[31] Recently, studies have shown its withanolides in combination with other herbs are effective against inflammation in OA, low back pain, limitations in walking, and high body mass index,[27,28,30,32] and in vitro studies show a novel chondroprotective effect that may explain its anti-rheumatic properties.[33] One case study reported reversible thyrotoxicosis in a pregnant woman.[34] Overall, its safety profile is excellent. Typical doses are 500–1000 mg daily to twice daily. For insomnia, prescribe it 30 minutes before bed.

A host of other Ayurvedic herbs, including cloves, cinnamon, cumin, coriander, cayenne, thyme, oregano, licorice, black pepper, shatavari, amla, harataki, bibhitaki, and guduchi[35–39] have all been studied and found to have at least initial, encouraging evidence that they may help to treat or sooth inflammation and diseases such as obesity, high cholesterol, heart disease, insomnia, anxiety, depression, and infections, which complicate rheumatic conditions.[17]

Recent data on the purity of Ayurvedic herbs were published in a JAMA article in August 2008. Twenty percent of the samples from the US and India contained arsenic, lead, or mercury at levels exceeding at least one standard for human safety.[40] In response, coalitions from the USA, UK, and Germany reanalyzed the data (www.ayurveda-nama.org), and concluded a 5% contamination level if supplements which were *meant* to contain these metals were excluded. Still, they recommended no more prescribing overtly heavy-metal-containing formulations until science can better elucidate the health effects. Organic and vertically-integrated growers/sellers may offer better standards.

Based on thousands of years of observation and 50 years of modern research, a picture of Ayurveda is emerging as an important approach to worldwide health, including the prevention and treatment of chronic disease. Ayurveda's principles may engage patients in reframing their illness, and Western practitioners can look to their Ayurvedically trained colleagues to oversee particular nutritional and herbal preparations and panchakarma.

Resources

Several excellent resources can be found at the following sites:

- www.chopra.com – books, products, Ayurvedic consults, conferences and residential retreats in California and around the world

- www.kripalu.com – products, workshops, training in Ayurveda, Ayurvedic consults, and residential retreats in Massachusetts
- www.banyanbotanicals.com – products, certified organic
- www.ayurveda-nama.org – research, conferences, networking with professionals
- www.ayurveda.com – training in Ayurveda, consults, in-patient programs
- www.vediccity.net – comprehensive services and training programs; residential options

REFERENCES

1. Chopra D. *Perfect Health: The Complete Mind-Body Guide*. New York, NY: Three Rivers Press; 2000:46–102, 122–133, 152–154, 244–249.
2. Simon D, Chopra D. *The Chopra Center Herbal Handbook: Forty Natural Prescriptions for Perfect Health*. New York, NY: Three Rivers Press; 2000:17, 44–45, 83–84, 158–159.
3. Babu PS, Prabuseenivasan S, Ignacimuthu S. Cinnamaldehyde: A potential antidiabetic agent. *Phytomedicine*. 2007;14:15–22.
4. Gray AM, Flatt PR. Insulin-releasing and insulin-like activity of the traditional antidiabetic plant *Coriandrum sativum* (coriander). *Br J Nutr*. 1999;81:203–209.
5. Hlebowicz J, Darwiche G, Björgell LO, Almér L. Effect of cinnamon on postprandial blood glucose, gastric emptying, and satiety in healthy subjects. *Am J Clin Nutr*. 2007;85(6):1552–1556.
6. Mang B, Wolters M, Schmitt B, et al. Effects of a cinnamon extract on plasma glucose, HbA1c, and serum lipids in diabetes mellitus type 2. *Eur J Clin Invest*. 2006;36:340–344.
7. Chitthra V, Leelamma S. Hypolipidemic effect of coriander seeds (*Coriandrum sativum*): Mechanism of action. *Plant Foods Hum Nutr*. 1997;51:167–172.
8. Koscielny J, Klüssendorf D, Latza R, et al. The antiatherosclerotic effect of *Allium sativum*. *Atherosclerosis*. 1999;144:237–249.
9. Shah, BH, Z Nawaz, Pertani SA, et al. Inhibitory effect of curcumin, a food spice from turmeric, on platelet-activating factor- and arachidonic acid-mediated platelet aggregation through inhibition of thromboxane formation and Ca2+ signaling. *Biochem Pharmacol*. 1990; 58(7):1167–1172.
10. Chauhan NB, Sandoval J. Amelioration of early cognitive deficits by aged garlic extract in Alzheimer's transgenic mice. *Phytother Res*. 2007;21:629–640.
11. Kim DSHL, Kim J-Y, Han YS. Alzheimer's disease drug discovery from herbs: Neuroprotectivity from amyloid insult. *J Altern Complement Med*. 2007;13:333–340.
12. Colic M, Vucevic D, Kilibarda V, et al. Modulatory effects of garlic extracts on proliferation of T-lymphocytes in vitro stimulated with concanavalin A. *Phytomedicine*. 2002;9:117–124.

13. Kimura I, Yoshikawa M, Kobayashi S, et al. New triterpenes, myrrhanol A and myrrhanone A, from guggul-gum resins, and their potent anti-inflammatory effect on adjuvant-induced air-pouch granuloma of mice. *Bioorg Med Chem Lett.* 2001;11(8):985–989.
14. Herron RE, Fagan JB. Lipophil-mediated reduction of toxicants in humans: An evaluation of an Ayurvedic detoxification procedure. *Altern Ther Health Med.* 2002;8:40–51.
15. Shankar TN, Shantha NV, Ramesh HP, et al. Toxicity studies on turmeric (Curcuma longa): acute toxicity studies in rats, guinea pigs, and monkeys. *Indian J Exp Biol.* 1980;18:73–75.
16. Sharma HM. *Maharishi Ayurveda.* In: Micozzi MS, ed. *Fundamentals of Complementary and Integrative Medicine, 3rd ed.* St. Louis: Saunders Elsevier, 2006:518–535.
17. Sharma H, Chandola H, Singh G, Basisht G. Utilization of Ayurveda in health care: an approach for prevention, health promotion, and treatment of disease. Part 1–Ayurveda, the science of life. *J Altern Comp Med.* 2007;13(9):1011–1019.
18. Prasher B, Negi S, Aggarwal S, et al. Whole genome expression and biochemical correlates of extreme constitutional types defined in Ayurveda. *J Transl Med.* 2008;6:48.
19. Zellweger M, Osterwalder R, Langewitz W, Pfisterer M. Coronary artery disease and depression. *Eur Heart J.* 2000;25(1):3–9.
20. Afsar B, Elsureer R, Eyileten T, Yilmaz M, Caglar K. Antibody response following hepatitis B vaccination in dialysis patients: Does depression and life quality matter? *Vaccine.* 2009;27(42):5865–5869.
21. Scherrer JF, Virgo KS, Zeringue A, et al. Depression increases risk of incident myocardial infarction among Veterans Administration patients with rheumatoid arthritis. *Gen Hosp Psychiatry.* 2009;31(4):353–359.
22. Khanna D, Sethi G, Kwang S, et al. Natural products as a gold mine for arthritis treatment. *Curr Opinion in Pharm.* 2007;7(3):344–351.
23. Deodhar, S; Sethi, R; Srimal, RC. Preliminary study on antirheumatic activity of curcumin (diferuloyl methane). *Ind J Med Res.* 1980;7:632–634.
24. Funk J, Oyarzo J, Frye J, et al. Turmeric extracts containing curcuminoids prevent experimental rheumatoid arthritis. *J Nat Prod.* 2006;69(3):351–355.
25. Kulkarni R, Patki P, Jog V, Gandage S, Patwardhan B. Treatment of osteoarthritis with a herbomineral formulation: a double-blind, placebo-controlled, cross-over study. *J Ethnopharmacol.* 1991;33:91–95.
26. Levy A, Simon O, Shelly J, Gardener M. 6-Shogaol reduced chronic inflammatory response in the knees of rats treated with complete Freund's adjuvant. *BMC Pharmacol.* 2006;6:12.
27. Srivastava KC and Mustafa T. Ginger (Zingiber officinale) and Rheumatic Disorders. *Med Hypothesis.* 1989;29:25–28.
28. Srivastava KC and Mustafa T. Ginger (Zingiber officinale) in Rheumatism and Musculoskeletal Disorders. *Med Hypothesis.* 1992;39:342–348.

29. Chrubasik J, Roufogalis B, Chrubasik S. Evidence of effectiveness of herbal antiinflammatory drugs in the treatment of painful osteoarthritis and chronic low back pain. *Phytother Res.* 2007;21(7):675–83.
30. Singh BB, Mishra L, Vinjamury S, Aquilina N, Singh VJ, Shepard N. The effectiveness of Commiphora mukul for osteoarthritis of the knee: an outcomes study. *Altern Ther Health Med.* 2003;9(3):74–9.
31. Singh B, Mishra L, Aquilina N, Kohlbeck F. Usefulness of guggul (Commiphora mukul) for osteoarthritis of the knee: An experimental case study. *Alt Ther in Health and Med.* 2001;7(2):120.
32. Kulkarni S, Dhir A. Withania somnifera: an Indian ginseng. Prog Neuropsychopharmacol *Biol Psychiatry.* 2008;32(5):1093–105.
33. Sumantran VN, Kulkarni A, Boddul S, et al. Chondroprotective potential of root extracts of Withania somnifera in osteoarthritis. *J Biosci.* 2007;32:299–307.
34. van der Hooft CS, Hoekstra A, Winter A, de Smet PA, Stricker BH. Thyrotoxicosis following the use of ashwagandha. *Ned Tijdschr Geneeskd.* 2005;149(47):2637–2638.
35. Mancini-Filho J, Van-Koiij A, Mancini DA. Antioxidant activity of cinnamon (Cinnamomum *zeylanicum*, Breyne) extracts. *Boll Chim Farm.* 1998;137:443–447.
36. Mujumdar, AM, Dhuley, JN, Deshmukh, VK. Anti-inflammatory Activity of Piperine. *Jpn J Med Sci Biol.* 1990;43(3):95–100.
37. Shan B, Cai YZ, Sun M, Corke H. Antioxidant capacity of 26 spice extracts and characterization of their phenolic constituents. *J Agric Food Chem.* 2005;53:7749–7759.
38. Sharma J. Comparison of the anti-inflammatory activity of Commiphora mukul (an indigenous drug) with those of phenylbutazone and ibuprofen in experimental arthritis induced by mycobacterial adjuvant. *Arzneimittelforschung.* 1977:Jul;27(7): 1455–1457.
39. Thomson M, Ali M. Garlic [Allium sativum]: A review of its potential use as an anti-cancer agent. Curr *Cancer Drug Targets.* 2003;3:67–81.
40. Saper R, Phillips R, Sehgal A, Khouri N, Davis R, Paguin J, Thuppil V, Kales S. Lead, Mercury, and Arsenic in US- and Indian-Manufactured Ayurvedic Medicines Sold via the Internet. *JAMA.* 2008;300(8):915–923.

13

Homeopathic Medicine and Rheumatologic Disorders

IRIS R. BELL, MD, MD(H), PhD

KEY CONCEPTS

- The systemic nature of many chronic rheumatologic and autoimmune conditions lends itself to the holistic, patient-centered diagnostic and treatment approach of classical homeopathy.
- Individually chosen homeopathic remedies are reportedly helpful for some patients with nonspecific joint and muscle pain, osteoarthritis, fibromyalgia, and rheumatoid arthritis. Case reports claim benefit in autoimmune diseases such as systemic lupus erythematosus, ankylosing spondylitis, and scleroderma.
- Clinical case series and observational studies, as well as most—but not all—randomized controlled trials of patients with joint and other musculoskeletal complaints, indicate significant patient benefit for polysymptom pictures and quality of life under homeopathic treatment, with low rates of adverse effects and high levels of patient satisfaction.
- Patient-perceived empathy during the initial visit with the homeopathic provider has been shown, likely via enablement, to account for a small but significant portion of the variance in subsequent overall clinical improvement.
- Scientific advances in physical chemistry, materials science, and other basic research offer theoretical and empirical evidence consistent with the plausibility and activity of homeopathically prepared medicines (remedies) apart from placebo effects.

■

Introduction

Homeopathy, one of the established historical whole systems of complementary and alternative medicine (CAM) of Western origin, was developed more than 200 years ago by a German physician and chemist, Samuel Hahnemann, MD.[1] In the 1990s, Kaul reported that over 500 million people worldwide had used homeopathy.[2] Countries such as England, India, Germany, France, Belgium, Israel, and much of Latin America utilize homeopathy much more commonly than does the US.

Homeopathic treatment encompasses not only first-aid and acute care, which consumers often use as part of self-care, but also treatment for chronic conditions. Such care is provided mainly by specially trained practitioners with any of a range of credentials—from health care professionals such as MDs, NDs, RNs, DOs, and DCs, to professional homeopaths (RSHom, CCH, etc). Certain states in the U.S., including Arizona, Nevada, and Connecticut, have specific licensing laws for homeopathic physicians.

Useful resources for homeopathic information and practitioner referrals include the National Center for Homeopathy, the American Institute of Homeopathy, the Homeopathic Academy of Naturopathic Physicians, and the North American Society of Homeopaths.

Surveys of homeopathic practices in the US suggest that symptoms of arthritis are among the top 10 conventional diagnoses for which patients seek homeopathic care.[3] A recent chart audit study of 102 patients with rheumatoid arthritis (RA) in India revealed that 20% of the 215 reported courses of CAM treatments involved homeopathy.[4] Among Israeli patients seen in rheumatology clinics, 44% of the CAM users (N=148) cited homeopathy as the most common form of CAM. Perceived effectiveness in the latter study was reported more often by patients with spondyloarthropathies and osteoarthritis than for those with rheumatoid arthritis.[5] Conditions such as rheumatoid arthritis, osteoarthritis, bursitis, tendonitis, Lyme disease, and fibromyalgia are among those reported to be treated successfully, with sustained improvements in hundreds of case reports by homeopaths.[6] Clinically, homeopaths claim that their system is more helpful in treating disturbances of function rather than of structure per se.

Homeopaths do not claim to be able to reverse end-stage tissue destruction. For a given arthritis patient, homeopaths might predict an ability to relieve pain and put the disease process into remission for extended periods, but not to restore previously damaged joints. Nonetheless, chronic pain is one of the leading reasons that consumers try CAM therapies of all types, including homeopathy.[7] Some,[8] but not all,[9,10] studies suggest that patients can substantially reduce their reliance on conventional medications and costs when they include homeopathy in their treatment programs.

Notably, evidence indicates that the overwhelming majority of people who use CAM also rely upon conventional medical treatment.[11] Consequently, the way in which most patients would use homeopathy for rheumatological problems would be complementary, rather than alternative to Western medical treatments. They may, however, not inform their conventional physicians of their use of other types of care.[12] Other studies suggest that patients who use CAM systems such as homeopathy may have different baseline personality traits (e.g., openness to experience), compared with nonusers.[13]

Conceptual Bases of Homeopathy

The core tenets of classical homeopathy include the Law of Similars, i.e., that a substance capable of producing a pattern of symptoms in a healthy person can cure the same pattern of symptoms in a sick person. Hippocrates had made comparable observations many years before Hahnemann formalized his clinical system of care, stating: "Through the like, disease is produced, and through the application of the like it is cured." Another key concept in homeopathy is the Law of the Minimum Dose, involving the preference to use the lowest possible dose of medicine ("remedy" in homeopathy) to produce a beneficial effect without harm.

Finally, a leading early American homeopath, Constantine Hering, MD, additionally articulated the Law of Cure. Hering's Law states that natural healing proceeds from within outward (from more important to less important organs), from above downwards (from head toward toes), and in reverse order in time of original appearance (more recently developed symptoms resolve sooner than longstanding problems). The latter concept implicitly invokes a holistic view of the human being as an indivisible self-organizing system, where change at any level of the system has indirect effects on all other levels of organization of the system.[14,15]

Homeopathic medicines derive from natural animal, mineral, and plant sources. More standardized than other forms of complementary and alternative medicine (CAM), homeopathic remedies are manufactured in accord with FDA-regulated guidelines in the Homeopathic Pharmacopoeia of the United States and, often, by regulatory agencies in other countries as well.

Manufacturers prepare remedies by performing serial dilutions in an ethanol/water solvent mixture and succussing (vigorously shaking) the solution after each dilution step. Dose designations include "x" (dilution factor of 1/10), "c" (dilution factor of 1/100), and "LM" (dilution factor of 1/50,000). Succussion, which may play an essential role in differentiating a remedy from a plain dilution, is typically performed between 20 and 100 times per dilution step.

Experienced homeopaths rely upon detailed clinical history and observation rather than laboratory tests to choose one out of thousands of possible remedies for treating a given patient. In the diagnostic and treatment process for chronic diseases, classical homeopathy involves an in-depth interview and analysis of the way in which a given patient experiences the symptom pattern of illness. The approach is a holistic, highly individualized, patient-centered care model that leads to prescription of a single remedy (medicine) to treat the totality of the patient's problems—mental, emotional, and physical. Homeopaths look for qualitative themes that permeate the case at every level of organization of the person as an indivisible system.

Skeptics propose that the homeopathic remedies per se are only placebos, and that the therapeutic effects of treatment relate entirely to the alliance between patient and provider. Preliminary studies support the notion that practitioner empathy has some influence on clinical outcomes in homeopathic patients, in part via enablement.[16] However, the correlation coefficients relating empathy ratings at the intake session with subsequent 3-month and 12-month outcomes are weak (roughly $r=0.2$ for chief complaint and global wellbeing at 3 months ($p<0.05$); and $r=0.03$ at 12 months [NS]). Still, a greater sense of self-efficacy is associated with improved quality of life for patients with arthritis.[17] Moreover, the body of data demonstrating in vitro, animal, adult self-care, and infant effects of homeopathic remedies suggests that the patient–provider relationship is a factor, but not itself a sufficient explanation for overall outcomes (see also below).[18]

Classical homeopathic diagnosis involves its own specific diagnostic approach at the whole-patient level that does not overlap with the more local, disease-oriented diagnostic labels of conventional Western medicine. The homeopathic practitioner looks at how the patient manifests his/her particular symptoms, with special attention to general (global) features, often considering the mental/emotional aspects of the symptoms. For instance, a patient with the flu who is dull and listless would receive a different remedy (e.g., gelsemium) from one who is anxious and restless (e.g., arsenicum album), even if the strain of influenza virus and common physical symptoms of flu were the same in both cases.

Treatment relies upon the single remedy whose documented effects on healthy people match the clinical picture of those manifested by the patient.

Homeopathic remedies reportedly useful for patients with acute inflammatory episodes of arthritis include aconite, belladonna, apis, bryonia, kalmia, and pulsatilla.[6]

Homeopathic remedies have extremely favorable safety records[8,10,19,20] with no significant concerns about drug–drug interactions, in contrast with other forms of CAM such as nutritional or herbal supplements.

Clinical Evidence for Homeopathic Remedy Effects in Rheumatologic Patients

Table 13.1 summarizes the significant set of large observational studies evaluating homeopathy in primary care on thousands of patients in multiple different countries. While the observational data cover a variety of clinical conditions from a Western medical perspective, chronic pain and affective disorders are common across most studies. The rates of reported benefit are generally 70%–90% for both psychological and physical symptoms, with as low or lower rates of adverse reactions from homeopathy compared with conventional care. Patient satisfaction with homeopathic treatment is also high, typically averaging around 80%.[21]

Table 13.2 gives an overview of major randomized controlled clinical trials (RCTs) of various homeopathic approaches in the treatment of rheumatoid arthritis, osteoarthritis, and fibromyalgia. As is common for many research areas in CAM,[22] homeopathic RCTs are small in number and limited in sample size per study. Thus, there are some positive[23] and a few negative studies[24] of individualized homeopathy for RA; one recent positive equivalence study of an externally-applied commercial homeopathic mixture in osteoarthritis of the knee;[25] and two positive studies of individualized homeopathy for fibromyalgia.[26,27] Previous systematic reviews of the controlled trial literature found that homeopathic remedies may have efficacy in rheumatic conditions overall,[28] or in osteoarthritis specifically,[29] but determined that the evidence was as yet insufficient for definitive conclusions.

Previous meta-analyses performed using the entire database of higher-quality controlled clinical trials on all forms of homeopathy used across

Remedies chosen more often by experienced homeopaths for fibromyalgia patients in a placebo-controlled, double-blind RCT of individualized homeopathy included rhus toxicodendron, calcarea carbonica, causticum, and cimicifuga.[26]

Table 13.1. Summary of Large-Scale Observational Trials on Homeopathy.

Authors	*Sample*	*Conclusions*
Witt et al[10]	N=3981 primary care patients with 97% chronic diagnoses homeopathically treated in Germany and Switzerland; prospective follow-up for 2 years	Significant reduction in disease severity and marked improvements in quality of life
Van Wassenhoven & Ives[8]	N=782 general medical practice patients homeopathically treated in Belgium; retrospective reports, with 78% reporting disease-related interference with activities of daily living	89% improved on homeopathic treatment, with 2.4% reported worsening; prescription drug costs were 1/3 of conventional medical practice costs
Guthlin et al[19]	N=900, general practice patients with chronic illnesses homeopathically treated in Germany; prospective follow-up for up to 4 years	Mid to large size effects for SF-36 quality of life rating scale improvements
Haidvogl et al., 2007	N=857 acute respiratory and/or ear complaints in primary care patients from 8 different countries receiving homeopathy versus conventional care	Homeopathy was equivalent to conventional care for overall improvement, but onset of improvement was faster with homeopathic treatment. Adverse events in adults were lower for homeopathy than for conventional care (3.1% vs. 7.6%). No difference for adverse event rates in children (homeopathy: 2.0%; conventional: 2.4%)

all conditions are themselves flawed, biased (at least from the point of view of whichever side was not supported by the conclusions), and mixed in terms of positive[30] and negative[31] conclusions. The net number of papers used in these meta-analyses is small and heterogeneous. For example, in the analysis by Shang and coworkers, only 8 studies were chosen out of 110 initially identified.[31] Such meta-analyses are of questionable value in determining applicability to a given rheumatologic patient considering a particular form of homeopathic treatment.

Several additional small-scale studies of homeopathy, in patients with symptoms that are often seen in rheumatologic conditions, are also promising.

Table 13.2. Randomized Controlled Trials of Homeopathy in Rheumatology-Relevant Conditions.

Authors	*Sample*	*Conclusions*
Fisher & Scott,[79]	N=112 RA patients (seropositive); with 58 completers at 6 months.	High drop-out rate. No evidence of benefit with homeopathy vs placebo.
Andrade et al.[24]	N=44 RA patients followed for 6 months	High drop-out rate. No significant differences between active and placebo for effects or side effects.
Gibson et al.[23]	N=46 RA patients followed for 3 months	Greater improvement in pain, articular index, stiffness, and grip strength with homeopathy vs placebo
Van Haselen & Fisher,[80]	N=184 radiographically confirmed osteoarthritis of knee patients, followed for 4 weeks	Externally applied homeopathic gel as effective and as well tolerated as nonsteroidal anti-inflammatory drug gel
Fisher et al.[27]	N=30 UK patients with fibromyalgia in 2-month crossover design	Pain and sleep improved significantly more in homeopathy vs placebo condition.
Bell et al.[70]	N=62 US patients with fibromyalgia in 3-month parallel group design	Significantly greater improvements in tender point pain, quality of life, global health ratings in individualized homeopathy vs placebo group

For example, RCTs have demonstrated positive findings for adjunctive homeopathic remedies in patients with xerostomia,[32] adults hospitalized for sepsis,[33] and children with stomatitis secondary to chemotherapy.[34] The literature on the acute use of the homeopathic remedy arnica for postsurgical edema and pain over a range of different surgical procedures reveals mixed findings, though a report on three RCTs in patients after knee surgery was positive in favor of arnica.[35] Common methodologic flaws in arnica studies are the lack of quality assessment for the choice, and dosing pattern of the remedy.

The lack of an extensive RCT literature on homeopathy specifically for rheumatology is problematic, though not unusual for the state of the science in CAM overall. Homeopathy is, historically, like other forms of CAM, a clinical discipline with little academic infrastructure or funding for researchers, as well as publication bias against the field.[36]

In short, a rheumatologist considering referral for homeopathy can find practitioners with nationally recognized credentials in the field, and extensive observational evidence for effectiveness and safety, but relatively little RCT data to guide decision-making. Some CAM investigators have argued that the historical and ongoing widespread utilization and safety records for many longstanding modalities (e.g., homeopathy, acupuncture and Ayurveda), support greater initial weighting for observational data from effectiveness designs (complex, multifactorial, real-world) over efficacy designs (mechanism-oriented, idealized),[37] especially when mechanisms are not as yet clearly defined. Thus, novel approaches of effectiveness measurement may be required to evaluate homeopathy.

As outlined in the section below, for appropriate design of efficacy studies in homeopathy, investigators still need to develop testable, non-pharmaceutically-oriented hypotheses concerning possible mechanisms of homeopathic action. Even the assumption that patient–provider relationship, not the remedies, is the primary operative factor in homeopathic outcomes, falls short as the sole mechanistic hypothesis when directly examined.[16]

Once adequate and testable models are available, then investigators can embark on more appropriately designed, efficacy-oriented research programs.[38–40] From a practical perspective, it may be more useful for clinicians and their patients to answer well-grounded effectiveness, rather than efficacy questions at present, using appropriate comparison groups.[41] Effectiveness studies examine the outcomes from the real-world intervention as an intact clinical whole, including interpersonal and remedy factors.

Recent Advances in the Basic and Preclinical Science Underlying Homeopathy

THE NATURE OF HOMEOPATHIC REMEDIES

Throughout its history, skeptics have attacked homeopathy from a variety of perspectives, most notably on the issue of the absence of remaining molecules of source material in the more dilute forms of the remedies.[42] Some homeopathic remedies are diluted beyond Avogadro's number. However, in dismissing the plausibility of generating an active agent, the skeptics typically overlook the potential contribution of the succussion process and the resultant changes from turbulence and pressure within the liquid during remedy preparation.

Recent developments in the modern scientific worlds of physical chemistry and materials science offer substantial evidence that the primary argument against the plausibility of homeopathy, an argument based on composition rather than of structure, is seriously flawed.[43] The data in the basic science, preclinical, and clinical arenas, all point to the likelihood that homeopathically prepared remedies do not act mechanistically like conventional pharmaceutical drugs, but that they nonetheless possess unique and measurable properties in vitro and in vivo.[25,44,45]

A detailed discussion of the relevant data is beyond the scope of this chapter. However, as the implausibility argument runs so strongly through the interpretation of any clinical data or case report findings,[46–48] it is necessary to address it in materials otherwise geared toward a clinical readership.[49–51] Studies using several different technologies, including calorimetry,[52–54] thermoluminescence,[55] and UV–Vis spectroscopy[56,57] have demonstrated that homeopathically prepared remedies differ from both diluted but unsuccussed materials, and from diluted and successed control solvents.

Technologies such as NMR spectroscopy and infrared spectroscopy appear unable to demonstrate unique characteristics of homeopathic remedies. Silicate contaminants from the walls of the glass containers in which manufacturers prepare remedies may serve as essential factors that stabilize the agent, but do not impart specificity to the remedy.[58] A leading working hypothesis is that the heterogeneous and dynamic-network organizational structure formed by multiple water molecules in interaction, rather than the structure of individual water molecules or the chemical composition of the original source agent, contributes to the unique remedy properties.[59]

POTENTIAL ACTIONS OF HOMEOPATHIC REMEDIES IN LIVING SYSTEMS

As noted elsewhere, it is unlikely that homeopathic remedies act by conventional mechanisms of local drug-receptor interactions. At the least, remedy effects appear to be state-dependent on the condition of the host. Consistent with the Law of Similars (above), for example, animal data show that a remedy can worsen edema if given *before* an experimentally induced injury, but lessen edema if given *after* the injury.[60]

The existence of nonlinear, host-state-dependent effects at low material doses, of a variety of chemically different substances, is well established in the toxicology research literature for the phenomenon of hormesis.[61,62] Hormesis refers to favorable biological responses, or adaptations, produced following exposures to chronic, low-dose toxins or other stressors. To date, hormesis has only been shown for agents at low, but still material, doses under the Avogadro number cut-off (i.e., source molecules remain in solution). Advocates of hormesis are quick to insist that the ultradilute/succussed remedies of homeopathy are not part of their field. Nevertheless, empirical tests of agents such as ultradilute acetylsalicylic acid suggest a parallel kind of nonlinear dose-response pattern (e.g., thrombogenesis rather than antithrombotic action), as seen in the dose-response curves for agents in the hormesis literature.[63] The state-dependent findings indicate that homeopathic remedies, if they do possess clinically relevant activity, might be a potential treatment (but not a preventive measure) in some patients with rheumatologic diseases.

One potential advantage of using homeopathy in the CAM armamentarium is that treatment involves a single agent for dysfunction over the whole system, rather than at a local body part. As such, homeopathy may be particularly well suited to address the polysymptomatic, systemic phenomenology of many rheumatologic conditions, especially those involving autoimmune processes.

Human physiology and behavior reflect nonlinear, dynamical, complex system or network organization.[15,63–68] Emerging work of clinical theoreticians in homeopathy suggests that homeopathic treatment acts at both global and local levels of organization across the organism, in a potentially bidirectional, state-dependent manner.[69] Consistent with a complex systems/network perspective, fibromyalgia patients who subsequently exhibited both global and local clinical improvements on individualized homeopathic treatment showed early, objective changes in quantitative electroencephalographic alpha responses to their own remedy, not seen in placebo-treated patients or in the subset of patients on active remedies, who later failed to show a comparably favorable clinical response under double-blind conditions.[70]

Such a holistic conceptualization is consistent with evidence that organisms are complex networks whose global and local levels interact iteratively and shape each other's properties; i.e., behavior.[71] Various homeopathic clinicians and researchers focus on the unifying behavioral themes of the system as a whole (generalities and mentals), as also expressed in symptoms manifest dynamically at local levels, in their choices of remedy treatment.[69,70,72–75]

How might these phenomena occur? Some theoretical work proposes that remedies act by inducing changes in the body water of the patient that lead to systemwide self-reorganization of functional biochemical and cellular networks.[15,59,76] Additional evidence outside homeopathy suggests, for example, that water network structures serving as hub molecules in biochemical reactions may interact with the configuration of proteins to produce the ordered functionality of living cells.[77,78]

Ultimately, if remedies can act physiologically, they must demonstrate measurable effects on markers of dysfunction involved in processes such as inflammation. One commercial homeopathic combination product used

Homeopaths claim that steroid and similar treatment that has suppressed disease activity successfully long-term can interfere with the actions of homeopathic remedies. Prior disease-modifying medication treatments may help account for some of the negative RCT findings for homeopathy seen more in RA more than in other rheumatologic conditions.

worldwide for arthritis pain (Zeel®) exhibits in vitro ability to inhibit cyclooxygenase-1 and -2 as well as 5-lipoxygenase pathways.[25]

Summary

Since its inception, homeopathy has survived, despite both rational and irrational medical skepticism and multiple political controversies. Convergent evidence from multiple laboratories around the world demonstrates that homeopathically prepared remedies have unique physicochemical properties not seen with plain, and especially unsuccussed, solvent controls. Large observational studies and hundreds of case reports suggest patient improvement rates of 70%–80%, high levels of patient satisfaction, lower rates of adverse events, and often, but not always, lower overall health care costs associated with homeopathic treatment.

A unique potential value of homeopathy is as an adjunctive strategy in polysymptomatic patients who need or want to reduce reliance on multiple symptomatic medications. On the one hand, if a clinician requires overwhelming randomized placebo-controlled clinical trial evidence before recommending a complementary therapy such as homeopathy, the available data are currently insufficient to decide for or against its inclusion. On the other hand, the consistently favorable findings on high levels of patient satisfaction and low levels of serious risks from homeopathic treatment, make this type of intervention a pragmatic option. Expert referral to qualified homeopathic practitioners is preferable for chronically ill patients. In this situation, homeopathic care would serve as a component of overall case management for patients with inadequate responsiveness to and/or tolerance for conventional pharmacological therapies in rheumatology.

ACKNOWLEDGEMENTS

Iris Bell is supported by NIH/NCCAM grants K24 AT000057, R21 AT003212, and R01 AT003314.

Conflict of Interest Statement

The author is a consultant for Standard Homeopathic Company/Hyland's Inc.

REFERENCES

1. Merrell WC, Shalts E. Homeopathy. *Med Clin N Am*. 2002;86(1):47–62.
2. Kaul PN. Alternative therapeutic modalities. Alternative medicine. *Prog Drug Res*. 1996;47:251–277.
3. Jacobs J, Chapman EH, Crothers D. Patient characteristics and practice patterns of physicians using homeopathy. *Arch Fam Med*. 1998;7(6):537–540.
4. Zaman T, Agarwal S, Handa R. Complementary and alternative medicine use in rheumatoid arthritis: an audit of patients visiting a tertiary care centre. *Natl Med J India*. 2007;20(5):236–239.
5. Breuer GS, Orbach H, Elkayam O et al. Perceived efficacy among patients of various methods of complementary alternative medicine for rheumatologic diseases. *Clin Exp Rheumatol*. 2005;23(5):693–696.
6. Hershoff A. *Homeopathy for Musculoskeletal Healing*. Berkeley, CA: North Atlantic Books; 1996.
7. Barnes PM, Powell-Griner E, McFann K et al. Complementary and alternative medicine use among adults: United States, 2002. *Adv Data*. 2004;27(343):1–19.
8. van Wassenhoven M, Ives G. An observational study of patients receiving homeopathic treatment. *Homeopathy*. 2004;93(1):3–11.
9. Bornhöft G, Wolf U, Ammon K, et al. Effectiveness, safety and cost-effectiveness of homeopathy in general practice – summarized health technology assessment. *Forsch Komplementarmed*. 2006;13(Suppl 2):19–29.
10. Witt C, Keil T, Selim D et al. Outcome and costs of homoeopathic and conventional treatment strategies: a comparative cohort study in patients with chronic disorders. *Complement Ther Med*. 2005;13(2):79–86.
11. Caspi O, Koithan M, Criddle MW. Alternative medicine or "alternative" patients: a qualitative study of patient-oriented decision-making processes with respect to complementary and alternative medicine. *Med Decis Making*. 2004;24(1):64–79.
12. Eisenberg DM, Davis RB, Ettner SL, Appel S, Wilkey S, Van Rompay M, Kessler RC. Trends in alternative medicine use in the US, 1990–1997. Results of a follow-up national survey. *JAMA*. 1998;280:1569–1575.
13. Honda K, Jacobson JS. Use of complementary and alternative medicine among United States adults: the influences of personality, coping strategies, and social support. *Prev Med*. 2005;40(1):46–53.
14. Bell IR, Baldwin CM, Schwartz GE. Translating a nonlinear systems theory model for homeopathy into empirical tests. *Altern Ther Health Med*. 2002;8(3):58–66.

15. Bell IR, Koithan M. Models for the study of whole systems. *Integr Cancer Ther.* 2006;5(4):293–307.
16. Bikker AP, Mercer SW, Reilly D. A pilot prospective study on the consultation and relational empathy, patient enablement, and health changes over 12 months in patients going to the Glasgow Homoeopathic Hospital. *J Altern Complement Med.* 2005;11(4):591–600.
17. Lorig K, Ritter P, Plant K. A disease-specific self-help program compared with a generalized chronic disease self-help program for arthritis patients. *Arthritis Rheum.* 2005;53(6):950–957.
18. Mathie RT. The research evidence base for homeopathy: a fresh assessment of the literature. *Homeopathy.* 2003;92:84–91.
19. Guthlin C, Lange O, Walach H. Measuring the effects of acupuncture and homoeopathy in general practice: an uncontrolled prospective documentation approach. *BMC Public Health.* 2004;4(1):6.
20. Riley D, Fischer M, Singh B et al. Homeopathy and conventional medicine: an outcomes study comparing effectiveness in a primary care setting. *J Altern Complement Med.* 2001;7(2):149–59.
21. Goldstein MS, Glik, D. Use of and satisfaction with homeopathy in a patient population. *Altern Ther Health Med.* 1998;4(2):60–65.
22. Aickin M. The importance of early phase research. *J Altern Complement Med.* 2007;13(4):447–450.
23. Gibson RG, Gibson SL, MacNeill AD et al. Homoeopathic therapy in rheumatoid arthritis: evaluation by double-blind clinical therapeutic trial. *Br J Clin Pharmacol.* 1980;9(5):453–459.
24. Andrade LE, Ferraz MB, Atra E et al. A randomized controlled trial to evaluate the effectiveness of homeopathy in rheumatoid arthritis. *Scand J Rheumatol.* 1991;20(3):204–208.
25. Birnesser H, Stolt P. The homeopathic antiarthitic preparation Zeel comp. N: a review of molecular and clinical data. *Explore.* 2007; 3(1):16–22.
26. Bell IR, Lewis DAI, Brooks AJ et al. Improved clinical status in fibromyalgia patients treated with individualized homeopathic remedies versus placebo. *Rheumatology.* 2004;43:577–582.
27. Fisher P, Greenwood A, Huskisson EC, Turner P, Belon P. Effect of homeopathic treatment on fibrositis (primary fibromyalgia). *BMJ.* 1989;299:365–366.
28. Jonas WB, Linde K, Ramirez G. Homeopathy and rheumatic disease. *Rheum Dis Clin North Am.* 2000;26(1):117–123.
29. Long L, Ernst E. Homeopathic remedies for the treatment of osteoarthritis: a systematic review. *Br Homeopath J.* 2001;90(1):37–43.
30. Linde K, Clausius N, Ramirez G et al. Are the clinical effects of homeopathy placebo effects? A meta-analysis of placebo-controlled trials. *Lancet.* 1997;350:834–843.
31. Shang A, Huwiler-Muntener K, Nartey L, et al. Are the clinical effects of homoeopathy placebo effects? Comparative study of placebo-controlled trials of homoeopathy and allopathy. *Lancet.* 2005;366(9487):726–732.

32. Haila S, Koskinen A, Tenovuo J. Effects of homeopathic treatment on salivary flow rate and subjective symptoms in patients with oral dryness: a randomized trial. *Homeopathy*. 2005;94(3):175–181.
33. Frass M, Linkesch M, Banyai S et al. Adjunctive homeopathic treatment in patients with severe sepsis: a randomized, double-blind, placebo-controlled trial in an intensive care unit. *Homeopathy*. 2005;94(2):75–80.
34. Oberbaum M, Yaniv I, Ben-Gal Y et al. A randomized, controlled clinical trial of the homeopathic medication TRAUMEEL S in the treatment of chemotherapy-induced stomatitis in children undergoing stem cell transplantation. *Cancer*. 2001;92(3):684–690.
35. Brinkhaus B, Wilkens JM, Lüdtke R, Hunger J, Witt CM, Willich SN. Homeopathic arnica therapy in patients receiving knee surgery: results of three randomised double-blind trials. *Complement Ther Med*. 2006;14(4):237–246.
36. Caulfield T, DeBow S. A systematic review of how homeopathy is represented in conventional and CAM peer reviewed journals. *BMC Complement Altern Med*. 2005;5(1):12.
37. Fønnebø V, Grimsgaard S, Walach H, et al. Researching complementary and alternative treatments–the gatekeepers are not at home. *BMC Med Res Methodol*. 2007;7:7.
38. Frei H, Everts R, von Ammon K et al. Randomised controlled trials of homeopathy in hyperactive children: treatment procedure leads to an unconventional study design Experience with open-label homeopathic treatment preceding the Swiss ADHD placebo controlled, randomised, double-blind, cross-over trial. *Homeopathy*. 2007;96(1):35–41.
39. Frei H, Everts R, von Ammon K, et al. Homeopathic treatment of children with attention deficit hyperactivity disorder: a randomised, double blind, placebo controlled crossover trial. *Eur J Pediatr*. 2005;164(12):7587–67.
40. Frei H, Thurneysen A, von Ammon K. Methodological difficulties in homeopathic treatment of children with ADD/ADHD. *J Altern Complement Med*. 2006;12(2):104; author reply.
41. Concato J, Shah N, Horwitz RI. Randomized, controlled trials, observational studies, and the hierarchy of research designs. *N Eng J Med*. 2000;342(25):1887–1892.
42. Barrett S. Homeopathy: the ultimate fake. Available at: http://www.quackwatch.com/01QuackeryRelatedTopics/homeo.html. Accessed on March 18, 2008.
43. Rustum R. The latest science on water: great advances for whole person health. Available at: http://www.rustumroy.com/structure%20of%20water.htm. Accessed on March 18, 2008.
44. Belon P, Cumps J, Ennis M, et al. Histamine dilutions modulate basophil activation. *Inflamm Res*. 2004;53(5):181–188.
45. Mathie RT, Hansen L, Elliott MF, Hoare J. Outcomes from homeopathic prescribing in veterinary practice: a prospective, research-targeted, pilot study. *Homeopathy*. 2007;96(1):27–34.
46. Lancet T. The end of homeopathy. *Lancet*. 2005;366:690.

47. Langman MJ. Homoeopathy trials: reason for good ones but are they warranted? *Lancet*. 1997;350(9081):825.
48. Vandenbroucke JP. Homeopathy trials: going nowhere. *Lancet*. 1997;350:824.
49. Aickin M. The end of biomedical journals: there is madness in their methods. *J Altern Complement Med*. 2005;11(5):755–757.
50. Bell IR. All evidence is equal, but some evidence is more equal than others: can logic prevail over emotion in the homeopathy debate? *J Altern Complement Med*. 2005;11(5):763–769.
51. Fisher P. Homeopathy and The Lancet. Evid Based *Complement Altern Med*. 2006;3(1):145–147.
52. Elia V, Napoli E, Germano R. The 'Memory of Water': an almost deciphered enigma. Dissipative structures in extremely dilute aqueous solutions. *Homeopathy*. 2007;96(3):163–169.
53. Elia V, Niccoli M. New physico-chemical properties of extremely diluted aqueous solutions. *J Therm Anal Calorim*. 2004;75:815–836.
54. Elia V, Niccoli M. Thermodynamics of extremely diluted aqueous solutions. *Ann N Y Acad Sci*. 1999; 879:241–248.
55. Rey L. Thermoluminescence of ultra-high dilutions of lithium chloride and sodium chloride. *Physica A*. 2003;323:67–74.
56. Rao M, Roy R, Bell IR. Characterization of the structure of ultra dilute sols with remarkable biological properties. *Materials Letters*. 2008;62:1487–1490.
57. Rao ML, Roy R, Bell IR. The defining role of structure (including epitaxy) in the plausibility of homeopathy. *Homeopathy*. 2007;96(3):175–182.
58. Anick DJ, Ives JA. The silica hypothesis for homeopathy: physical chemistry. *Homeopathy*. 2007;96(3):189–195.
59. Roy R, Tiller W, Bell IR et al. The Structure of Liquid Water: Novel Insights from Materials Research and Potential Relevance to Homeopathy. *Materials Research Innovation*. 2005;9(4):557–608.
60. Bertani S, Lussignoli S, Andrioli G et al. Dual effects of a homeopathic mineral complex on carrageenan-induced oedema in rats. *Br Homoeopath J*. 1999;88(3):101–105.
61. Calabrese EJ. Toxicological awakenings: the rebirth of hormesis as a central pillar of toxicology. *Toxicol Appl Pharmacol*. 2005;204(1):1–8.
62. Calabrese EJ, Baldwin LA. Hormesis: a generalizable and unifying hypothesis. *Crit Rev Toxicol*. 2001;31:353–424.
63. Doutremepuich C, Aguejouf O, Pintigny D et al. Thrombogenic properties of ultra-low-dose of acetylsalicylic acid in a vessel model of laser-induced thrombus formation. *Thromb Res*. 1994;76(2):225–229.
64. Bar-Yam Y. *Dynamics of Complex Systems*. Reading, MA: Perseus Books; 1997.
65. Fredrickson BL, Losada MF. Positive affect and the complex dynamics of human flourishing. *Am Psychol*. 2005;60(7):678–686.
66. Goldberger AL. Non-linear dynamics for clinicians: chaos theory, fractals, and complexity at the bedside. *Lancet*. 1996;347:1312–1314.
67. Lipsitz LA, Goldberger AL. Loss of 'complexity' and aging. Potential applications of fractals and chaos theory to senescence. *JAMA*. 1992;267:1806–1809.

68. Mandell AJ, Selz KA. Nonlinear dynamical patterns as personality theory for neurobiology and psychiatry. *Psychiatry*. 1995;58:371–90.
69. Sankaran R. *Sensation Refined*. Mumbai, India: Homeopathic Medical Publishers; 2007.
70. Bell IR, Lewis DA, 2nd, Schwartz GE et al. Electroencephalographic cordance patterns distinguish exceptional clinical responders with fibromyalgia to individualized homeopathic medicines. *J Altern Complement Med*. 2004;10(2):285–99.
71. Vasquez A, Dobrin R, Sergi D et al. The topological relationship between the large-scale attributes and local interaction patterns of complex networks. *Proc Natl Acad Sci U S A*. 2004;101(52):17940–17945.
72. Bell IR, Lewis DA, 2nd, Brooks AJ et al. Individual differences in response to randomly assigned active individualized homeopathic and placebo treatment in fibromyalgia: implications of a double-blinded optional crossover design. *J Altern Complement Med*. 2004;10(2):269–283.
73. Bellavite P. Complexity science and homeopathy: a synthetic overview. *Homeopathy*. 2003;92(4):203–212.
74. Hyland ME, Lewith GT. Oscillatory effects in a homeopathic clinical trial: an explanation using complexity theory, and implications for clinical practice. *Homeopathy*. 2002;91(3):145–149.
75. Sherr J. Dynamic Materia Medica. Syphilis: A Study of Syphilitic Miasm through Remedies. Great Malvern Worcestershire, England: Dynamis Books; 2002.
76. Torres JL. Homeopathic effect: a network perspective. *Homeopathy*. 2002;91(2): 89–94.
77. Barabasi AL, Bonabeau E. Scale-free networks. *Sci Am*. 2003;288(5):60–69.
78. Watterson JG. The pressure pixel – unit of life? *Biosystems*. 1997;41(3):141–152.
79. Fisher P, Scott DL. A randomized controlled trial of homeopathy in rheumatoid arthritis. *Rheumatology*. 2001;40(9):1052–1055.
80. van Haselen RA, Fisher PA. A randomized controlled trial comparing topical piroxicam gel with a homeopathic gel in osteoarthritis of the knee. *Rheumatology*. 2000;39(7):714–719.

14

Rheumatoid Arthritis

DANIEL MULLER, MD, PhD

KEY CONCEPTS

- Rheumatoid arthritis is common, affecting 1 out of every 100 persons
- The mainstay of therapy is allopathic using disease modifying agents to stop the progression of the disease
- Complementary therapy can be of immense help in managing disease, particularly exercise, mind-body therapies, and anti-inflammatory diet and supplements
- A single joint affected beyond the rest is presumed to be septic arthritis until proven otherwise

■

Case

A 43-year old woman presents with a history of a sudden onset of joint pain. Affected are all small joints of the hands, wrists, knees, and forefeet. A steroid dose-pack relieved all symptoms for one month, but was followed by a slow return of joint pain, now with minor swelling, and morning stiffness lasting 2 hours. There is no back pain. Her symptoms were moderately well-controlled for 3 more months on maximum doses of ibuprofen. She is now having a return of the pain, swelling, and stiffness. Of note, her father died unexpectedly 1 week prior to the onset of symptoms. She has 3 children ages 13-16, her husband is a busy attorney. She works half-time in a flower shop, and is having difficulty cutting flowers and picking up anything over 5 pounds. She eats mostly meat and potatoes, due to the dietary wishes of her husband and children. She has no regular exercise program. She is active in her church and has several close friends.

Physical exam reveals minimal boggy synovitis at the metacarpal phalengeal joints with tenderness. There is tenderness but no synovitis at the knees and metatarsal phalengeal joints. The rest of the joints are normal, as is the rest of the exam. Her BMI is in the normal range.

Laboratory evaluation revealed that she is rheumatoid factor positive, anti-cyclic citrullinated peptide (CCP) negative, and has only minimal elevations of her sedimentation rate. All other routine laboratory findings were negative. X-rays of her affected joints show minimal periarticular osteopenia and no erosions. MRI of her hands reveal minimal synovitis and no erosive disease.

Pathophysiology

Rheumatoid arthritis (RA) affects about 1 out of every 100 adults worldwide, and without treatment usually progresses to disability.[1] RA is likely caused by a pathologic immune response in a genetically predisposed person to an environmental insult, likely a viral or bacterial infection.[2] Epidemiologic studies show that genes encoding the class II major histocompatibility antigens are linked to clinical features of RA. The HLADR4 and DR1 proteins present foreign and self-antigens to T cells. These molecules are presumed to play a direct role in the etiology of this autoimmune disease by presenting an "arthritogenic" viral or bacterial antigen to T cells. However, no organism has been definitively linked to the etiology of RA. Antibiotic therapy with minocycline is helpful in mild disease, owing mainly to its direct immunomodulatory/anti-inflammatory effects, as opposed to its antibacterial activity. Other genes of the immune, endocrine, and neural systems may contribute to the pathogenesis of RA, while the precise pathophysiologic cascade is not yet defined.

RA is an autoimmune inflammatory disease in which immunosuppressive drugs constitute the mainstay of therapy. Certain cytokines, such as tumor necrosis factor (TNF), interleukins 1 and 6 (IL-1, IL-6), appear to play important roles, as inhibitors of these molecules decrease disease activity.[3–6] Similarly, the importance of the roles of cell surface molecules on B and T cells can be shown when used as targets for immunomodulatory therapy.[3–5,7,8]

Nonsteroidal anti-inflammatory drugs (NSAIDs) act to inhibit the enzymes that produce inflammatory prostaglandins, particularly thromboxanes and leukotrienes. The newer NSAIDs preferentially inhibit the cyclo-oxygenase-2 (COX-2) enzyme that produces certain of these inflammatory molecules. Unfortunately, these COX-2 inhibitors may have increased thrombotic and, hence, cardiovascular risks, and may have only moderate gastroprotection.[9,10] Celecoxib (Celebrex) is still on the market, albeit, with increased warnings, the other COX-2 inhibitors have been withdrawn from the market. Omega-3 fatty acids and certain botanicals such as ginger and turmeric also may act by decreasing the production or activity of inflammatory prostaglandins.[11–15]

The neural, endocrine, and immune systems all share "communication molecules" that interact extensively. Compounds from the hypothalamic-pituitary-adrenal axis (such as cortisol and corticotropin-releasing factor) and from the sympathetic-adrenal-medullary system, are linked to disease activity in RA.[16] Corticosteroid drugs have powerful disease-suppressing activity, with equally powerful adverse side effects, including osteoporosis.[17,18] Prolactin and the estrogenic and androgenic sex hormones have been postulated to play roles as well. Other environmental factors such as nutrition, coffee, and tobacco may also contribute to the increased risk of RA.[19–21]

Stress and psychological factors have been linked to the etiology of RA and to disease exacerbations.[22] In one study, psychological factors and depression accounted for at least 20% of disability in patients with RA, greater than the 14% attributable to articular signs and symptoms.[23] In another study, helplessness had a direct effect on disease activity.[24]

Integrative Therapy

EXERCISE

Joint pain can inhibit activity, leading to muscle disuse and atrophy. In turn, muscle atrophy can lead to decreased stability of joints. A variety of exercise activities are unseful in mitigating the effects of RA. Light weight training can maintain or even increase muscle strength around joints, leading to increased joint stability. Stretching muscles can help to decrease flexion contractures. Aerobic exercise improves mood, decreases fatigue, and helps to control weight gain. Water exercise can be helpful as it is less stressful on joints, but weight training and walking work better to decrease bone loss (osteoporosis). Finally, Asian exercise disciplines such as tai chi and yoga can also be extremely beneficial. A form of tai chi called the range of motion (ROM) dance is particularly suited to persons with disabilities (http://www.taichihealth.com). The Arthritis Foundation has extensive information on useful exercise programs around the country (www.arthritis.org).

PHYSICAL THERAPY AND OCCUPATIONAL THERAPY

Physical therapy and occupational therapy programs can be invaluable in the treatment of RA. Goals are to improve range of motion and strengthen muscles. Joint protection from deformities can be aided by education, and the judicious use of splints, orthotics, ambulatory aids, and other devices. Massage and local heat and cold applications decrease inflammation, increase circulation, and relax muscles.

MIND-BODY THERAPY

Meditation has been shown to be helpful for chronic pain.[25] A study of meditation in psoriasis, an autoimmune inflammatory skin disease, showed decreased time to clearing the skin disease.[26] There are 2 published studies investigating the role of meditation in RA. Pradhan and colleagues[27] reported improvements in psychological stress and well-being even after 6 months. Zartua and colleagues[28] reported that both cognitive therapy and meditation were helpful in RA, with better responses in subjects with depression.

Both cognitive-behavioral therapy and a coping intervention are useful in RA.[29,30] Self-help courses given through the Arthritis Foundation provide information about diseases and medication and can help in developing coping skills. Simply writing in a journal about positive and negative emotions for 15 minutes a day can be powerful medicine, relieving symptoms by 25% or more.[31]

NUTRITION

Food Triggers

Fasting clearly decreases symptoms in RA, especially during flares of the disease; however, symptoms usually recur with the resumption of food intake.[32] A small percentage of people with RA appear to have a food intolerance that exacerbates their disease. A much larger number believe that certain foods exacerbate symptoms, but this effect cannot be shown in blinded trials of food exposure. The offending foods are usually dairy products, wheat, citrus, or nuts. An elimination diet for 2 weeks, with the reintroduction of the suspected food, can be done with or without the supervision of a physician or a nutritionist.

Omega-3 and Omega-9 Fatty Acids

Increased intake of omega-3 fatty acids from cold water fish, such as salmon, and from nuts, such as walnuts, flaxseed, or hempseed, can provide modest improvement in the control of RA.[11,12,32] The role of saturated fatty acids (TRANS-fats) in increasing symptoms is unproved; however, in view of their association with cardiovascular disease, reduction in intake is worthwhile (see Chapters 2 and 3 for details).

Cooked vegetables and olive oil have been found to be independently protective for the development of RA. Omega-9 fatty acids in olive oil may confer anti-RA activity.[33]

Coffee

A high intake of coffee, 4 or more cups a day, has been linked to an increased risk of RA.[19,21] Intake should be decreased to below this level, or the patient can switch to green tea, which provides some caffeine, but with a benefit from its antioxidant polyphenols.

ELIMINATION OF TOBACCO USE

In addition to its inherent lung cancer risk, smoking also causes oxidant stress on connective tissue, as evident from the increased wrinkles seen in long-term smokers. One study has shown an association between smoking and increased risk of RA; therefore, RA patients should be counseled to avoid tobacco.[20]

SUPPLEMENTS

Essential Fatty Acids

Omega-3 fatty acids can be increased by dietary means or through supplementation. Approximate doses for supplementation are eicosapentaenoic acid 30 mg/kg per day and docosahexaenoic acid 50 mg/kg per day equivalent to 2-4 grams of fish oil daily.[11,32]

Gamma-linolenic acid (GLA), 1.4 to 2.8 g per day, the equivalent of 6 to 11 g of borage oil daily, also has been shown to be helpful.[11] Effects may not be felt for 6 weeks or more, and continued improvement may occur after many months.

Antioxidants

Antioxidant vitamins may be helpful in RA, as they seem to be in osteoarthritis. Additionally, vitamin E has some analgesic effects.[13] Vitamin E should be taken at 800-1600 international units (IU) daily as mixed tocopherols, and vitamin C at 250 mg twice per day. Selenium can be found in many foods including Brazil nuts; intake should be at least 100 μg daily, not to exceed 400 μg daily.

Recommended intake of calcium to prevent osteoporosis is 1500 mg daily. It is probably prudent to add magnesium at 400 to 750 mg daily and a vitamin D3 supplement at 1,000 to 4,000 IU per day.[34] Persons with darker skin color in northern climates will need higher doses of vitamin D. For a more in depth discussion of vitamin D therapy see the chapter 17 (Fibromyalgia).

BOTANICALS

Ginger

Ginger (*Zingiber officinale*) may have efficacy in RA by inhibiting inflammatory prostaglandins.[14]

- **Dosage.** As the dried root, 1g 2 to 3 times per day to start; increase up to 4 g daily. As a tea, 1 g of dried root steeped in 150 mL of boiling water for 5 to 10 minutes and strained; use 1 cup up to 4 times daily.
- **Precautions.** Ginger may stimulate bile flow, which can cause pain in the presence of cholelithiasis. Other risks include bleeding, hypertension or hypotension, and hypoglycemia.

Turmeric

Turmeric (*curcumin*) in an open trial has been shown to be similar to NSAIDs in efficacy.[15]

- **Dosage.** As powdered root, 0.5 to 1 g 2 to 3 times daily.
- **Precautions.** Risks include bleeding, gastrointestinal intolerance, and impaired fertility.

NOTE

Echinacea should be avoided by patients with rheumatoid arthritis, as there have been anecdotal reports of increased symptoms in persons with autoimmune disease.

PHARMACEUTICALS

Nonsteroidal Anti-inflammatory Drugs

NSAIDs can be used short-term with minor risk of gastrointestinal toxicity. The long-term use of NSAIDs, particularly in the elderly, poses significant risks for gastrointestinal bleeding. There are many NSAIDs, and many of the newer ones are restricted on some formularies. The popular classic NSAIDs include ibuprofen, used in a dose of 800 mg 3 times daily, and naproxen used in a dose of 500 mg twice daily. Both have antiplatelet activity. The advantage of using the COX-2 inhibitor, celecoxib, for possible decreased gastrointestinal toxicity, has been called into question.[10] Note, celecoxib shares a lack of antiplatelet effects with other newer NSAIDs. It should be kept in mind that these drugs also have the potential for renal toxicity and are no more effective than older NSAIDs. Recent data point to the risk of increased thrombosis in patients taking COX-2 inhibitors who have a preexisting increased risk of thrombosis or cardiovascular disease.[9] Two other COX-2 inhibitors have been withdrawn from the market. Celecoxib is used in a dose of 200 mg twice daily.

Corticosteroids

Corticosteroids can rapidly decrease RA symptoms, often within a few hours when used at high doses. However, both short-term and long-term toxic effects are well known. High and even moderate doses can lead to avascular necrosis of joints such as the hip, knee, or shoulder; fortunately, this is a rare occurrence. With proper care and early diagnosis of avascular necrosis, disability and joint replacement may be avoided. With long-term use, osteoporosis is a significant risk with doses above 7.5 mg daily of prednisone or equivalent. Due to risks of osteoporosis it is recommended that patients taking greater than 5 mg of prednisone or equivalent for greater than 3 months be started on a bisphosphonate.[35]

Other risks include atherosclerosis, diabetes mellitus, cushingoid features, acne, and infection. Often a minor disease flare can be treated with a moderately high dose such as 30 to 40 mg of prednisone orally and a rapid taper over the course of 1 to 2 weeks. In some patients, a low dose of corticosteroids appears necessary for optional function; prednisone 5 to 7.5 mg daily is often used for this purpose.[17,18] A common method of treating an RA flare is to give a long-acting depot preparation such as triamcinolone acetonide (Kenalog) 80 mg intramuscularly. This approach can often control disease for 1 to 2 months, long enough for the slower acting disease-modifying antirheumatic drugs (DMARDs) to start working. For disease flares in isolated joints, once infection is ruled out, an intra-articular injection of triamcinolone (Kenalog) 2.5 to 40 mg can be given to control local disease.

NOTE

Remember: *A single joint with severely decreased range of motion and increased pain is presumed to be infected until proven otherwise. The patient should be hospitalized overnight for joint aspiration to obtain culture specimens; blood should also be drawn for cultures, followed by administration of intravenous antibiotics until results of culture are known.*

Antibiotics

Antibiotics, particularly minocycline (Minocin) in a twice-daily dose of 100 mg, may be useful in patients with less severe disease.[36] Side effects include gastrointestinal intolerance, dizziness, photosensitivity rash, vaginitis, skin and gingival discoloration, and rarely hepatic, lung, and kidney injury. The salutary effects of these agents may not be due to their antibacterial activity, because the tetracyclines also show immunomodulatory and anti-inflammatory activities.

Disease-Modifying Antirheumatic Drugs

Disease-modifying antirheumatic drugs (DMARDs) are also referred to as slow-acting antirheumatic drugs (SAARDs) because they usually take 6 weeks to 3 months to show activity. The use of most FDA approved DMARDs are supported by Cochrane reviews including low dose steroids, hydroxychloroqine, sulfasalazine, methotrexate (with folic acid), azathioprine, leflunomide, cyclophosphamide, entanercept, adalimumab, and infliximab.

Hydroxychloroquine and Sulfasalazine

Hydroxychloroquine and sulfasalazine each are used early in disease when a diagnosis may not be clear or there is no characteristic erosive disease. Both drugs have little short-term and long-term toxicity.

- **Dosage.** The current accepted dose of hydroxychloroquine is 200 mg twice daily, which carries little risk of toxicity; nevertheless, an ophthalmologic examination to test for retinal toxicity (see precautions) is recommended every 6 to 12 months. To reduce gastrointestinal intolerance, sulfasalazine is usually used in an enteric-coated form; dosing is started at 500 mg a day and raised by 1 tablet every few days until a dose of 1 g twice daily is reached.
- **Precautions.** Hydroxychloroquine when used in high doses carries a risk of retinal toxicity due to deposition of the drug into the retina. Sulfasalazine can uncommonly cause rash, hepatotoxicity, and leukopenia.

Methotrexate

Of all of the so-called DMARDs, methotrexate has been shown to be tolerated for longer periods of treatment than any other drug.[37] Methotrexate is a folate antagonist and has a multitude of immunomodulatory activities, but its exact mechanism of action in RA is unknown. Doses of methotrexate for RA are usually between 5 and 25 mg given once per week. The dose is usually given orally in tablet form; however, the liquid form can be used orally and is sometimes less expensive. A former common practice was to start with 7.5 mg orally once per week and then increase. Today, most practitioners, including myself, recommend starting at a higher dose such as 15 mg once per week. With use of higher doses of 20 mg and above, patients are often taught to self-administer the dose subcutanously once per week to avoid possible problems with gastrointestinal absorption. To decrease side effects, I always prescribe folic acid 1 to 2 mg to be taken each day. A decision to start methotrexate therapy or to raise or decrease the dose should be placed in the hands of a practitioner with extensive experience. Methotrexate is the standard by which all other drugs are judged, yet few patients achieve remission, and less than a majority achieve a 50% improvement on composite scores.

Contraindications to use of methotrexate include preexisting hepatic, renal, or pulmonary disease; unwillingness to discontinue alcoholic beverages; and recent malignancy. There are many side effects, the most prominent being hepatitis, bone marrow suppression, pneumonitis, mouth sores, nausea, and headache. A complete blood count, platelet count, and determination of aspartate transaminase, albumin, and creatinine levels are done initially and then every 2 weeks for 6 weeks after methotrexate therapy is begun. Thereafter, monitoring can be done every 4 to 8 weeks. A baseline hepatitis screen and chest radiography are recommended. Tuberculosis skin testing is reserved for patients with strong risk factors or abnormal appearance on chest x-ray film.

Other Immunosuppressive Drugs

Many other immunosuppressive drugs are used in RA. Leflunomide is a newer drug that is similar in efficacy to methotrexate.[38] Leflunomide interferes with pyrimidine synthesis, whereas methotrexate interferes with purine synthesis. Leflunomide has fewer hepatotoxic effects and possibly less bone marrow toxicity but is much more likely to cause diarrhea. Azathioprine is metabolized to 6-mercaptopurine and interferes with inosinic acid synthesis. It is often is substituted for methotrexate; however, its use is associated with gastrointestinal and bone marrow toxicity. Other immunosuppressive drugs less commonly used are mycophenolate mofetil, cyclosporine, tacrolimus, and chlorambucil. Cyclophosphamide is often used to treat rheumatoid vasculitis.

RECOMBINANT BIOLOGICS

Recent advances in the therapy of RA targets cytokines and cell surface molecules used to communicate between cells of the immune system.[3–5] Etanercept (Enbrel), adalimumab (Humira), and infliximab (Remicade) are tumor necrosis factor (TNF) inhibitors.[39–41] Etanercept is given subcutaneously once or twice per week, adalimumab is given subcutaneously once every 2 weeks, whereas infliximab is usually given intravenously once every 2 months. Two newer TNF inhibitors, certolizumab (Cimzia) and golimumab (Simponi), were recently approved and can be given subcutaneously once per month.[42] These drugs are most often used with a cytotoxic agent, usually methotrexate, to reduce the development of antibodies toward these monoclonal proteins. Short-term safety is very high, with little toxicity. As many as 30% of patients may show almost complete remission of symptoms with the combination of methotrexate and a anti-TNF agent. Currently, there is about 10-years of data on long-term safety and efficacy.[43] Use of these agents carries a risk of life-threatening exacerbations of severe infections, especially sepsis. Patients should temporarily discontinue the anti-TNF therapy duing presumed infections and restart the therapy when the infection has resolved. All patients must be tested for latent tuberculosis using the PPD skin test before beginning therapy. These drugs also may exacerbate demyelinating disorders; therefore, they should be avoided in patients with suspected or proven multiple sclerosis or optic neuritis. An IL-1 receptor antagonist, anakinra (Kineret), is approved for the treatment of RA. It is given subcutaneously daily and also increases the risk of serious infection. Anakinra is generally thought to have lower efficacy in RA than other biologics. Agents directed toward a cell surface molecule on B-cells (rituximab, Rituxin),[7] and a costimulatory molecule on T cells (abatacept)[8] are both recently approved for treatment of RA. Another anti-cytokine biologic, directed toward IL-6,[7] tocilizumab (Actemra) is the most recently approved agent for use in RA.

NOTE

There are more than 170 possible dual-DMARD or triple-DMARD combinations among the 5 non-biologics; methotrexate, leflunomide, hydroxychloroquine, minocycline, and sulfasalazine. Add to this the five currently approved biologics, and you have a complicated set of decisions. There is some simplicity to this latter addition, since no two biologics can be used together due to unacceptable risks of infection. An excellent review has recently been published on the evidence supporting the use of these medications in different clinical scenarios (Saag, et al, 2008).

ACUPUNCTURE

Several small controlled trials of acupuncture in RA showed decreased knee pain for an average of 1 to 3 months.[44] For a detailed discussion, please refer to Chapter 10.

LOW LEVEL LASER THERAPY

Low Level Laser Therapy (LLLT) uses a single wavelength laser source that likely has photochemical effects, and not thermal effects, on cells. A recent Cochrane review suggests that LLLT could be considered for short-term relief of pain and morning stiffness for RA patients, particularly since it has few side-effects.[45]

SURGERY

Loss of joint function and intractable pain may be indications for surgical intervention. Synovectomy can be helpful when systemic therapy and intra-articular corticosteroids are ineffective. Joint replacement can help to restore function and to increase independent activity. Patients with RA have an increased risk of surgical and postoperative complications. Cervical spine disease can lead to spinal instability and risk of neurologic injury. Replacement of one joint can result in increased stress on other joints during recovery and rehabilitation. Note that long-term corticosteroid use can cause fragility of vessels and connective tissue, hence, increasing the risks of surgery.

OTHER THERAPIES TO CONSIDER

There have not been adequate studies on the role of traditional Chinese medicine, Ayurveda, homeopathy, or spiritual therapies in the management of RA. Patients should learn about several different modalities and then record their feelings about these modalities in a journal. They may then choose to visit a practitioner of a selected modality for a trial of the techniques. If the economic burden is not too great, further exploration of that therapeutic modality may be in order.

Summary

Evidence is accumulating that current allopathic treatments are successful in slowing joint destruction and in decreasing the mortality associated with RA.[37,39–41,42,43,46] In addition, the rates of extra-articular manifestations of RA, such as Felty's syndrome and rheumatoid vasculitis, seem to be decreasing. Therefore, in any but the mildest cases of RA, an integrated approach should include the so-called DMARDs, usually starting with methotrexate, particularly if erosive disease is seen. NSAIDs are used as little as possible owing to gastrointestinal toxicity. The classic NSAIDs are ibuprofen and naproxen at maximal doses. The COX-2 inhibitors decrease but do not eliminate the risk of gastrointestinal bleeding.

A majority of patients with RA are receiving combinations of drugs. Most patients are given methotrexate therapy unless there are contraindications or side effects. A common combination is methotrexate and hydroxychloroquine.

Corticosteroids in moderately high doses with a rapid taper are often used for exacerbations. Commonly, a TNF inhibitor such as etanercept, adalimumab, or infliximab is added if methotrexate is only partially effective. Leflunomide or azathioprine is often substituted for methotrexate if there are intolerable side effects with methotrexate. Methotrexate and leflunomide can be used together with only a modest increase in risk of side effects. The DMARDs and the recombinant biologics have many varied side effects, some of which are only now being defined. New biologics seem to be coming on the market at an increasing rate. The immunosuppressive pharmaceuticals should be used only with input from a subspecialist rheumatologist.

All patients should be counseled about exercise and mind-body techniques, and journaling should be encouraged. Exacerbating factors such as smoking should be eliminated. With suspected intolerance to dairy products, wheat, citrus, or nuts, a trial of an elimination diet for 2 weeks with the reintroduction of the suspected food can be undertaken. Encourage a diet rich in omega-3 fatty acids or use supplements. Vitamin E should be taken as mixed tocopherols, and vitamin C should be added. Maintain adequate selenium intake as Brazil nuts or supplements. Recommend adequate intake of calcium and, perhaps, magnesium, and a vitamin D supplement is strongly recommended. Try botanicals such as ginger and turmeric. Avoid Echinacea.

Acupuncture can be tried for any patient with RA. This modality may be less effective in patients taking corticosteroids. Low Level Laser Therapy (LLLT) can be tried with little risk of side effects.

Loss of joint function and intractable pain may be indications for surgical intervention. Synovectomy can be helpful when systemic therapy and intra-articular corticosteroids are ineffective. Joint replacement can help to restore function and to increase independent activity.

Case Revisited

This 43-year old woman has mild, non-erosive RA. She needs to find time to rest as well as increase her physical activity. I would start with the mild DMARD hydroxychloquine and perhaps a systemic steroid depot injection to decrease symptoms quickly and allow for the 6-12 weeks that the the DMARD will need to take effect. We can recommend warm water pool aerobics and physical therapy. Consider adding fish oil at 2-4 grams per day, as well as ginger and tumeric. Encourage her to eat more fresh fruits and vegetables and decrease red meat, trans-fats, and corn syrup. Evaluate her calcium and vitamin D intake and sun exposure. Approach the use of mind-body therapies, journaling, and other complementary therapies, keeping in mind the patient's openness to new ideas, and possible barriers. Counsel her on the the supporting evidence for these modalities. Encourage her to create her own path toward healing.

See chapters on mind-body therapies, herbal medicine, nutrition, fatty-acids, homeopathy, and ayruvedic for further ideas and more in-depth reviews. Keep in mind that many patients have coexistant osteoarthritis either as a primary problem or secondary to RA; the chapter on osteoarthritis (17) provides further ideas for integrative treatment.

REFERENCES

1. Jantti J, Aho K, Kaarela K, Kautiainen H. Work disability in an inception cohort of patients with seropositive rheumatoid arthritis: a 20 year study. *Rheumatol.* 1999;38:1138–1141.
2. Muller D. The molecular biology of autoimmunity. *Immunol Allergy Clin North Am.* 1996;16:659–682.
3. Choy E, Panayi G. Cytokine pathways and inflammation in rheumatoid arthritis. *N Engl J Med.* 2001;344:907–916.
4. Olsen N, Stein CM. New drugs for rheumatoid arthritis. *N Engl J Med.* 2004;350:2167–2179.
5. Singh R, Robinson DB, El-Gabalawy HS. Emerging biologic therapies in rheumatoid arthritis: cell targets and cytokines. *Curr Opin Rheumatol.* 2005;17:274–279.
6. Choy E. Clinical experience with inhibition of interleukin-6. *Rheum Dis Clin NA.* 2004;30:405–415.
7. Edwards J, Szczepanski L, Szechinski J, et al. Efficacy of B-cell-targeted therapy with rituximab in patients with rheumatoid arthritis. *N Eng J Med.* 2004;350:2572–2581.
8. Genovese M, Becker J, Schiff M, et al. Abatacept for rheumatoid arthritis refractory to tumor necrosis factor alpha inhibition. *N Eng J Med.* 2005;353:1114–1123.
9. Kimmel S, Berlin J, Reilly M, et al. Patients exposed to rofecoxib and celecoxib have different odds of nonfatal myocardial infarction. *Ann Int Med.* 2005;142:157–164.
10. Stockl K, Cypren L, Chang E. Gastrointestinal bleeding rates among managed care patients newly started on COX-2 inhibitors or nonselective NSAIDs. *J Manag Care Pharm.* 2005;11:550–558.
11. Mangge H, Herman J, Schauenstein K. Diet and rheumatoid arthritis–a review. *Scand J Rheumatol.* 1999;28:201–209.
12. Ernst E, Chrubasik S. Phyto-anti-inflammatories: A systemic review of randomized, placebo-controlled, double-blind trials. *Rheum Dis Clin North Am.* 2000; 26:13–27.
13. Edmonds SE, Winyard PG, Guo R, et al. Putative analgesic activity of repeated doses of vitamin E in the treatment of rheumatoid arthritis. Results of a placebo-controlled double-blind trial. *Ann Rheum Dis.* 1997;56:649–655.
14. Sirivastava KC, Mustafa T. Ginger (*Zingiber officinale*) and rheumatic disorders. *Med Hypotheses.* 1989;29:25–28.

15. Deodhar SD, Sethi R, Srimal RC. Preliminary studies on antirheumatic activity of curcumin (deferaloyl methane). *Indian J Med Res.* 1980;71:632–634.
16. Straub R, Cutolo M. Involvement of the hypothalamic-pituitary-adrenal/gonadal axis and the peripheral nervous system in rheumatoid arthritis. *Arthritis Rheum.* 2001;44:493–507.
17. Kirwan JR, and the Arthritis and Rheumatism Council Low-Dose Glucocorticoid Study Group. The effect of glucocorticoids on joint destruction in rheumatoid arthritis. *N Engl J Med.* 1995;333:142–146.
18. van Everdingen A, Jacobs J, van Reesema D, Bijlsma J. Low-dose prednisone therapy for patients with early active rheumatoid arthritis: clinical efficacy, disease modifying properties, and side-effects. *Ann Intern Med.* 2002;136:1–12.
19. Heliovaara M, Aho K, Knekt P, et al. Coffee consumption, rheumatoid factor, and the risk of rheumatoid arthritis. *Ann Rheum Dis.* 2000;59:631–635.
20. Hutchinson D, Shepstone L, Moots R, et al. Heavy cigarette smoking is strongly associated with rheumatoid arthritis (RA), particularly in patients without a family history of RA. *Ann Rheum Dis.* 2001;60:223–227.
21. Mikuls T, Cerhan J, Criswell L, et al. Coffee, tea, and caffeine consumption and risk of rheumatoid arthritis: Results from the Iowa Women's Health Study. *Arthritis Rheum.* 2002;46:83–91.
22. Huyser B, Parker J. Stress and rheumatoid arthritis: An integrated review. *Arthritis Care Res.* 1998;11:135–145.
23. Escalante A, Del Rincon I. How much disability in rheumatoid arthritis is explained by rheumatoid arthritis? *Arthritis Rheum.* 1999;42:1712–1721.
24. Parker J, Smarr K, Angelone E, et al. Psychological factors, immunologic activation, and disease activity in rheumatoid arthritis. *Arthritis Care Res.* 1992;5:196–201.
25. Kabat-Zinn J, Lipworth L, Burney R. The clinical use of mindfulness meditation for the self-regulation of chronic pain. *J Behav Med.* 1985;8:163–190.
26. Kabat-Zinn J, Wheeler W, Light T, et al. Influence of a mindfulness meditation-based stress reduction intervention on rates of skin clearing in patients with moderate to severe psoriasis undergoing phototherapy (UVB) and photochemotherapy. *Psychosom Med.* 1998;60:625–632.
27. Pradhan EK, Baumgarten M, Langenberg P, et al. Effect of Mindfulness-Based Stress Reduction in rheumatoid arthritis patients. *Arthritis Rheum.* 2007;57:1134–4112.
28. Zautra A, Davis M, Reich J, et al. Comparison of cognitive behavioral and mindfulness meditation interventions on adaptation to rheumatoid arthritis for patients with and without history of recurrent depression. *J Consult Clin Psychol.* 2008;76:408–421.
29. Bradley L, Turner R, Young L, et al. Effects of cognitive-behavioral therapy on pain behavior of rheumatoid arthritis (RA) patients: preliminary outcomes. *Scad J Behav Ther.* 1985;14:51–64.
30. Savelkoul M, De Witte L, Candel M, et al. Effects of a coping intervention on patients with rheumatic diseases: Results of a randomized controlled trial. *Arth Care Res.* 2001;45:69–76.

31. Smyth J, Stone AA, Hurewitz A, Kaell A. Effects of writing about stressful experiences on symptom reduction in patients with asthma or rheumatoid arthritis. *JAMA*. 1999;281:1304–1309.
32. Henderson CJ, Panush RS. Diets, nutritional supplements, and nutritional therapies in rheumatic diseases. *Rheum Dis Clin North Am*. 1999;25:937–968.
33. Linos A, Kaklamani VG, Kaklamani E, et al. Dietary factors in relation to rheumatoid arthritis: A role for olive oil and cooked vegetables? *Am J Clin Nutr*. 1999;70: 1077–1082.
34. Merlino L, Curtis J, Mikuls T, Cerhan J, Criswell L, Saag K. Vitamin D intake is inversely associated with rheumatoid arthritis: Results from the Iowa Women's Health Study. *Arthritis Rheum*. 2004;50:72–77.
35. Canalis E, Mazzioti G, Giustina A, Bilezikian J. Glucocorticoid induced osteoporosis: pathophysiology and treatment. *Osteoporos Int*. 2007;18:1319–1328.
36. Alarcon GS. Minocycline for the treatment of rheumatoid arthritis. *Rheum Dis Clin North Am*. 1998;24:489–499.
37. Pincus T. Assessment of long-term outcomes of rheumatoid arthritis. *Rheum Dis Clin North Am*. 1995;21:619–654.
38. Breedveld FC, Dayer JM. Leflunomide: Mode of action in the treatment of rheumatoid arthritis. *Ann Rheum Dis*. 2000;59:841–849.
39. Blumenauer B, Judd M, Cranney A et al. Etanercept for the treatment of rheumatoid arthritis. [Systematic Review] Cochrane Musculoskeletal Group Cochrane Database of Systematic Reviews. 3, 2005.
40. Navarro-Sarabia F, Ariza-Ariza R, Hernandez-Cruz B, Villanueva I. Adalimumab for treating rheumatoid arthritis. [Systematic Review] Cochrane Musculoskeletal Group Cochrane Database of Systematic Reviews. 3, 2005.
41. Blumenauer B, Judd M, Cranney A, et al. Infliximab for the treatment of rheumatoid arthritis. [Systematic Review] Cochrane Musculoskeletal Group Cochrane Database of Systematic Reviews. 3, 2005.
42. Feely M, Erickson A, O'Dell J. Therapeutic options for rheumatoid arthritis. *Expert Opin Pharmacother*. 2009;13:2095–2106.
43. Saag K, Teng G, Patkar N, et al. American College of Rheumatology 2008 recommendations for the use of nonbiologic and biologic disease-modifying antirheumatic drugs in rheumatoid arthritis. *Arth Rheum*. 2008;59:762–784.
44. Wang C, de Pablo P, Chen X, Scmid C, McAlindon T. Acupuncture for pain relief in patients with rheumatoid arthritis: A systemic review. *Arth Rheum*. 2008;59: 1249–1256.
45. Brosseau L, Welch V, Wells, G, et al. Low level laser therapy (Classes I, II and III) for treating rheumatoid arthritis. [Systematic Review] Cochrane Musculoskeletal Group Cochrane Database of Systematic Reviews. 3, 2005.
46. Krause D, Schleusser B, Herborn G, Rau R. Response to methotrexate treatment is associated with reduced mortality in patients with severe rheumatoid arthritis. *Arthritis Rheum*. 2000;43:14–21.

15

Fibromyalgia Syndrome

DANIEL MULLER, MD, PhD AND NANCY SELFRIDGE, MD

KEY CONCEPTS

- The diagnostic criteria for the fibromyalgia syndrome includes widespread pain present for greater than 3 months, and tenderness in at least 11 of 18 defined points.
- These patients may be the "canaries in the coal mine" as a consequence of highly sensitive individuals living in a society that expects high productivity at the expense of self-care.
- Self-motivated exercise and mind-body therapies are central to successful outcomes.
- Passive treatments such as psychotherapy, medications, supplements, acupuncture, and massage may be useful to help patients develop self-motivated pathways toward healing.
- Often, fibromyalgia coexists with autoimmune diseases such as rheumatoid arthritis and lupus; care must be taken to avoid treating the fibromyalgia symptoms with increasing doses of immunosuppressive medications.

■

Cases

Case 1: A 45-year-old woman presents with 2 hours of morning stiffness, upper and lower back pain, fatigue, nausea, and difficulty at her administrative job over the past year. She is married with a supportive husband, and 3 children ages 8–18. She is a previous triathlete, out of training for 15 years. She takes over-the-counter anti-inflammatory medications without relief. No history of depression or abuse, or other diagnosed illnesses. She gained 20 pounds in the past 3 years. Physical exam only shows 14 of 18 tender points, and laboratory screenings are all normal. X-rays show mild degenerative disease of the lumbar spine.

Case 2: A 45-year-old woman presents with 2 hours of morning stiffness, upper and lower back pain, fatigue, and nausea, for 15 years. She is divorced, unemployed, and receiving disability. She has 3 children ages 8–18. She is being treated for depression and pain with 2 antidepressants and oxycodone with little relief of symptoms. She has a history of childhood sexual abuse and abuse in her past marriage. She gained 50 pounds in the past 15 years. Physical exam only shows 14 of 18 tender points and laboratory screenings are all normal. X-rays show mild degenerative disease of the lumbar spine.

Pathophysiology

The diagnostic criteria for fibromyalgia syndrome (FMS) include widespread pain present for greater than 3 months, and tenderness in at least 11 of 18 defined points.[1] In practice, there are many other characteristic signs and symptoms, including nonrestorative sleep, chronic fatigue, stiffness, headache, migraine, irritable bowel syndrome, temporomandibular joint syndrome, and mood disorders.[2] Autonomic nervous system dysfunction is common, including orthostatic hypotension, with tilt-table test abnormalities and decreased heart rate variability.[3,4] The degree to which psychological components contribute to pain sensitivity and symptom expression in fibromyalgia remains controversial. However, there is evidence that mood disorders may modulate pain processing in patients with and without fibromyalgia.[5–7] Some investigators have noted a high frequency of FMS patients with post-traumatic stress disorder (PTSD).[8,9] In fact, careful history-taking will often reveal a stressful trigger event or period (e.g., an accident, a flu-like illness, emotional stress, or a period of overwork) preceding the onset of symptoms. Therefore, we do not feel it is a dangerous intuitive leap to assume that stress, trauma, and emotions play a role in the pathogenesis of fibromyalgia and, therefore, must be taken into consideration in the comprehensive management of symptoms.

In our practices, FMS patients often appear to have sensitive temperaments even before they develop physical symptoms. This is characterized by high levels of empathy, a tendency to adopt caretaker roles, and a higher than average sensitivity to environmental factors and emotional cues from others.[10,11] These patients may be the "canaries in the coal mine," exhibiting these symptoms as a consequence of living in a society that expects high productivity at the expense of self care. It is possible that this temperament describes a way of processing information that creates a vulnerability to stress and trauma, and subsequent increased central nervous system (CNS) sensitivity to pain. Our understanding of inter-individual differences in personality and temperament, then, would suggest that eventually we may find genetic differences in neurotransmitter pathways in people with fibromyalgia that confer susceptibility to this complex chronic pain problem. Genetic[12–14] and environmental factors likely both contribute to the development of this syndrome.

FMS often presents as a form of allodynia, in which normally painless stimuli are perceived as painful, and studies find little abnormality in the peripheral musculature but do point to increased CNS sensitivity to pain.[15–17] Because this is not a disease of autoimmune function per se, or of tissue inflammation, it probably does not actually qualify as a "rheumatologic disorder," though rheumatologists will likely continue to see many of these patients. In fact, fibromyalgia and most chronic pain syndromes likely represent primarily a disorder of neurologic function, notwithstanding the more subtle changes in the immune and endocrine systems. Patients with fibromyalgia have increased spatial and temporal summation of mechanically-induced muscle pain compared to normal controls.[18] Neuroimaging and neurobiology studies provide direct and indirect evidence for the increased central pain sensitivity in patients with fibromyalgia.[19–22] In two similar fMRI studies, a nonpainful level of stimulation for control subjects was perceived as painful in patients with fibromyalgia, and blood flow increased in the specific brain areas shown to be associated with painful stimuli.[23,24] Additionally, SPECT perfusion has been shown to correlate with clinical severity.[25]

FMS also can coexist with a variety of autoimmune diseases. The increased prevalence of FMS in females may point to a hormonal influence, although the increased sensitivity to pain does not correlate with menstrual cycle.[26] In addition, sex hormones do not seem to be altered in fibromyalgia.[27] Cerebrospinal fluid levels of substance P are elevated, and additional abnormalities in the regulation of cortisol, and in the adrenergic and serotonin systems, have been noted.[28,29] Antidepressant use is directed at raising CNS levels of serotonin and norepinephrine, as well as restoring sleep.

Hypothyroidism must be ruled out as a treatable cause of similar symptoms. However, a number of other abnormalities of the hypothalamic-pituitary-adrenal (HPA) axis have been found, suggesting physiologic hyperactivity of the stress response.[30–34] Although these physiologic abnormalities, such as decreased levels of growth hormone and somatomedin, do not appear to be critical in the etiology of FMS, they may contribute to the persistence of symptoms and an increasing central pain sensitivity.[35]

Vitamin D deficiency has also been associated with chronic nonspecific pain.[36] Checking 25-OH vitamin D levels in all fibromyalgia patients is prudent. Levels below 30 ng/ml are common at northern hemisphere latitudes above 30 degrees, but severely deficient single-digit levels are not uncommon. We have noted some pain improvement with corrections of D deficiency.

Alterations in the pituitary-adrenal axis in FMS appear to be quite different than are seen in clinical depression, which is somewhat surprising given the frequent concurrence of the two conditions.[37] The affinity and function of corticosteroid receptors on lymphocytes appear to be altered in FMS, which changes the cellular response when they are incubated with hormones in the laboratory.[38] There are reports of decreased numbers of T cells expressing activation markers, as well as a deficiency of interleukin-2 release.[39] Although these immunologic changes in FMS do not meet criteria for an immunodeficiency or autoimmune disease, the lymphocyte abnormalities may reflect an altered response to hormone feedback, and altered patterns of cytokine release may contribute to fatigue and inflammatory-type symptoms.

Integrative Therapy

GENERAL CONSIDERATIONS

Fibromyalgia patients are often viewed as difficult and burdensome in busy practices, whether in family practice, internal medicine, or rheumatology clinics. It is our observation that parallel syndromes are found in many of the subspecialties; eg, chronic chest wall pain, chronic abdominal pain of undertermined etiology, and irritable bowel syndrome, interstitial cystitis, chronic pelvic pain, dyspareunia, and vulvodynia. In our practices, patients with these problems often report experiences of feeling dismissed and disrespected in their encounters with physicians. Since FMS is a syndrome diagnosis, and we have not clearly identified the etiology or pathophysiology, well-meaning physicians will often tell patients that they "don't believe in FMS." We feel this is an error for two reasons. First, there is clear evidence of altered physiology in this disorder, particularly in the realm of neuroscience research. Second, patients experience statements like this as harmful, judging, and implying that their symptoms are not real or valid. It is important to affirm the patient's experiences of what often appear to be bizarre symptoms, even when we cannot fully understand them. Because there is so little evidence of efficacy for allopathic interventions in fibromyalgia, we want to emphasize the importance of generous listening in the healing relationship. Patients experience this affirmation as therapeutic, and it is something that all caregivers can provide, even when we feel we have little else to offer. Finally, it is important to not "hex" the patient. Though a conventionally difficult disorder to treat, it is unwise to make statements to patients such as "there is nothing we can do for you" or "you are likely to have this forever" or "you will eventually be disabled by this." Certainly, there are some patients who will do poorly, but many will become galvanized by a sense of empowerment when they are presented with all of the approaches that can be explored as symptom-relieving strategies. In fact, as our understanding of neurological function is perfected over time, it is not inconceivable that effective drug therapy may finally be developed.

Many patients remain concerned that something is seriously wrong with them, and that a serious diagnosis has been missed during evaluation, until a sensible explanation for their symptoms is presented to them. Explaining that the emerging evidence points to increased central nervous system sensitivity as a reason for physical symptoms helps patients to develop a sense of understanding and acceptance toward their physical symptoms. Obtaining a careful trauma and stress history can be very helpful in increasing the patient's awareness and understanding that the physiology of the stress response is potentially and intimately involved in the development of the disorder. Some patients will initially respond to questions about stressors and trauma with no recollection of any particularly traumatic events in their lives. It pays to revisit this line of questioning, however. Some trauma experts believe that the trauma events with the most significant potential for pathology are often associated with the "freeze" response.[40] In mammals this is associated with apparent paralysis or immobility, whereas in humans, there is often some degree of altered consciousness, amnesia, or dissociation temporally associated with the trauma. Because of this, patients often do not bring to mind the event when questioned initially, but may with repeated encouragement. It may often help to ask about traumas and stressors with a spouse, friend, or family member present. As clinicians, we also need to think of stress and trauma very broadly. Certainly accidents, illnesses, and childhood abuse are inarguably traumatic. But our culturally commonplace events, such as elective surgeries, medical procedures, divorce, job loss, or even caring for a sick family member, can be equally traumatic for the sensitive soul—especially if the events are accompanied by a sense of helplessness or powerlessness. The therapeutic benefit in this simple practice of our history-taking and making sense of the disease may be that the decrease in worry about physical symptoms might help diminish the stress response that tends to add to autonomic dysfunction and increased pain sensitivity.[41] Treating FMS patients can be a growth experience for the integrative practitioner, helping us to accept our own limitations in alleviating patients' suffering. We are taught to compassionately support a patient in a treatment plan that largely rests on the patient's thoughts and activity, rather than prescriptions from the physician.

EXERCISE

Exercise helps to decrease the symptoms of FMS.[42] However, overuse results in increased symptoms—often severe—and can lead to a cycle of muscle disuse. Patients may report feeling like they "ran a marathon" after only a few minutes of exercise. In one study, 9 of 16 subjects were worse or unchanged after a 14-week aerobic training intervention. However, the 3 subjects able to maintain a program of aerobic exercise no longer fulfilled criteria for FMS diagnosis 4 years later.[43] In a 21-week study of strength training, neck pain, fatigue, and depression decreased.[44] Warm-water pool aerobic therapy may be helpful, particularly in severe cases.[45] The Arthritis Foundation has further information on exercise programs. Asian exercise disciplines such as tai chi and yoga can also be beneficial. A form of tai chi called the range of motion (ROM) dance is particularly suited to persons with disabilities, requires little time commitment and incorporates a meditation/relaxation practice as well.

Physical therapy can restore muscle balance, and local therapy with stretching, heat, and cold can be beneficial. Massage therapy has been shown to be more useful than transcutaneous nerve stimulation (TENS), but TENS was better than sham TENS, and also may be helpful in some cases.[46] Treatment and exercises for all forms of soft tissue rheumatic pain are outlined in an excellent textbook by Sheon, et al.[47]

Though "activation" of the patient through exercise is a most desirable treatment goal, many patients demonstrate resistance. We have found it useful to explore with the patients the reasons for resistance by asking, sometimes repeatedly over a long relationship, "What is hard about starting or sticking with an exercise program?" Severe post-exercise pain is often cited, but many patients are similar to our usual primary care patients in that they have never embraced an active, exercise-oriented lifestyle. Exploring all the ways that one can move the body, rather than selectively focusing on a structured exercise program, can be useful. We often tell people to abandon the idea of "working out" and think more in terms of "playing." After all, who wants to have more work assigned to them?

MIND–BODY THERAPY

Meditation

Meditation has been shown to be helpful in FMS.[48–50] This training increases the ability to be comfortable in the present, which can lessen the fear of future pain and, with practice, can help the patient to transform the sensation of pain. Meditation is also useful for personal growth. We recommend training with a nondenominational teacher using a program such as "Mindfulness Meditation," pioneered by Dr. Jon Kabat-Zinn.[51] If no teacher is available, tapes can be helpful. It is interesting to note that the focus on the present moment and deep levels of personal inquiry that are cultivated in a meditation practice are actually quite useful to the practitioner working with FMS patients. Therefore, we endorse this practice for people working with FMS patients, as well.

PSYCHOTHERAPEUTIC INTERVENTIONS

In one study, 10 of 15 subjects responded to a 14-week cognitive-behavioral and relaxation training intervention.[43] However, no patients remained improved on 4-year follow-up evaluation. Electromyographic biofeedback[52] and hypnotherapy[53] have been helpful in controlled studies. Biofeedback training can be useful for people who find difficulty with meditation.

Increasing disability should prompt examination of basic aspects of the patient's quality of life. A framework for such a review is the "Four Rs."[54]

- **Roles**: The patient's ability to maintain self-esteem through normal roles as spouse, parent, provider, and so on, may be impaired. The work role requires very careful evaluation and is often problematic in people who are becoming progressively more symptomatic and disabled. We focus on a simple question: "In all of your roles, are you living for your heart's desire?" as a way of exploring where problems may exist.
- **Reactions**: The emotional reaction to events such as the diagnosis of FMS often follows a grieving process as outlined by Kübler-Ross.[55] These stages are denial, anger, bargaining, depression, and acceptance. Patients are often stuck in anger and depression. In addition, the sensitive temperament of many of these patients is often associated with a greater physiologic reaction to all emotions.[10/11] Meditation practice and journaling can be uniquely helpful for decreasing neurohormonal reactivity by increasing the time from stimulus to reaction.
- **Relationships**: The patient may often face seemingly insurmountable problems at home or in relationships at work, creating repeated stress triggers for symptoms.
- **Resources**: Psychotherapy, ministers, community programs, and self-help groups may each become a key for altering this progressive

decrease in ability to function; guided imagery is particularly useful. Isolation and alienation clearly make patients symptomatically worse.

Dr. John Sarno, a physiatrist at New York University, has written a book that some patients may find to be quite useful.[56] Dr. Sarno calls FMS, and all chronic tendonitis-bursitis disorders, "tension-myalgia syndrome." The short summary is that the patient may substitute physical pain for emotional pain. He believes that this simple realization can abrogate pain in certain persons. We have seen this happen in FMS, in multiple bursitis-tendinitis syndrome, and in chronic low back pain. A recent study documented decreased pain scores for chronic back pain patients using a mind-body treatment intervention aimed at educating patients how psychological factors can manifest as physical pain, and supporting patients in developing insight into their own emotional issues as causes of physical pain.[57] Our experience suggests that a certain level of self-awareness and acceptance of the power of the mind are required to experience symptom improvement just with this insight. One of us (NS) has written a book for patients applying Dr. Sarno's principles to fibromyalgia using journaling, meditation, and other workbook format exercises.[58] One controlled trial found guided imagery more effective than amitriptyline at reducing pain scores after one month of treatment.[59]

Another area of potential benefit for FMS patients is emerging from the new and growing field of energy psychology. Emotional Freedom Technique (EFT), or "tapping," as it is sometimes called, and Eye Movement, Desensitization and Reprocessing (EMDR) are showing anecdotal evidence of value in alleviating physical and psychological symptoms in FMS patients. It remains to be determined how these therapies work, but they are simple, quite harmless, and EFT can be taught to the patient to use at home for self-treatment. A good description and several anecdotes about EFT can be reviewed on the website www.emofree.com. Descriptions of EMDR, its history, and evidence of efficacy can be reviewed at www.emdr.com. These therapies fit descriptions of what Dietrich Klinghardt, MD, calls "uncoupling" techniques that may bypass cognitive-level processes to diminish or eliminate the CNS connection between

Note

Early and aggressive use of exercise, which likely can include any form, including aerobic, yoga, or tai chi, is an important, evidence-based, key to decreasing the symptoms of FMS. A combination of exercise with "mindfulness meditation" affords the best chance of achieving a remission.

the neurophysiology of traumatic memory and emotions, and the physiology of bodily felt symptoms (see www.neuraltherapy.com). We hope the future will bring research directed at examining in depth the efficacy and possible mechanisms for these therapies, since many fibromyalgia patients will give us trauma histories and yet, may not fit the diagnostic criteria for PTSD. Further, the efficacy of conventional drug and psychotherapy interventions for traumatic stress remain limited.

NUTRITION

Though no specific diet has been shown to be very effective in FMS, an anti-inflammatory diet may be helpful and likely benefits the patient's health in a more general way. This is a plant-based, whole foods diet that limits animal proteins, animal fats and processed foods. We emphasize complete avoidance of trans fats (partially hydrogenated oils, margarine, and shortening) and corn syrup, and addressing the common nutritional deficiencies in the standard American diet. Details can be found in Chapter 2.

Chlorella

Chlorella pyrenoidosa (a freshwater green alga) is a source of many nutrients, including protein, lipids, vitamins, and minerals. Preliminary studies in vitro and in animals have shown anti-tumor, immune-enhancing, and anti-viral activities for chlorella at a dose of 10 grams per day. A double-blind, crossover study has shown significant reduction in the number of FMS tender points after 3 months of supplementation.[60] Note, chlorella contains iodine and allergic reactions have been reported. As a significant source of vitamin K, chlorella supplementation can antagonize the anticoagulant activity of Coumadin (warfarin).

HOMEOPATHY

A controversial placebo-controlled trial of a homeopathic treatment (R toxicodendron 6c) decreased tender points.[61] A second study using individualized therapy for 3 months also showed modest positive effects compared to placebo.[62] We recommend referral to a homeopathic physician for evaluation and treatment. Note that homeopathic remedies are reported to be less effective in the presence of certain pharmaceuticals.

SUPPLEMENTS

Calcium and Magnesium

The effects of calcium and magnesium supplementation have not been studied adequately; nevertheless, in anecdotal reports, supplementation has been helpful. We recommend 1500 mg of calcium and 400 to 750 mg of magnesium daily. Calcium supplements cannot be adequately utilized without vitamin D; thus our recommendations for vitamin D supplementation (below). Patients can easily titrate their magnesium dose—too much for a given individual commonly increases the frequency of bowel movements.

Antioxidants

Antioxidant vitamins may be helpful in FMS, particularly to relieve muscle cramping. Vitamin E as mixed tocopherols should be taken in a dose of 400 to 1600 (IU) daily, and vitamin C in a dose of 250 mg twice per day. Selenium can be found in many foods, including Brazil nuts; intake should be at least 100 μg daily but should not exceed 400 μg daily.

Other Supplements

A high-potency multivitamin with minerals containing at least 400 IU of Vitamin D3 is recommended. Additional vitamin D3 (cholecalciferol) up to 4000 IU daily can be recommended based on assessed 25-OH vitamin D levels. Aim to restore levels to 40 ng/ml or higher, and check levels periodically to assess peak levels in summer and nadir levels in mid-winter. Vitamin D is most effectively produced in the skin with UVB exposure, so patients' levels and supplementation requirement may vary seasonally depending on their UVB exposure to spring and summer sunlight, especially at higher latitudes, and depending upon skin color. Though tanning beds do raise vitamin D levels (possibly at exposures that do not result in much skin tan or increased risk of skin cancer), we cannot promote their use; many continue to emit electromagnetic radiation, and the proportion of UVA may contribute to skin collagen breakdown and photo-aging. When patients do choose to try to maintain their vitamin D levels with sun exposure, remind them that it does not take more than a minimal "erythema dose" to produce large amounts of vitamin D in the skin, so tanning and burning are neither necessary nor recommended. Getting 10 minutes of midday sun before applying sunscreen, three or more times per week, is likely sufficient. Blood level testing will help patients determine the strategy that works best for them. Patients can stay up to date on vitamin D research and recommendations at www.vitamindcouncil.org. Persons with darker skin color in northern climates will need higher doses of vitamin D.

S-Adenosylmethionine (SAMe) acts as a mild antidepressant and pain reliever, and has shown moderate efficacy in FMS.[63] The recommended dose is 400 mg, two to three times per day, taken 30 minutes before meals. It tends to be expensive.

Omega-3 fatty acids have not been tested in FMS, but can have moderate analgesic activity and increase levels of anti-inflammatory prostaglandins. Omega-3 fatty acid intake can be increased by dietary means or through supplementation. Common sources include fish oil and flaxseed oil, though flax oil may not have the same biologic effect as fish oil.[64] The Environmental Protection Agency has recommended limits for dietary consumption of fish to avoid mercury toxicity.[65] At the present time, it is likely that this safe limit of fish weekly will not achieve the therapeutic doses of Omega 3 that we recommend. Thus, patients are advised to use fish oil supplements and are advised to purchase a product that is of pharmaceutical grade, thus free of mercury, other heavy metals, and PCBs. Approximate doses for supplementation are eicosapentaenoic acid 30 mg/kg per day and docosahexaenoic acid 50 mg/kg per day. We will simplify this for patients by telling them that they may take 2–4 grams of high-quality fish oil daily. A common complaint about fish oil supplementation is "fish burps," as most products now are made from sardines and anchovies. Ways to mitigate this problem are to take the entire dose at bedtime, or to purchase a product made from salmon or krill. Alternatively, as the fish oil may become rancid, store it in the refrigerator or freezer. We also tell patients that there is evidence that Omega 3 supplementation may be beneficial for many conditions and for overall health. Gamma-linolenic acid (GLA) in a dose of 1.4 to 2.8 g per day, the equivalent of 6 to 11 g of borage oil daily, may have similar analgesic effects.

BOTANICALS

There are no adequate controlled trials of botanical treatments in FMS. In anecdotal reports, many treatments lead to a benefit that wanes with time, which may indicate a short-term placebo effect.

Sleep-Promoting Agents

The tricyclic antidepressants (TCAs) are used to promote sleep, because they have been shown to be helpful in double-blind studies.[66–68] Patients who would rather avoid TCAs can try St. John's wort, keeping in mind the multiple interactions with other drugs. Some patients prefer to promote sleep by using kava; if they choose this therapy, patients should be monitored for dermopathy and liver toxicity. Higher doses of kava can be detrimental to driving and can potentiate the effects of alcohol and other sedating botanicals and drugs. We no longer recommend kava, because of concerns of abuse and liver toxicity, plus potential for diminished commercial availability. Valerian is another possibility for promoting sleep; the patient should be warned about benzodiazepine-withdrawal type symptoms after extended use. In rare cases, valerian causes hepatotoxicity. German chamomile is widely used as a tea, has a very mild sedative activity, and is safe. Chamomile tea can be used when other botanicals are too sedating. Any of these also can be used for an anxiolytic effect.

DOSAGE

- St. John's wort: As extract standardized to 0.3% hypericin content, use 300 mg up to three times daily; or as tea, steep 2–4 g of the dried herb in 150 ml of boiling water for 5 to 10 minutes and strain; take 1 cup up to three times daily.
- Valerian: As tea, steep 2–3 g of root in 150 ml of boiling water for 5 to 10 minutes and strain; take 1 cup up to three times daily; or, as a tincture, 1–3 ml, one to 3 times daily, or as valerian extract, 400–900 mg 2 hours before bedtime.
- German chamomile: As tea, steep 3 g of dried flower heads in 150 ml of boiling water for 5 to 10 minutes and strain; take 1 cup up to three times daily; 2–8 g of dried flower heads can be taken three times daily.

Anti-inflammatory Agents

Ginger, turmeric (curcumin), and an Ayurvedic herb, boswellia, have not been tested in FMS, but may exert some analgesic activity by inhibiting inflammatory prostaglandins.

DOSAGE

- Ginger: As dried root, 1 g two to three times per day to start: increase to up to 4 g daily; as tea, 1 g dried root steeped in 150 ml of boiling water for 5 to 10 minutes and strain; take 1 cup up to four times daily.
- Turmeric: As powdered root, 0.5 to 1 g two or three times daily.
- Boswellia: As standardized extract (boswellin) 500 mg three times daily.

Precautions. Ginger may increased bile flow and cause pain in the presence of cholelithiasis. Other risks include bleeding, hypertension or hypotension, and hypoglycemia. Turmeric-associated risks include bleeding, gastrointestinal intolerance, and impaired fertility. Boswellia may inhibit platelet activity and is relatively contraindicated for patients on anticoagulants. All three of these agents need to be discontinued at least 2 weeks before elective surgery.

Energy-Increasing Agents

Ginseng and gotu kola have not been tested properly in FMS or chronic fatigue syndrome (CFS) but may provide increased energy. Ginseng products are used for 2 to 8 weeks and then discontinued for 2 weeks. There are three types of ginseng: Asian, or panax ginseng (*Panax ginseng*), American ginseng (*Panax quinquefolius*), and Siberian ginseng (*Eleutherococcus Aconthopanax senticosus*). Asian ginseng and Siberian ginseng appear to have a more stimulating effect, and may be more beneficial in treating fatigue. The German Commission E monographs state that ginseng root is helpful in counteracting weakness and fatigue, in restoring stamina, and in reversing impaired concentration. Ginseng is classified as an adaptogen, which is a term used to suggest that a substance can act to strengthen the body and increase general resistance.

Gotu kola (*Centella asiatica*) is often used in venous insufficiency, and has also been used for fatigue.

DOSAGE

- Asian or panax ginseng (Panax ginseng): As powdered root, 0.6–3.0 g one to 3 times per day. A capsule extract comes in 100, 250, and 500 mg doses; average capsule dose: 200 to 600 mg.

- Siberian ginseng (*Eleutherococcus senticosus*): As powdered root, 0.6–3 g one to 3 times per day. As ethanolic extract, 0.56 ml one to 3 times per day. Note: The demand for this herb exceeds the supply, which invites products that may not have appropriate content. Recommend standardized extracts that state the content of eleutherosides, the active component. The higher the percentage the better.
- American ginseng (*Panax quinquefolius*): As powdered root, 0.6–3 g one to 3 times per day; as tea, 3 g of root steeped in 150 ml of boiling water for 5 to 10 minutes and strained; take 1 cup up to 3 times daily; as capsules, 200 to 600 mg per day.
- Gotu kola (*Centella asiatica*): As dried leaves, 600 mg three times per day; as tea; 600 mg of dried leaves steeped in 150 ml of boiling water for 5 to 10 minutes and strained; take 1 cup 3 times per day.

Precautions. Ginseng can cause insomnia, increase bleeding, and contribute to hypoglycemia. Gotu kola in large doses can increase cholesterol, elevate blood pressure, and cause photosensitivity, sedation, and abortion.

PHARMACEUTICALS

Antidepressants

Patients with a new diagnosis of FMS are usually started on treatment including a sedating tricyclic antidepressant (TCA) at night, often with an activating antidepressant in the morning, as well as low-level aerobic exercise and physical therapy. Selection and dosage of antidepressants are tailored to minimize side effects and to balance the fatigue and sleep problems for each patient. Therapeutic benefit is associated with improvements in sleep.[66–68]

Initial drug therapy for FMS is a low dose of a sedating TCA, usually amitriptyline (Elavil) 5 to 10 mg, 1 hour before bedtime. The dose is titrated upward every 5 to 14 days as tolerated, using the minimal dose necessary to achieve restorative sleep. Excessive sedation can be an adverse effect of TCAs; therefore, an agent such as sertraline (Zoloft) 25 mg in the morning, or another of the more activating antidepressants such as fluoxetine (Prozac), can be added. Other, less sedating TCAs, such as nortriptyline, can be substituted for amitriptyline in the evening. Doxepin (Sinequan), a non-TCA antidepressant, can be particularly useful in liquid form to titrate at low doses, 2 to 5 mg, for sedation at night. Trazodone hydrochloride (Desyrel) 25 to 300 mg also can be helpful for promoting sleep. Cyclobenzaprine (Flexeril) 2.5 to 40 mg in divided doses has muscle relaxant and sedative effects. Our favorite sedating antidepressant, also favored by many of our patients, is trazodone. Perhaps this is because trazodone produces less suppression of REM sleep than other antidepressants. Meta-analyses have supported the use of antidepressants and cyclobenzaprine. Two new dual serotonin and norepinephrine reuptake inhibitors, milnacipran and duloxetine, have shown benefits in FMS in randomized controlled trials.[69,70] Both have recently received FDA approval. The practitioner should develop a familiarity with several different antidepressants in order to feel comfortable managing the myriad side effects. For a systematic review see Uceyler.[71]

Nonsteroidal Anti-inflammatory Drugs

Nonsteroidal anti-inflammatory drugs (NSAIDs) had a poor showing in a controlled trial testing their analgesic efficiency in fibromyalgia.[72] It may be better to try supplements or botanicals such as omega-3 fatty acids, gamma-linolenic acid (GLA), higher doses of vitamin E, ginger, tumeric, or boswellia for their modest analgesic effects.

Anticonvulsant

Gabapentin has been used off-label for fibromyalgia because of its indication for use in chronic pain. A similar pharmaceutical, pregabalin, has been studied at a dose of 450 mg/day in an 8-week placebo-controlled trial and showed significant, but quite modest, efficacy for improvement of pain, sleep, and fatigue.[73] Pregabalin has been recently approved by the FDA for treatment of fibromyalgia.

Tramadol

One controlled trial showed a beneficial effect of tramadol (Ultram) 50 to 400 mg given in divided doses;[74] however, use of tramadol with antidepressants can cause the potentially serious side effect of serotonin syndrome. Tramadol can also cause excessive sedation. It may be useful in allowing a 4-week drug holiday from antidepressant therapy, to reset neural receptors, and in intermittent therapy for exacerbations. In general, we avoid the chronic use of benzodiazepines and narcotics. Our observation has been that patients with fibromyalgia rarely, if ever, achieve significant relief of pain and reduction of pain behaviors with chronic opioid use. In addition, a recent large study suggests that chronic opioid therapy for noncancer pain did not meet any of the key outcome opioid treatment goals, including pain relief, improved quality of life, or improved functional capacity.[75]

Sodium oxybate is a schedule III drug dispensed by a single specialty pharmacy, and is FDA approved for narcolepsy. It shows evidence for increasing sleep quality, and some efficacy in fibromyalgia.[76]

Note

Often FMS can coexist with diagnosable autoimmune diseases such as rheumatoid arthritis or systemic lupus erthrythematosus. Identification of such disorder as the cause of pain is important to avoid treating the FMS with escalating doses of immunosuppressive medications.

ACUPUNCTURE

One high-quality, short-term trial of electroacupuncture showed almost complete remission in 20%, satisfactory benefit in 40%, and no effect in 40% of patients with FMS.[77] But a review of several trials concluded that benefits were reduced with time.[78] Still another recent study of acupuncture showed no significant effect compared to 3 sham acupuncture treatments.[79] However, a limitation of this latter study was that it used directed acupuncture at fixed points, pointing out the difficulty of blinding that may have affected the outcome of many reports (including the original cited electroacupuncture study). Acupuncturists often define fibromyalgia as a disharmony of spirit. One of us (NS) works closely with several MSOM (Masters of Oriental Medicine) acupuncturists in an integrative clinical setting. Needle placement for the fibromyalgia patients referred to these practitioners varies widely from patient to patient, with subtle differences in pain quality and location, mood, and associated symptoms influencing the precise treatment quite dramatically. It is this lack of a "one size fits all" approach to treating patients that makes acupuncture outcome studies so difficult to perform and interpret. It is our belief that an acupuncture trial is appropriate for most patients interested in exploring this intervention, given personal financial constraints.

SOFT TISSUE INJECTION

The use of subcutaneous tender point injections may be helpful, particularly if they are given into palpable areas of muscle spasm. These injections are often given as 0.5 to 1 ml of 1% lidocaine per site, although dry needling or saline may work as well. The use of corticosteroids for injection does not add any benefit, has risks, and should be avoided.

SURGERY

There are no surgical treatments for FMS.[80] Chiari malformations and cervical stenosis can cause symptoms that can mimic FMS. However, FMS does not cause defined focal neurologic changes. A neurologic examination by a primary care physician can rule out neurologic abnormalities. If mild abnormalities are found, referral to a neurologist, not a neurosurgeon, is recommended.

OTHER THERAPIES TO CONSIDER

There have not been adequate studies on the roles of traditional Chinese, Ayurvedic, or spiritual medicine in the management of FMS. We counsel our patients to learn about several different modalities and then record in a journal their feelings about these modalities. Then, after discussion, the patient can visit a practitioner of the selected therapy to explore the approach further. If the economic burden is not too great, addition of the therapeutic modality may be in order.

Prevention

There are no proven methods of preventing FMS. However, the following can be recommended:

- Laugh as much as possible. Watch funny movies, read funny books, get up every morning and force yourself to laugh, you'll find it is awkward at first, but, it works anyway!
- Journal about stressful events. Make a list of 25 things for which you are grateful.
- Be creative. Do art, dance, play an instrument, beat a drum, write poetry or prose.
- Meditate, we recommend mindfulness meditation.
- Find meaning in life. Ask what gives you the energy to get up in the morning.
- Investigate your personality (Keirsey, 1998). Try new things that you are afraid to do.
- If you feel "stuck," find a good psychotherapist who understands fibromyalgia.

- **Exercise. Combine aerobics, core exercisies, strength training, and stretching. Make it a time to play!**
- **Love people. Hang out with "positive people," make sure they outweigh the "negative" people in your life. Find "positive" support groups.**
- **Eat well. Try a vegetarian diet. Make sure to balance your protein intake and make sure you have an adequate vitamin intake.**
- **Eliminate smoking, and alcohol. consider your use of caffeinated beverages. make high sugar desserts a small rare treat.**

Summary and Cases

There is no documented "cure" for FMS. Studies have reported an improvement in 5% to 53% of patients, although 47% to 100% continue to meet criteria for FMS 2 to 5 years after diagnosis.[80] Only a small minority of patients experience complete resolution of symptoms. Despite these dismal statistics, we cannot emphasize enough the therapeutic benefit of generous listening and affirming the patient's felt experience. In our practices about 75% of patients report "some" relief of symptoms with treatment. Better response to treatment is seen in patients of younger age, and in those with continued employment, supportive families, and an absence of litigation and of affective disorders.[81] Simply giving a diagnosis of fibromyalgia can decrease total costs of health care.[82,83]

LIFESTYLE INTERVENTIONS

We have observed a few remissions following complete self reevaluation and transformation of the patient's previous life style. These changes often involved several of the following:

- Taking up practice of an Asian discipline including movement and meditation (meditation with yoga, Qigong, or tai chi, or an intensive aerobic exercise program).
- Changes in relationships at home and at work that promote taking control of the patient's life, and support a belief system that endorses self care rather than self sacrifice as a virtue (paradoxically, part of having more control is also "letting go" of the way things "should" be).
- Psychotherapy to investigate and change ingrained habits and beliefs that maintain adverse relationships and roles, and increase self esteem and self care principles.

- Using treatments from complementary and alternative medicine such as acupuncture, massage, and even spiritual therapies to help the patient overcome particular problems.
- Spending a significant portion of time helping others perceived as more needy than the patient, usually on a voluntary basis.

EXERCISE

Aerobic training, along with muscle strengthening and stretching, can be invaluable to maintaining function. Physical therapy can be used initially for instruction; the "ROM dance" form of tai chi can be helpful (www.taichihealth.com). Warm water pool aerobics is sometimes the only tolerable exercise. As much exercise as can be tolerated should be encouraged.

MIND-BODY MODALITIES

The practice of meditation, particularly mindfulness meditation, is highly recommended. However, a strong daily commitment of time devoted to scrutiny of body, mind, and spirit is required. Also recommended are biofeedback, relaxation exercises, and other methods to cope with stress. Tai chi and yoga training also may include a meditative component. Psychotherapy, especially guided visualization, can be helpful. We suggest that all patients read *The Mind-Body Prescription* by Dr. John Sarno[56] if the mind-body model makes sense to them, and that they consider working through the exercises in the text, Freedom From Fibromyalgia.[58]

Patients are often quite resourceful in using insight and intuition to help manage their disease, once they understand how they may have developed their fibromyalgia. To this end we often recommend additional helpful reading including *The Trauma Spectrum* by Robert Scaer, MD;[84] *Waking the Tiger* by Peter Levine, PhD;[85] and *They Can't Find Anything Wrong* by David Clarke, MD.[86] A trial of EMG-biofeedback or hypnotherapy or guided imagery can be recommended.

REMOVAL OF EXACERBATING FACTORS

Eliminate consumption of coffee, smoking, and alcohol. Aggravating factors include improper body mechanics at work or play, structural features such as flat feet, and anxiety and depression. Patients, families, and appropriate personnel in the workplace must be involved in identifying goals and limitations.

NUTRITION

No specific diet has been shown to be effective. An anti-inflammatory diet may be helpful, essentially a diet full of whole foods, multiple daily servings of fruits, vegetables, whole grains, nuts and legumes, and limited in the volume of animal and dairy protein, fat and processed foods. The book *Super Foods Rx* by Steven Pratt, MD, is a good resource for patients. *Chlorella pyrenoidosa*, freshwater green alga, 10 g daily, can be used for a 3-month trial.

SUPPLEMENTS

- Vitamin E as mixed tocopherols, 400 to 1600 IU daily
- Vitamin C 250 mg twice per day
- Selenium intake as nuts or supplements: at least 100 μg daily; not to exceed 400 μg daily
- Calcium 1.5 g daily; magnesium 600–750 mg daily
- A vitamin D3 supplement 1000–4000 IU per day
- A high-potency multivitamin with minerals and extra B vitamins
- S-adernosylmethionine (SAMe) 400 mg 2–3 times per day, 30 minutes before meals, for pain, anxiety, or depression

BOTANICALS

Botanical sedatives can be used to promote sleep or treat anxiety.

- St. John's wort 300 mg up to 3 times daily
- Valerian: as extract, 400–900 mg 2 hours before bedtime
- German chamomile: as tea, steep 3 g of dried flower heads in 150 ml boiling water for 5 to 10 minutes and strain; take one cup up to 3 times daily

Ginger and tumeric (curcumin) may show some analgesic effects.

- Ginger: As dried root, 1 g 2 to 3 times per day to start, increased up to 4 g daily
- Turmeric: As powdered root, 0.5–1 g, 2 to 3 times daily
- Boswellia: As standardized extract (boswellin), 500 mg 3 times daily

Ginseng and gotu kola may provide some increased energy.

- Siberian ginseng: As powdered root, 0.6–3 g, 1 to 3 times per day, or ethanolic extract, 0.56 ml one to 3 times a day; use for 2 to 8 weeks, then abstain for 2 weeks
- Gotu kola: As dried leaves, 600 mg 3 times per day; as tea, 600 mg dried leaves steeped in 150 ml of boiling water for 5 to 10 minutes and strain; take one cup 3 times per day

PHARMACEUTICALS

Therapeutic benefit is associated with improvements in sleep. Use low doses of a sedating antidepressant such as amitriptyline or nortriptyline 5 to 10 mg, 1 hour before bedtime, titrated upward every 5 to 14 days as tolerated. Trazodone 25 to 300 mg can also be used. For excessive sedation, add sertraline 25 mg or fluoxetine in the morning. Cyclobenzaprine, 2.5 to 40 mg in divided doses, has muscle relaxant and sedative effects. Treat depression with full doses of antidepressants. Gabapentin or pregababalin can be tried, and tramadol can be used short term for exacerbations.

We avoid the chronic use of benzodiazapines and narcotics.

ACUPUNCTURE

A trial is worthwhile; short-term effects can be seen in as many as 60% of patients, and long-term improvements also occur. If the patient can afford the treatments, the true reduction in pain may enable them to increase their aerobic exercise.

SOFT TISSUE INJECTION

The use of subcutaneous tender point injections may be helpful, particularly if injections are given into palpable areas of muscle spasm. Use 0.5–1 ml of 1% lidocaine per site, using a 23 gauge needle; steroids should be avoided.

Caution. Studies have not been done on the possible additive effects of ginger, tumeric, vitamin E, and an NSAID for increased risk of hemorrhage. Other commonly used supplements or botanicals such as ginkgo may add further risk. Particular care must be used in patients receiving other anti-platelet agents or Coumadin. Mixing multiple sedating botanicals and pharmaceuticals must be avoided.

Cases Revisited

These cases exemplify two ends of a spectrum for fibromyalgia. Obviously, the patient in the first case, epidemiologically, has a better chance of becoming fully functional. However, one should not presume that Case 2 has no chance for recovery. There are many factors that may be hidden from view. Starting with the use of some of the above modalities may be helpful for either patient. Also, perhaps time may reveal that the first patient has more family problems than one can see at first glance, and may require extensive social and psychotherapeutic support for recovery. The patient in the second case may on her way up from a low point. She may, with the proper support, find a way for stopping her cycle of abuse. She may eventually get off her narcotics and develop a program of improved diet, mindfulness meditation, and exercise. Warn that there is no "Magic Bullet," and empower the patient to make her own decisions as to treatment. Your own ability to be mindful, drop your adverse judgments, be open to your intuition, and to meet the patient just where they are, may be the key to helping each patient on the path toward their own recovery.

REFERENCES

1. Wolfe F, Smythe H, Yunus M, et al. The American College of Rheumatology 1990 criteria for the classification of fibromyalgia. *Arthritis Rheum*. 1990;33:160–172.
2. Yunus M, Masai A, Calabro J, et al. Primary fibromyalgia (fibrositis): Clinical study of 50 patients with matched normal controls. *Semin Arthritis Rheum*. 1981;11:151–171.
3. Cohen H, Neumann L, Shore M, et al. Autonomic dysfunction in patients with fibromyalgia; application of power spectral analysis of heart rate variability. *Semin Arthritis Rheum*. 2000;29:217–227.
4. Cohen H, Neumann L, Alhosshle A, et al. Abnormal sympathovagal balance in mend with fibromyalgia. *J Rheumatol*. 2001;28:581–589.
5. Abeles AN, Pillinger MH, Solitar, BM, Abeles, M. Narrative review: the pathophysiology of fibromyalgia. *Ann Intern Med*. 2007;146:726–734.
6. Giesecke T, Gracely RH, Williams DA, et al. The relationship between depression, clinical pain, and experimental pain in a chronic pain cohort. *Arthritis Rheum*. 2005;52:1577–1584.

7. Yunus MB. Fibromyalgia and overlapping disorders: the unifying concept of central sensitivity syndromes. *Semin Arthritis Rheum.* 2007;36:339–356.
8. Amir M, Kaplan Z, Neumann L, et al. Posttraumatic stress disorder, tenderness, and fibromyalgia. *J Psychosomat Res.* 1997;42:607–613.
9. Cohen H, Neumann L, Haiman Y, et al. Prevalence of post-traumatic stress disorder in fibromyalgia patients: overlapping syndromes or post-traumatic fibromyalgia syndrome? *Semin Arthritis Rheum.* 2002;32:38–50.
10. Aron EN, Aron A. Sensory-processing sensitivity and its relation to introversion and emotionality. *J Personality and Soc Psy.* 1997;73:345–368.
11. Aron EN. Revisiting Jung's concept of innate sensitiveness. *J Anal Psych.* 1997;49:337–367.
12. Buskila D, Neumann L. Genetics of fibromyalgia. *Curr Pain and Headache Rep.* 2005;9:313–315.
13. Buskila D, Sarzi-Puttini P, Ablin JN. The genetics of fibromyalgia syndrome. *Pharmacogenomics.* 2007;8:67–74.
14. Arnold LM, Hudson JI, Hess EV, et al. Family study of fibromyalgia. *Arthritis Rheum.* 2004;50:944–952.
15. Staud R. Evidence of involvement of central neural mechanisms in generating fibromyalgia pain. *Curr Rheumatol Rep.* 2002;4:299–305.
16. Desmeules JA, Cedraschi C, Rapiti E, et al. Neurophysiologic evidence for a central sensitization in patients with fibromyalgia. *Arthirits Rheum.* 2003;48:1420–1429.
17. Meeus M, Nijs J. Central sensitization: a biopsycholscial explanation for chronic widespread pain in patients with fibromyalgia and chronic fatigue syndrome. *Clin Rheum.* 2007; 26:465–473.
18. Staud R, Koo E, Robinson ME, Price DD. Spatial summation of mechanically evoked muscle pain and painful alters sensations in normal subjects and fibromyalgia patients. *Pain.* 2007;130:177–187.
19. Kwiatek R, Barnden L, Tedman R, et al. Regional cerebral blood flow in fibromyalgia: single photon-emission computed tomography evidence of reduction in the pontine tegmentum and thalami. *Arthritis Rheum.* 2000;43:2823–2833.
20. Chen JJ, Wang JY, Chang YM, et al. Regional cerebral blood flow between primary and concomitant fibromyalgia patients: a possible way to differentiate concomitant fibromyalgia from the primary disease. *Scand J Rheumatol.* 2007;36:226–232.
21. Wood PB, Schweinhardt P, Jaeger E, et al. Fibromyalgia patients show an abnormal dopamine response to pain. *Eur J Neurosci.* 2007;25:3576–3582.
22. Montoya P, Sitges C, Garcia-Herrera M, et al. Reduced brain habituation to somatosensory stimulation in patients with fibromyalgia. *Arthritis Rheum.* 2006;54:1995–2000.
23. Gracely R, Petzke F, Wolf J, Clauw D. Functional magnetic resonance imaging evidence of augmented pain processing in fibromyalgia. *Arthritis Rheum.* 2002;46:1333–1343.
24. Cook D, Lange G, Ciccone D, Liu W, Steffener J, Natelson B. Functional imaging of pain in patients with primary fibromyalgia. *J Rheumatol.* 2004;31:364–378.

25. Guedj E, Cammilleri S, Niboyet J, et al. Clinical correlate of brain SPECT perfusion abnormalities in fibromyalgia. *J Nucl Med.* 2008;49:1798–1803.
26. Alonso C, Loveinger B, Muller D, Coe C. Menstrual cycle influences on pain and emotion in women with fibromyalgia. *J Psychosomatic Res.* 2004;57:451–458.
27. El Maghraoui A, Tellal S, Achemlal L, et al. Bone turnover and hormonal perturbations in patients with fibromyalgia. *Clin Exp Rheumatol.* 2006;24:428–431.
28. Russell I, Orr M, Littman B et al. Elevated cerebrospinal fluid levels of substance P in patients with the fibromyalgia syndrome. *Arthritis Rheum.* 1994;37:1593–1601.
29. Neeck G, Crofford L. Neuroendocrine perturbations in fibromyalgia and chronic fatigue syndrome. *Rheum Dis Clin NA.* 2000;26:989–10002.
30. Adler GK, Kinsley BT, Hurwitz S, et al. Reduced hyothalamic-pituitary and sympathoadrenal responses to hypoglycemia in women with fibromyalgia syndrome. *Am J Med.* 1999;106:534–543.
31. Torpy DJ, Papanicolau DA, Lotsikas AJ, et al. Responses of the sympathetic nervous system and the hypothalamic-pituitary-adrenal axis to interleukin-6. *Arthritis Rheum.* 2000;43:872–880.
32. McLean SA, Williams DA, Stein PK, et al. Cerebrospinal fluid corticotropin-releasing factor concentration is associated with pain but not fatigue symptoms in patients with fibromyalgia. *Neuropsychopharmacology.* 2006;31:2776–2782.
33. Weissbecker I, Floyd A, Dedert E, et al. Childhood trauma and diurnal cortisol disruption in fibromyalgia syndrome. *Psychoneuroendocrinology.* 2006;31:312–324.
34. Jones KD, Deodhar P, Lorentzen A, et al. Growth hormone perturbations in fibromyalgia: a review. *Semin Arthritis Rheum.* 2007;36:357–379.
35. Neeck G. Pathogenic mechanisms of fibromyalgia. *Ageing Res Rev.* 2002;1: 243–255.
36. Plotnikoff GA, Quigley BA. Prevalence of severe hypovitaminosis D in patients with persistent nonspecific musculoskeletal pain. *Mayo Clin Proc.* 2003;78:1463–1470.
37. Hudson J, Pope H. The relationship between fibromyalgia and major depressive disorder. *Rheum Dis Clin North Am.* 1996;22:285–303.
38. Lentjes E, Griep E. Boersma J, et al. Glucocorticoid receptors, fibromyalgia and low back pain. *Psychoneuroendocrinol.* 1997;22:603–614.
39. Hader N, Rimon D, Kinarty A, Lahat N. Altered interleukin-2 secretion in patients with primary fibromyalgia syndrome. *Arthritis Rheum.* 1991;34:866–872.
40. Scaer RC. *The Spectrum.* New York: WW Norton & Company; 2005.
41. Brosschot J, Pieper S, Thayer J. Expanding stress theory: prolonged activation and perserverative cognition. *Psychoneuroendocrinol.* 2005;30:1043–1049.
42. Busch A, Schachter CL, Peloso PM, Bombardier C. Exercise for treating fibromyalgia syndrome. *Cochrane Database Syst Rev.* 2007;(4):CD003786.
43. Wiger SH, Stiles TC, Vogel PA. Effects of aerobic exercise versus stress management treatment in fibromyalgia. *Scand J Rheum.* 1996;25:77–86.
44. Hakkinen A, Hakkinen K, Hannonen P, Alen M. Strength training-induced adaptations in neuromuscular function of premenopausal women with fibromyalgia: Comparisons with healthy women. *Ann Rheum Dis.* 2001;60:21–26.

45. Jentoft ES, Kvalvik AG, Mengshoel AM. Effects of pool-based and land-based aerobic exercise on women with fibromyalgia/chronic widespread muscle pain. *Arth Care Res.* 2001;45:42–47.
46. Sunshine W, Field TM, Quintino O, et al. Fibromyalgia benefits from massage therapy and transcutaneous electrical stimulation. *J Clin Rheumatol.* 1996;2:18–22.
47. Sheon RP, Moskowitz RW, Goldberg VM. *Soft Tissue Rheumatic Pain: Recognition, Management, and Prevention, 3rd ed.* Baltimore: Williams & Wilkins; 1996.
48. Kaplan KH, Goldenberg DL, Galvin-Nadeau M. The impact of a meditation-based stress reduction program on fibromyalgia. *Gen Hosp Psych.* 1993;15:284–289.
49. Grossman P, Tiefenthaler-Gilmer U, Raysz A, Kesper U. Minfulness training as an intervention for fibromyalgia: Evidence of postintervention and 3-year follow-up benefits well-being. *Psychther Psycosom.* 2007;76:226–233.
50. Stephton S, Salmon P, Weissbecker I, et al. Mindfulness meditation alleviates depressive symptoms in women with fibromyalgia: Results of a randomized clinical trial. 2002;57:77–85.
51. Kabat-Zinn J. *Full Catastrophe Living: Using the Wisdom of Your Body and Mind to Face Stress, Pain, Illness.* New York: Bantam Doubleday Dell; 1990.
52. Ferraccioli G, Ghirelli L, Scita F, et al. EMG-biofeedback training in fibromyalgia syndrome. *J Rheumatol.* 1987;14:820–825.
53. Haanen HCM, Hoenderdos HTW, van Romunde LKJ, et al. Controlled trial of hypnotherapy in the treatment of refractory fibromyalgia. *J Rheumatol.* 1991;8: 72–75.
54. Neustadt DH. Commentary. Psychosocial factors in rheumatic disease. *Orthop Rev.* 1984;13:114–115.
55. Kübler-Ross E. *On Death and Dying.* New York: Macmillan Publishing; 1996.
56. Sarno JE. *The Mind-Body Prescription.* New York: Warner Books; 1998.
57. Schecter D, Smith A, Beck J, Roach J, et al. Outcomes of a mind-body treatment program for chronic back pain with no distinct structural pathology-a case series of patients diagnosed and treated as tension myositis syndrome. *Alt Ther.* 2007;13:5:26–35.
58. Selfridge N, Peterson F. *Freedom from Fibromyalgia.* New York: Three Rivers Press; 2001.
59. Fors EA, Sexton H, Gotestam KG. The effect of guided imagery and amitriptyline on daily fibromyalgia pain: a prospective, randomized, controlled trial. *J Psychiatr Res.* 2002;36:3:179–187.
60. Merchant RE, Carmack CA, Wise CM. Nutritional supplementation with Chlorella pyrenoidosa for patients with fibromyalgia syndrome: A pilot study. *Phytother Res.* 2000;14:167–173.
61. Fisher P, Greenwood A, Huskisson EC, et al. Effect of homeopathic treatment on fibrositis (primary fibromyalgia). *BMJ.* 1989;299:365–366.
62. Bell I, Lewis D, Brooks A, Schwartz G, Lewis S, Walsh B, Baldwin C. Improved clinical status in fibromyalgia patients treated with individualized homeopathic remedies versus placebo. *Rheumatology.* 2004;43:577–582.

63. Jacobsen S, Danneskiold-Samose B, Anderson RB. Oral S-adenosylmethionine in primary fibromyalgia. Double-blind clinical evaluation. *Scand J Rheumatol.* 1991;20:294–302.
64. Simopoulos, AP. Evolutionary aspects of diet, the omega-6/omega-3 ratio and genetic variation: nutritional implications for chronic diseases. *Biomed Pharmacother.* 2006;9:502–507.
65. Fish consumption advisories: Mercury: http://www.epa.gov/mercury/advisories.htm.
66. Simms R. Fibromyalgia syndrome: Current concepts in pathophysiology, clinical features, and management. *Arthritis Care Res.* 1996;9:315–328.
67. McCain G. A cost-effective approach to the diagnosis and treatment of fibromyalgia. *Rheum Dis Clin North Am.* 1996;22:323–349.
68. Goldenberg D, Smith N. Management of the fibromyalgia syndrome. *JAMA.* 2004;292:2388–2395.
69. Gendreau R, Mease P, Rao S, et al. Milnacipran: a potential new treatment of fibromyalgia. *Arthritis Rheum.* 2003;48:S616.
70. Arnold L, Lu Y, Crofford L, et al. A double-blind, multi-center trial comparing duloxetine to placebo in the treatment of fibromyalgia with or without major depressive disorder. *Arthritis Rheum.* 2004;50:2974–2984.
71. Uceyler N, Hauser W, Sommer C. A systematic review on the effectiveness of treatment with antidepressants in fibromyaglia syndrome. *Arth Rheum.* 2008;59: 1279–1298.
72. Goldenberg D, Felson D, Dinerman HA. Randomized, controlled trial of amitriptyline and naproxen in the treatment of patients with fibromyalgia. *Arthritis Rheum.* 1986;29:655–659.
73. Crofford L, Rowbotham M, Mease P, et al. Pregabalin for the treatment of fibromyalgia syndrome: results of a randomized, double-blind, placebo-controlled trial. *Arthritis Rheum.* 2005;52:1264–1273.
74. Russell IJ, Kamin M, Bennett RM, et al. Efficacy of tramadol in treatment of pain in fibromyalgia. *J Clin Rheumatol.* 2000;6:250–257.
75. Eriksen J, Sjogren P, et al. Critical issues on opioids in chronic non-cancer pain: an epidemiologic study. *Pain.* 2006;125(1–2):172–179.
76. Russel I, Perkins A, Michalek J, et al. Sodium oxybate relieves pain and improves function in fibromyalgia syndrome. *Arth Rheum.* 2009;60:299–309.
77. Deluze C, Bosia L, Zirbs A, et al. Electroacupuncture in fibromyalgia: Results of a controlled trial. *BMJ.* 1992;305:1249–1252.
78. Berman BM, Ezzo J, Handhazy V, Swyers JP. Is acupuncture effective in the treatment of fibromyalgia? *J Fam Pract.* 1999;48:213–218.
79. Assefi N, Sherman K, Jacobsen C, et al. A randomized clinical trial of acupuncture compared with sham acupuncture in fibromyalgia. *Ann Intern Med.* 2005;143:10–19.
80. Horstman J. Chiari surgery. Arthritis Today 2000;Sep–Oct:78–82.
81. Yunus M, Bennett R, Romano, et al. Fibromyalgia consensus report: Additional comments. *J Clin Rheum.* 1997;3:324–327.

82. Turk DC, Okifuji A, Sinclair JD, Starz T. Pain, disability, and physical functioning in subgroups of patients with fibromyalgia. *J Rheumatol.* 1996;23:1255–1262.
83. Annemans L, Wessely S, Spaepen E, et al. Health economic consequences related to diagnosis of fibromyalgia syndrome. *Arthritis Rheum.* 2008;58:895–902.
84. Scaer R. *The Trauma Spectrum: Hidden Wounds and Human Resiliency.* London: Norton; 2005.
85. Levine P, Frederick A. *Waking the Tiger–Healing Trauma.* Berkeley, CA: North Atlantic Books; 1999.
86. Clarke D. *They Can't Find Anything Wrong.* Boulder, Colorado: Sentient Publications; 2007.
87. Pratt SG, Matthews K. *Super Foods Rx: Fourteen Foods That Will Change Your Life.* New York: HarperCollins Publishers Inc.; 2004.

16

Systemic Lupus Erythematosus

MICHELLE PETRI, MD, MPH

KEY CONCEPTS

- SLE is a female predominant disease (9:1), with onset usually in the 20s to 30s. It is more common and more severe in African Americans than Caucasians. The incidence has likely tripled since the 1950s–1970s.
- The pathogenesis of SLE is complex, involving a genetic predisposition, hormonal factors, and environmental factors. It is usually a multisystem disease, with skin, joints, and kidneys most commonly involved.
- Most patients with SLE are antinuclear antibody (ANA) positive. However, a positive ANA is not sufficient to make a diagnosis of SLE. Common autoantibodies in SLE include anti-dsDNA, anti-Sm, anti RNP, anti-Ro, anti-La, anticardiolipin, lupus anticoagulant, and direct Coombs test. Low complement (C3 or C4) levels are also frequent.
- Treatment includes hydroxychloroquine, NSAIDs, prednisone, and immunosuppressive drugs.
- The majority of organ damage in SLE is either directly or indirectly tied to corticosteroids. Corticosteroid sparing is a key part of management.
- The major cause of death in SLE is accelerated atherosclerosis. Traditional cardiovascular risk factors are increased, but cannot totally explain the higher risk.

■

Introduction

Systemic lupus erythematosus (SLE) is a systemic autoimmune disease primarily affecting females, with onset in the 20s and 30s. Its pathogenesis is complex, involving a polygenic predisposition, hormonal factors, and multiple environmental precipitants. Although SLE is thought of as a B cell disease, with production of autoantibodies, the immunopathogenesis is much more complex—including plasmacytoid dendritic cells, myeloid dendritic cells, macrophages, T cells, B cells, immune complexes, cytokines and chemokines.

The diagnosis of SLE may be delayed, because initial symptoms and signs may be nonspecific. Common presentations include photosensitive rashes, polyarthritis, and nephritis. Treatment includes hydroxychloroquine, prednisone, and often other immunosuppressive drugs. Unfortunately, treatment often leads to side effects and organ damage. Surprisingly, the major cause of death in SLE is accelerated atherosclerosis—not lupus activity, infections, or renal failure. This chapter will explore all of these concepts.

Epidemiology

SLE is much more common in women than in men and in African-Americans than in Caucasians.

SLE has a strong gender bias, with the female:male ratio being 9:1. The onset is usually after puberty. Most women are diagnosed in their 20s and 30s. SLE does occur in children, where the male:female ratio is more nearly equal. In younger patients, nephritis is more common.

SLE is more common in African Americans than in Caucasians. It is more severe in both African Americans and Hispanic Americans than in Caucasians.[1]

It is estimated that there are 161,000 to 322,000 SLE patients in the United States.[2] The incidence of lupus appears to have tripled since the 1950s–1970s.[3] This increase cannot be explained by recognition of mild disease, because the frequency of nephritis is equal.

Pathogenesis

GENETIC PREDISPOSITION

There is a genetic predisposition to SLE. Concordance in identical twins is 50% or higher. A shared genetic predisposition leads to multiple related autoimmune diseases, such that family members of a SLE patient may have autoimmune thyroid disease, Sjogren's syndrome, rheumatoid arthritis, or myasthenia gravis—not just SLE. Some of the genes predisposing to SLE have been identified. HLA-DR and DQ alleles, and null complement alleles, predispose to lupus. Recently identified genes include the interferon regulatory factor (IRF5) and STAT-4 (involved in intracellular signaling).

HORMONAL FACTORS

The female gender bias of SLE points towards a role of sex hormones in SLE. Estrogen has multiple effects on immune function, including increasing the production of autoantibodies. However, multiple sex hormone interactions are instrumental in SLE. Both women and men with SLE have lower androgen levels. Women with SLE have lower levels of dehydroepiandrosterone, a mild androgen produced by the adrenal glands. Some women with SLE have increased levels of prolactin.

ENVIRONMENTAL PRECIPITANTS

> The classic precipitant of SLE is ultraviolet light – both UV-A and UV-B activate disease.

The classic environmental precipitant of SLE is ultraviolet light. Other precipitants include infection, especially Epstein Barr Virus (EBV). In multi-case families, children with SLE have a very strong association with EBV exposure.[4] In adults, antibodies to EBV appear before SLE autoantibodies.[5] Medications can induce idiopathic SLE. The classic culprit is trimethoprim-sulfa.[6]

Table 16.1. Classification Criteria for SLE.

Systemic lupus erythematosus may be classified if 4 or more of the following 11 disorders are present:

- Malar rash
- Discoid rash
- Photosensitivity
- Oral ulcers
- Arthritis
- Serositis

Renal disorder

- a. > 0.5 g/d proteinuria, *or*
- b. ≥ 3+ dipstick proteinuria, *or*
- c. Cellular casts

Neurologic disorder

- a. Seizures, *or*
- b. Psychosis (without other cause)

Hematologic disorder

- a. Hemolytic anemia, *or*
- b. Leukopenia (< 4000/mL), *or*
- c. Lymphopenia (< 1500/mL), *or*
- d. Thrombocytopenia (< 100,000/mL)

Immunologic disorder

- a. Antibody to native DNA, *or*
- b. Antibody to Sm (Smith), *or*
- c. Anticardiolipin antibodies, lupus anticoagulant, or false-positive serologic test for syphilis

Positive antinuclear antibodies

Adapted from Tan et al[7] *and Hochberg.*[8]

Classification Criteria

Four of the 11 American College of Rheumatology classification criteria (Table 16.1) are needed to confirm a classification of SLE.[7,8] Although not developed for diagnostic purposes, the criteria are frequently used as such. The criteria do emphasize the multisystem nature of lupus; however, it is possible to classify as SLE a patient with 4 cutaneous criteria (photosensitivity, malar rash, discoid rash, and oral ulcers) but no systemic disease. Lupus nephritis alone would be sufficient to diagnose lupus, even in the absence of any other criteria. The neurologic criterion is limited to seizures and psychosis, even though the neurologic manifestations of SLE are much more varied.[9]

Organ Systems

MUCOCUTANEOUS

Lupus rashes include malar rash, discoid rash, maculopapular rash, alopecia, cutaneous vasculitis, subacute cutaneous lupus, bullous lupus and erythema.

Most lupus rashes are photosensitive. Typical lupus rashes include the malar rash (over the cheeks and bridge of the nose) and a maculopapular rash in sun-exposed area, such as the neck, v-area of the chest, and forearms. Acute cutaneous lupus can also cause erythema and even a desquamating rash of the fingertips.

Subacute cutaneous lupus (SCLE) presents more slowly. Patients who don't have SLE can have SCLE. In fact, a frequent cause of SCLE is drugs. There are two clinical types of SCLE: an annular form (often mistaken as fungal) and a psoriaform (often mistaken as psoriasis).

Chronic cutaneous lupus is also called discoid lupus. It can occur as part of SLE, or as a "stand alone" type of lupus. Because it involves the deeper layer—the dermis—it is more likely to scar (either as hyperpigmentation or hypopigmentation). When it occurs on the scalp, it can lead to permanent scarring alopecia.

Bullous lupus is a rare blistering rash of SLE. Panniculitis (fat inflammation) is a rare manifestation of lupus, occurring most often on the face or upper arms. Cutaneous vasculitis (palpable purpura) can also occur.

Mucous membrane involvement in SLE includes oral ulcers and nasal ulcers. Discoid lupus can occur in the mouth and palate, as well.

MUSCULOSKELETAL

Lupus arthritis is not erosive. Joint deformities are reducible (called Jaccouds arthritis).

SLE causes both arthralgias and true arthritis (synovitis). The joint distribution overlaps that of rheumatoid arthritis (proximal interphalangeal joints (PIPs), metacarpophalangeal joints (MCPs), wrists, knees), but SLE arthritis is rarely erosive. Because of tendon and ligament laxity, there can be reversible joint deformities, called *Jaccoud's arthropathy*. Myositis can also occur in SLE. Surprisingly, however, the major cause of muscle pain in SLE is fibromyalgia.

SEROSITIS

Inflammation of serosal surfaces, including pleurisy (with or without pleural effusion), pericarditis (with or without pericardial effusion) and peritonitis (very rare, with or without ascites), occurs in SLE.

RENAL

Proteinuria occurs in about 40% to 50% of SLE patients, and is more common in African Americans than in Caucasians. Hematuria and red blood cell casts can also occur with nephritis. Renal biopsy identifies 5 types of nephritis by ISN class: mild mesangial, mesangial, focal, diffuse, and membranous. The most serious presentation, diffuse proliferative glomerulonephritis, can rapidly lead to renal failure.

NEUROLOGIC

The American College of Rheumatology has summarized neuropsychiatric syndromes that can occur in SLE.[9] The most common is cognitive impairment, which occurs in 80% by ten years after diagnosis.[10] Other neurologic manifestations include seizures, psychosis, cranial neuropathy, transverse myelitis, peripheral neuropathy, mononeuritis multiplex, and encephalopathy.

HEMATOLOGIC

Cytopenias are common in SLE. Leukopenia occurs, but rarely is the white blood count below 1.8 (it is largely lymphopenia; neutropenia is rare). Thrombocytopenia can occur from SLE directly, but also from antiphospholipid antibodies or drugs. The most common anemia related to lupus is anemia of chronic inflammation. Hemolytic anemia (with positive Coombs' test) is rare.

CONSTITUTIONAL

Fever can be part of a SLE flare, but infection must always be ruled out. Lymphadenopathy, especially in the cervical chain, can be found. Hepatomegaly and splenomegaly are rare. Weight loss sometimes occurs early in SLE.

IMMUNOLOGIC

A positive antinuclear antibody (ANA) is found in most SLE patients; the titer is often greater than 640, but need not be. Autoantibodies specific for SLE include anti-dsDNA and anti-Sm (for "Smith"). Other common autoantibodies are anti-Ro, anti-La, and anti-RNP. Low complement (C3 and/or C4) can occur.

ANTIPHOSPHOLIPID ANTIBODIES

About 50% of SLE patients will have an antiphospholipid antibody (although they can be intermittently positive): lupus anticoagulant, anticardiolipin or anti-β_2 glycoprotein 1. These antibodies are associated with hypercoagulability, pregnancy loss, and thrombocytopenia.[11]

Organ Damage

> The majority of organ damage in SLE is directly or indirectly tied to corticosteroid treatment.

There is a new emphasis in SLE on prevention of organ damage. One third of patients end up on disability. The major surprise is that 80% of permanent organ damage is directly or indirectly due to corticosteroid treatment.[12] High dose oral corticosteroids are associated with osteonecrosis and cataract. Even low-dose steroids are associated with osteoporotic fractures and with cataracts. The patients with the highest risk of coronary artery disease are those maintained on low-dose prednisone (but, of course, this is because of ongoing activity of disease).[13]

SLE itself is still a cause of renal failure, in spite of treatment with intravenous cyclophosphamide or mycophenolate mofetil. Discoid lupus continues to cause scarring and permanent alopecia. Antiphospholipid syndrome can cause stroke and venous stasis ulcers after deep venous thrombosis.

Much organ damage, though, is multifactorial, due to SLE and to comorbidity. This is especially apparent with the major cause of death in SLE: premature atherosclerosis. The risk of myocardial infarction in women with SLE between 35 and 44 years is increased 50-fold.[14] Not all of the risk is explained by traditional cardiovascular risk factors: SLE itself is a risk factor.[15] However, attention to traditional cardiovascular risk factors is mandatory in SLE.

Osteoporosis is another example of multifactoral causation. Corticosteroid use is the major risk factor. Inflammation, however, is also a risk factor. SLE patients, because of the need for sun avoidance, may also be vitamin D deficient. African Americans, with a greater risk of SLE, are more likely to be vitamin D deficient.

Malignancy is increased in SLE, even without exposure to immunosuppressive drugs.[16] This increase in malignancy is not limited to those exposed to immunosuppressive therapy.

Quality of Life

The quality of life of an average SLE patient is poor, on par with someone with HIV infection. All domains of quality-of-life can be affected, including mental and physical components.

Treatment

SLE remains an unpredictable disease. About half of patients have chronically active disease, and another have a “flare” pattern with sudden exacerbations.[17] Very few patients have remissions requiring no therapy.

Hydroxychloroquine is the mainstay of SLE treatment – not just for skin and joint lupus, but to prevent flares.

A major goal is prevention of flares. Hydroxychloroquine should be the cornerstone of SLE management, because it can reduce flares by 50%, and prevent progression of disease.[18] All patients should avoid known precipitants of flares, including ultraviolet light, echinacea, and trimethoprin sulfa.[6]

The treatment of active lupus is dictated by the organ system. Photosensitive rashes are treated by sun avoidance, UV-A and UV-B sunblock, and hydroxychloroquine. A second antimalarial drug, quinacrine, can be added in recalcitrant cases. Severe discoid lupus, unresponsive to combination antimalarial drugs, often responds to thalidomide. However, the toxicity of thalidomide (fetal malformation, premature ovarian failure, thrombosis, and peripheral neuropathy) makes it a difficult choice. Some patients may need oral corticosteroids. If, after initial response, there is reoccurrence of disease activity with taper, corticosteroid-sparing immunosuppressive drugs such as mycophenolate mofetil, azathioprine, and methotrexate may be added.

Lupus arthritis requires hydroxychloroquine. NSAIDs are used, but all NSAIDs now carry the warning of increased cardiovascular risk. Low-dose corticosteroids may be necessary. Immunosuppressive drugs approved for rheumatoid arthritis, including methotrexate and leflunomide, are often effective in SLE arthritis as well. However, anti- tumor necrosis factor biologics, which have been such a revolution in rheumatoid arthritis, are not favored in SLE because, although effective, they can increase the titers of SLE autoantibodies, including anti-dsDNA and anticardiolipin.[19]

The gold standard for the treatment of lupus nephritis is mycophenolate mofetil.

The treatment of renal lupus has drastically changed in the last 5 years. Because mycophenolate mofetil is equivalent (and, perhaps in African Americans, superior) to intravenous cyclophosphamide,[20,21] it is usually the first choice for the treatment of focal, diffuse, and membranous lupus nephritis. A "renal sparing regimen" is an essential adjunct, using ACE-inhibitors, angiotensin receptor blockers, and/or sprionolactone to reduce proteinuria and retard renal sclerosis.

The most common neurologic manifestation of SLE is cognitive impairment.

Central nervous system (CNS) lupus is varied in both presentation and severity. Severe CNS-lupus syndromes, such as encephalopathy, transverse myelitis, and mononeuritis multiplex, will usually require high-dose intravenous or oral corticosteroids. Lack of quick improvement may necessitate the need for monthly intravenous cyclophosphamide. "Last resort" treatments may include plasmapheresis or intravenous rituximab.

Hematologic lupus, such as mild leucopenia, thrombocytopenia above 30,000, or anemia of chronic disease, may not require treatment. Severe thrombocytopenia or hemolytic anemia will require high-dose corticosteroids and often intravenous immunoglobulin. Intravenous rituximab can be considered in recalcitrant cases. Splenectomy is not curative in all and, thus, should not be a first choice. Granulocyte colony stimulating factor has caused fatal SLE flares, and should not be the first choice for neutropenia due to intravenous cyclophosphamide.[22]

Serositis, when mild, may be treated with NSAIDs and, often, a one-time dose of intramuscular corticosteroids.[23] Severe serositis may require high-dose corticosteroids and maintenance immunosuppressive drugs, such as azathioprine or mycophenolate mofetil.

One alternative therapy, dihydroepiandrosterone (DHEA) has been extensively studied in SLE clinical trials and has benefit for mild to moderate SLE.[24,25] Other alternative therapies have been studied in murine models,[26] with little human data available.[27]

Complications of SLE Treatments

Hydroxychloroquine is the safest SLE treatment. Retinopathy is rare, and is estimated at one out of 5,000 patients. Yearly ophthalmology monitoring is recommended. The dose should be reduced with severe renal insufficiency. Hydroxychloroquine can be used in pregnancy.[28]

Corticosteroids are fraught with difficult side effects, including weight gain, depression, psychosis, insomnia, acne, hirsutism, diabetes mellitus, hypertension, hyperlipidemia, osteoporosis, osteonecrosis, infections, poor wound healing, cataracts, and glaucoma. The minimal dose should be used for the shortest period of time.

Immunosuppressive drugs can cause cytopenias, infection, and increased risk of malignancy. Cyclophosphamide, especially, is associated with nausea, vomiting, alopecia, hemorrhagic cystitis, malignancy, and premature ovarian failure. Lupron given 2 weeks before each infusion can help to protect ovarian function.[29] Mycophenolate mofetil can cause abdominal discomfort and diarrhea. Mycophenolate mofetil is not allowed in pregnancy. Genetic testing thiopurine methyl transferase (TPMT) can identify in advance SLE patients at risk for cytopenias from azathioprine.

Health Maintenance

SLE patients should be up to date on inactivated vaccines, including influenza vaccine, pneumococcal vaccine, and tetanus-diphtheria. Meningococcal vaccine should be considered, especially before college. However, the use of live viral vaccines is contraindicated in SLE patients.

SLE patients on corticosteroids should have Dual X-Ray Absorptiometry (DEXA) scans every 2 years. SLE patients on corticosteroids or on hydroxychloroquine must have yearly ophthalmology examinations.

Because of the increased risk of malignancy, American Cancer Society guidelines should be followed, including PAP smears, mammograms, and colonoscopy screening.

Closely Related Syndromes

UNDIFFERENTIATED CONNECTIVE TISSUE DISEASE

Mild autoimmunity is more common than SLE. Several groups have proposed criteria for "undifferentiated connective tissue disease."[30] A typical patient might be a young woman with positive ANA, Raynaud's, and arthralgias. If autoantibodies for a specific disease (such as anti-dsDNA for lupus, anti-centromere for Calcinosis Cutis, Raynaud's Phenomenon, Esophageal Dysfunction, Sclerodactyly and Telangiectasia Syndrome (CREST) are present, the risk of progression to a "named" disease is increased. On average, however, over the following 10 years, only 10% will progress.[31]

MIXED CONNECTIVE TISSUE DISEASE

The term "mixed connective tissue disease" was coined by Gordon Sharp and colleagues[32] to describe an overlap of lupus, myositis and scleroderma found in patients with high-titer anti-ribonucleoprotein. This term has fallen into disfavor because, over time, most patients will declare themselves as having SLE or scleroderma.[33]

REFERENCES

1. Alarcon GS, Roseman JM, Bartolucci AA, et al. Systemic lupus erythematosus in three ethnic groups: II. Features predictive of disease activity early in its course. LUMINA Study Group. Lupus in minority populations: nature vs nurture. *Arthritis Rheum.* 1998;41:1173–1180.
2. Helmick CG, Felson DT, Lawrence RC, et al. Estimates of the prevalence of arthritis and other rheumatic conditions in the United States: Part I. *Arthritis Rheum.* 2008;58(1):15–25.
3. Uramoto KM, Michet CJJ, Thumboo J, Sunku J, O'Fallon WM, Gabriel SE. Trends in the incidence and mortality of systemic lupus erythematosus, 1950–1992. *Arthritis Rheum.* 1999;42:46–50.
4. Harley JB, James JA. Epstein-Barr virus infection may be an environmental risk factor for systemic lupus erythematosus in children and teenagers [letter]. *Arthritis Rheum.* 1999;42(8):1782–1783.
5. James JA, Neas BR, Moser KL, et al. Systemic lupus erythematosus in adults is associated with previous Epstein-Barr virus exposure. *Arthritis Rheum.* 2001;44(5):1122–1126.
6. Petri M, Allbritton J. Antibiotic allergy in SLE: a case-control study. *J Rheumatol.* 1992;19:265–269.
7. Tan EM, Cohen AS, Fries JF, et al. The 1982 revised criteria for the classification of systemic lupus erythematosus. *Arthritis Rheum.* 1982;25:1271–1277.
8. Hochberg MC. Updating the American College of Rheumatology revised criteria for the classification of systemic lupus erythematosus [letter]. *Arthritis Rheum.* 1997;40:1725.
9. The American College of Rheumatology nomenclature and case definitions for neuropsychiatric lupus syndromes. *Arthritis Rheum.* 1999;42(4):599–608.
10. Brey RL, Holliday SL, Saklad AR, et al. Neuropsychiatric syndromes in SLE: Prevalence using standardized definitions in the San Antonio Study of Neuropsychiatric Disease Cohort. *Neurology.* 2002;58:1214–1220.
11. Petri M. Clinical and management aspects of the antiphospholipid syndrome. In: Wallace DJ, Hahn BH, eds. *Dubois' Lupus Erythematosus. 7th ed.* Philadelphia: Lippincott Williams & Wilkins; 2006: 1262–1297.
12. Gladman DD, Urowitz MB, Rahman P, Ibanez D, Tam LS. Accrual of organ damage over time in patients with systemic lupus erythematosus. *J Rheumatol.* 2003;30(9):1955–1959.
13. Zonana-Nacach A, Barr SG, Magder LS, Petri M. Damage in systemic lupus erythematosus and its association with corticosteroids. *Arthritis Rheum.* 2000;43:1801–1808.
14. Manzi S, Meilahn EN, Rairie JE, et al. Age-specific incidence rates of myocardial infarction and angina in women with systemic lupus erythematosus: comparison with the Framingham Study. *Am J Epidemiol.* 1997;145(5):408–415.

15. Esdaile JM, Abrahamowicz M, Grodzicky T, et al. Traditional Framingham risk factors fail to fully account for accelerated atherosclerosis in systemic lupus erythematosus. *Arthritis Rheum.* 2001;44(10):2331–2337.
16. Bernatsky S, Joseph L, Boivin JF, et al. The relationship between cancer and medication exposures in systemic lupus erythaematosus: a case-cohort study. *Ann Rheum Dis.* 2008;67(1):74–79.
17. Barr S, Zonana-Nacach A, Magder L, Petri M. Patterns of disease activity in systemic lupus erythematosus. *Arthritis Rheum.* 1999;42:2682–2688.
18. Canadian Hydroxychloroquine Study Group. A randomized study of the effect of withdrawing hydroxychloroquine sulfate in systemic lupus erythematosus. *N Engl J Med.* 1991;324:150–154.
19. Aringer M, Graninger WB, Steiner G, Smolen JS. Safety and efficacy of tumor necrosis factor alpha blockade in systemic lupus erythematosus: an open-label study. *Arthritis Rheum.* 2004;50(10):3161–3169.
20. Ginzler EM, Dooley MA, Aranow C, Kim MY, Buyon J, Merrill JT, et al. Mycophenolate mofetil or intravenous cyclophosphamide for lupus nephritis. *N Engl J Med.* 2005;353(21):2219–2228.
21. Contreras G, Pardo V, Leclercq B, Lenz O, Tozman E, O'Nan P, et al. Sequential therapies for proliferative lupus nephritis. *N Engl J Med.* 2004;350(10):971–980.
22. Vasiliu IM, Petri MA, Baer AN. Therapy with Granulocyte Colony-Stimulating Factor in Systemic Lupus Erythematosus May Be Associated with Severe Flares *J Rheumatol.* 2006;33(9):1878–1880.
23. Danowski A, Magder L, Petri M. Flares in lupus: Outcome Assessment Trial (FLOAT), a comparison between oral methylprednisolone and intramuscular triamcinolone. *J Rheumatol.* 2006;33(1):57–60.
24. Petri M. Sex hormones and systemic lupus erythematosus. *Lupus.* 2008;17(5): 412–415.
25. Petri MA, Lahita RG, Van Vollenhoven RF, et al. Effects of prasterone on corticosteroid requirements of women with systemic lupus erythematosus: a double-blind, randomized, placebo-controlled trial. *Arthritis Rheum.* 2002;46(7):1820–1829.
26. Petri M. Diet and systemic lupus erythematosus: from mouse and monkey to woman? *Lupus.* 2001;10:775–777.
27. Moore AD, Petri MA, Manzi S, Isenberg DA, Gordon C, Senecal JL, et al. The use of alternative medical therapies in patients with systemic lupus erythematosus. Trination Study Group. *Arthritis Rheum.* 2000;43(6):1410–1418.
28. Parke A, West B. Hydroxychloroquine in pregnant patients with systemic lupus erythematosus. *J Rheumatol.* 1996;23:1715–1718.
29. Somers EC, Marder W, Christman GM, Ognenovski V, McCune WJ. Use of a gonadotropin-releasing hormone analog for protection against premature ovarian failure during cyclophosphamide therapy in women with severe lupus. *Arthritis Rheum.* 2005;52(9):2761–2767.
30. Doria A, Mosca M, Gambari PF, Bombardieri S. Defining unclassifiable connective tissue diseases: incomplete, undifferentiated, or both?. *J Rheumatol.* 2005;32(2): 213–215.

31. Williams HJ, Alarcon GS, Joks R, Steen VD, Bulpitt K, Clegg DO, et al. Early undifferentiated connective tissue disease (CTD). VI. An inception cohort after 10 years: disease remissions and changes in diagnoses in well established and undifferentiated CTD. *J Rheumatol.* 1999;26(4):816–825.
32. Sharp GC, Irvin WS, May CM, Holman HR, McDuffie FC, Hess EV, et al. Association of antibodies to ribonucleoprotein and Sm antigens with mixed connective-tissue disease, systematic lupus erythematosus and other rheumatic diseases. *N Engl J Med.* 1976;295(21):1149–1154.
33. Black C, Isenberg DA. Mixed connective tissue disease—goodbye to all that. *Br J Rheumatol.* 1992;31(10):695–700.

17

Osteoarthritis

NISHA MANEK, MD, MRCP (UK)

KEY CONCEPTS

- Osteoarthritis is the most prevalent form of arthritis worldwide, and a significant cost burden for health care in the developed countries.
- The etiology of osteoarthritis is multifactorial, and epidemiological studies have shown a strong association of obesity with risk for incident and progression of knee osteoarthritis (OA). Weight reduction, therefore, is a modifiable risk factor for knee OA.
- The popular nutraceuticals glucosamine sulfate and chondroitin sulfate, alone or in combination, merit a trial in patients with symptomatic knee OA.
- There is some evidence for the analgesic effects of *Harpagophytum procumbens*, or Devil's claw, in the treatment of back pain, and S-adenosylmethionine (SAMe) in treatment of knee OA.
- Acupuncture has a measurable, although modest, benefit in treating pain from knee OA.
- Exercise such as Tai Chi has preliminary evidence for benefit in symptomatic knee OA, and has the added benefit of improved balance and quality of life.

■

Introduction

Osteoarthritis (OA) is a major cause of morbidity, physical limitation, and increased healthcare utilization among the elderly in developed countries, and the burden of disease is predicted to increase substantially in the next 2 decades.[1–4] The etiology of OA is complex. Aging, genetics,[5] and modifiable risk factors such as obesity[6] have been shown to be strong associations in epidemiological studies.[7]

Baseline Assessment and Management Objectives

Management of OA is to a large extent site-specific (Table 17.1, Figure 17.1). The main guiding principles of treatment can be outlined as follows: to base patient management decisions on the severity of pain, disability and distress, rather than on the severity of joint damage or radiographic changes; to empower people by providing them with advice about simple measures that they can take to help themselves; and to progress to interventions that require supervision or specialist knowledge only if simple measures fail.[8–10] Other aspects of the patient's disease at baseline must be established (Table 17.2, 17.3, and 17.4). Because OA has no cure, the main conventional strategy has been to manage pain with pharmacological agents, such as nonsteroidal anti-inflammatory drugs (NSAIDs), which can have significant adverse effects.[11,12]

According to the 2002 National Health Interview Survey (N = 30,785), which included integrative medicine (termed complementary and alternative medicine, or CAM), 41% of those who reported having arthritis had used some form of CAM.[13] Other community surveys have shown similar results.[14,15]

Table 17.1. The Descriptive Epidemiology of Osteoarthritis.

- The most common form of arthritis
- Occurs most frequently in the knee joints, hands (distal interphalangeal joints, DIP's; proximal interphalageal joints, PIP's; and carpo-metacarpal joint, CMC at the thumb base), hips, neck and lower back (cervical spine, and lumbar spine) (See Figure 17.1)
- Incidence and prevalence higher in women than in men, especially after the age of 50 years
- Many have joint symptoms without radiographic changes and vice versa

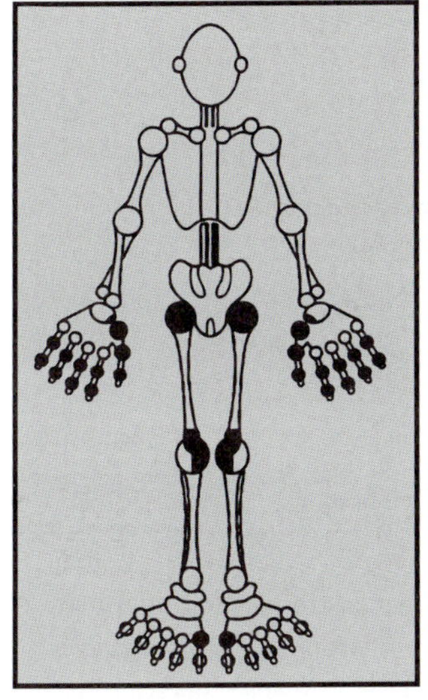

Common pattern of joint pain involvement in primary osteoarthritis
Upper extremities: Carpo-metacarpal joints (CMC), and distal interphalangeal joints (DIP)
Lower extremities: Knee (especially medial compartment), hip, and first metatarsal joint (MTP)
Axial: cervical and lumbar spine

FIGURE 17.1. Joint Distribution of Primary Osteoarthristis.

Whereas high-quality scientific evaluations of integrative therapies have been sparse, evidence is increasing as more randomized trials are conducted (Table 17.6). A suggested protocol for using integrative therapies is provided at the end of the chapter, and is based upon the severity of OA symptoms (Figure 17.6, and Table 17.6).

Table 17.2. Common Symptoms and Signs of Osteoarthritis.

Symptoms	*Signs*
Pain	Crepitus
Stiffness	Restricted movement
Alteration in shape	Tenderness
Functional impairment	-joint line
± anxiety, depression	-peri-articular
	Bony swelling
	Defromity
	Muscle wasting/weakness
	± effusions, increased warmth
	± instability

Table 17.3. Establishing a Baseline Program.

Relevant History

- Duration of OA
- Location and number of symptomatic joints
- Duration of symptoms as well as exacerbating and remitting factors
- Prior treatments for OA and success of these treatments
- Adverse effects, if any, from these treatments
- Clear account of over-the-counter medication use
- Understanding by the patient of the condition
- Prior intra-articular steroid or hyaluronate injections
- Surgical procedures performed on the joints
- Use of assistive devices such as canes, crutches, and knee braces

Other relevant medical information at baseline evaluation

- History of peptic ulcer disease, and any episodes of upper gastrointestinal bleeding episodes, coronary artery disease and heart failure, hypertension, renal disease, liver disease, and any chronic skin condition if use of topical agents (capsaicin cream) is considered
- Concomitant chronic diseases, especially chondrocalcinosis and thyroid disease
- Concomitant warfarin and anti-coagulant therapy
- Concomitant oral steroid use

Table 17.4. Possible needs of the patient with osteoarthritis.*

Physical	*Educational*	*Psychological*	*Social*
Diagnostic procedures Medication Exercise Diet Splinting Adaptive equipment Surgery	Instruction regarding medication (dosages, side effects) Methods of compliance Joint positioning Use of orthotics/ adaptive equipment Weight control	Aid in coping with: Depression Anxiety Anger Low self-esteem Changes in lifestyle	Finances for medical and daily living Avoidance of isolation Employment counseling Home care Sexual counseling

*Adapted from Manek NJ. Osteoarthritis Baseline Program In: Osteoarthritis Medical/Surgical Management Chapter 17 pp361–369

The Evidence for Integrative Therapies in OA

ACUPUNCTURE

Millions of Americans use acupuncture for pain-related symptoms,[16] and the medical community of rheumatologists and pain specialists consider acupuncture a legitimate medical practice.[17,18] Four large RCTs that comprise most of the evidence in treatment of knee osteoarthritis used a minimum of 10 to as many as 23 acupuncture treatments. The difference in WOMAC pain scale was modest but significant.[19–23]

Despite the evidence, the role of acupuncture in the management of knee OA is still unclear, particularly if a patient is already undertaking exercise.[24,22] It is possible that acupuncture will be most beneficial in those who cannot or do not exercise. Safety considerations, cost, and choosing an acupuncture practitioner have been discussed in an excellent review.[25] Further information regarding the role of acupuncture in arthritis can be found in Chapter 10.

AVOCADO SOYBEAN UNSAPONIFIABLES (ASU)

Avocado soybean unsaponifiables (often referred to as ASU) are a natural blended vegetable extract made from avocado and soybean oils, which have recently been popularized as therapy for OA. ASU are formed following hydrolysis, and are roughly composed of one-third avocado oil and two-thirds soybean oil. The mechanism of action of ASU is complex, and more recent work demonstrates this compound's effect on type 2 collagen synthesis.[26] Data from 4 key trials are summarized in Table 17.5.[27–30] Although the data are not uniform, the majority of studies suggest a beneficial effect of ASU in knee or hip OA of least 6 months duration.[31] The only long-term study[30] showed no difference in pain, functional ability, or daily NSAID use over 24 months, but it examined only patients with OA of the hip, with low initial daily use of NSAID. No serious adverse effects of ASU have been noted in any of the 4 trials. Although the volume of evidence is not large, it seems reasonable to suggest a course of ASU 300 mg daily for a minimum of 3 months in patients with moderate symptomatic OA of the hip or knee.[32]

NUTRACEUTICALS – GLUCOSAMINE AND CHONDROITIN SULFATE

Glucosamine: Glucosamine is a naturally occurring amino sugar which, in a sulfated form, is a normal constituent of glycoaminoglycans in cartilage matrix

Table 17.5. Randomized Controlled Trials of ASU for Osteoarthritis.**

Author (year)	*Study design**	*Sample size*	*Diagnosis*	*Intervention protocol*	*Outcome measure*	*Main results*	*Comment*
Blotman (1997)	2 Parallel groups	163	Knee or hip OA	300mg ASU or placebo daily for 3 months	Proportion taking NSAIDs during 2nd half of trial	ASU better than placebo	Secondary outcome measure (patients' overall ratings or functional index) also favored ASU. No inter-group differences in pain
Maheu (1998)	2 Parallel groups	164	Knee or hip OA	300mg ASU or placebo daily for 6 months	Lequesne index	ASU superior to placebo	Secondary outcome measures (global assessment, pain, function, NSAIDs requirements) favored ASU
Appelboom (2001)	3 Parallel groups	260	Knee OA	300mg ASU vs 600mg ASU vs placebo daily for 3 months	NSAID and analgesic intake	ASU superior to placebo, trend for dose dependent effects	Secondary outcome measures (Lequesne's index, pain) favored ASU
Lequesne (2002)	2 Parallel groups	163	Hip OA	300mg ASU or placebo (daily for 2 years)	Joint space width on radiographs	No significant inter-group differences. Subgroup analysis shows favorable results in most severely affected patients	No differences in secondary outcome measures, including Lequesne's index, pain, NSAID use, patients' global assessment, hip replacement surgery, sick leave (1 year data only)

**Adapted from Ernst E. Clinical Rheumatology 2003

ASU, Avocado Soybean Unsaponifiables; NSAIDs, non-steroidal anti-inflammatory drugs

*All studies randomized, double-blind, placebo-controlled

and synovial fluid. Numerous trials have investigated the effect of oral supplemental glucosamine in the treatment of knee OA. A Cochrane review assessed 20 studies including 2,570 patients[33] and found that the results varied depending on the assessment scale used, and whether or not the glucosamine sulfate was manufactured by the Italian pharmaceutical group, Rottapharm (Figure 17.2 and 17.3). The NIH funded a much-anticipated US trial, Glucosamine/chondroitin Arthritis Intervention Trial (GAIT).[34] The primary objective of the study was to compare the efficacy of treatment with glucosamine, chondroitin sulfate, or the two in combination, in patients with knee OA. Results of the GAIT trial were noteworthy in that over 60% of the patients in the placebo group demonstrated a positive outcome. In addition, a subgroup of patients with moderate to severe pain who received combination therapy with glucosamine and chondroitin had significantly higher rates of response than placebo therapy: rate of response with combination treatment was 79.2%, compared with 54.3% in patients treated with placebo ($p=0.002$) (Figure 17.4). The editorial accompanying the study results raised concerns that the preparation of glucosamine used in GAIT, glucosamine hydrochloride, might be less efficacious than glucosamine sulfate. On the basis of the results from GAIT, it seems prudent to tell patients with moderate to severe knee OA that neither glucosamine hydrochloride nor chondroitin sulfate alone has been shown to be more efficacious, but that the combination may afford more pain relief. Most importantly, the GAIT study confirmed previous trial data that both glucosamine and chondroitin were safe to use, with a side effect profile similar to that of placebo. Therefore, if patients who are using these nutraceuticals perceive benefit, I am reluctant to withdraw their use. An analysis of the structural effects of glucosamine and chondroitin will emerge from the GAIT study.

Chondroitin sulfate: Chondroitin sulfate is a naturally occurring complex carbohydrate that helps cartilage retain water. Biochemically, it is a glycosaminoglycan (GAG) which is usually found attached to proteins as part of a proteoglycan. Oral chondroitin alone, or in combination with glucosamine (usually glucosamine hydrochloride), has become a very popular treatment for OA. A previous meta-analysis reported significant relief of pain in patients using chondroitin.[35] However, the GAIT results[34] and another high-quality trial in knee OA[36] found conflicting results. Reichenbach and colleagues[37] undertook a meta-analysis to determine the effects of chondroitin alone on pain in patients with OA, and found the symptomatic benefit minimal or non-existent (Figure 17.5). Because chondroitin, at least in the United States, is almost always sold in a combination pill with glucosamine, the results of this meta-analysis may not apply to the combined product. What can clinicians take away from this study? Some patients are convinced that chondroitin helps their joints

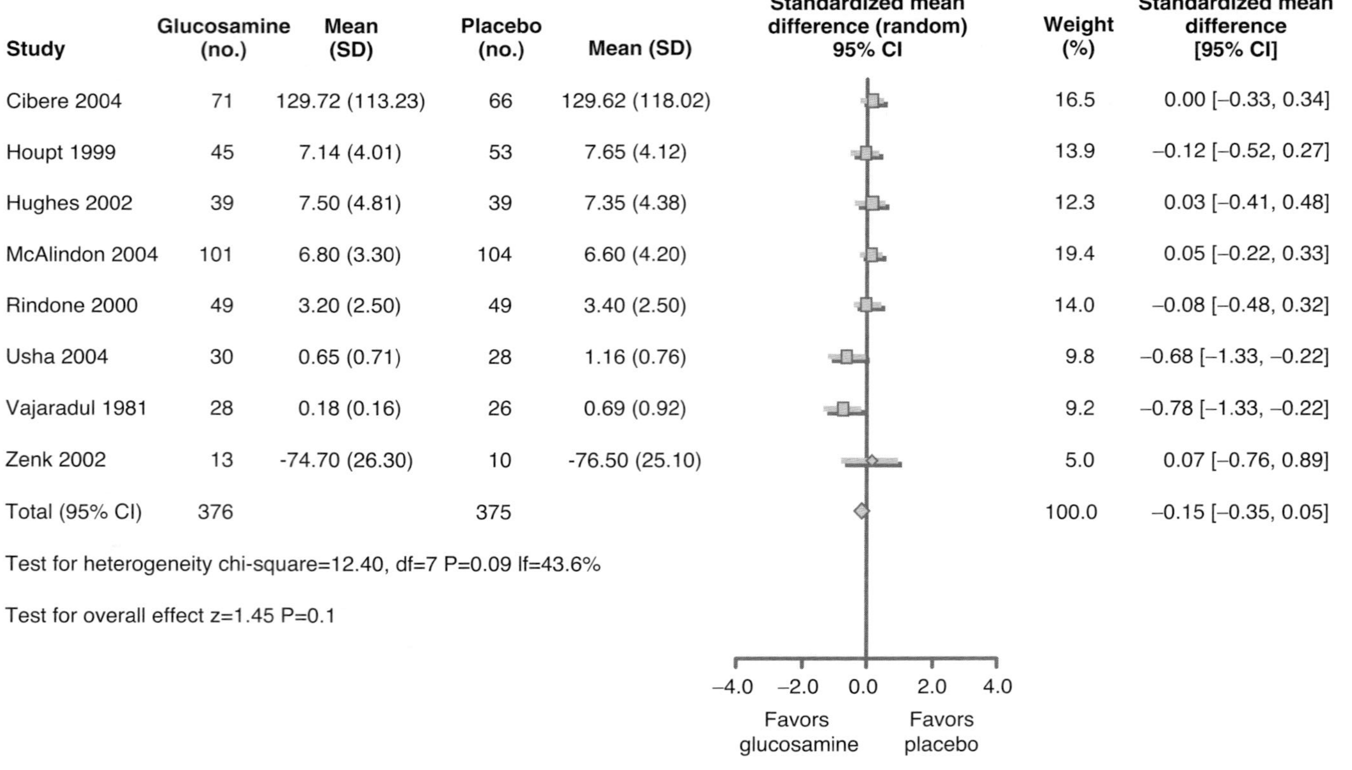

Study	Glucosamine (no.)	Mean (SD)	Placebo (no.)	Mean (SD)	Standardized mean difference (random) 95% CI	Weight (%)	Standardized mean difference [95% CI]
Cibere 2004	71	129.72 (113.23)	66	129.62 (118.02)		16.5	0.00 [–0.33, 0.34]
Houpt 1999	45	7.14 (4.01)	53	7.65 (4.12)		13.9	–0.12 [–0.52, 0.27]
Hughes 2002	39	7.50 (4.81)	39	7.35 (4.38)		12.3	0.03 [–0.41, 0.48]
McAlindon 2004	101	6.80 (3.30)	104	6.60 (4.20)		19.4	0.05 [–0.22, 0.33]
Rindone 2000	49	3.20 (2.50)	49	3.40 (2.50)		14.0	–0.08 [–0.48, 0.32]
Usha 2004	30	0.65 (0.71)	28	1.16 (0.76)		9.8	–0.68 [–1.33, –0.22]
Vajaradul 1981	28	0.18 (0.16)	26	0.69 (0.92)		9.2	–0.78 [–1.33, –0.22]
Zenk 2002	13	-74.70 (26.30)	10	-76.50 (25.10)		5.0	0.07 [–0.76, 0.89]
Total (95% CI)	376		375			100.0	–0.15 [–0.35, 0.05]

Test for heterogeneity chi-square=12.40, df=7 P=0.09 If=43.6%

Test for overall effect z=1.45 P=0.1

FIGURE 17.2. Meta-Analysis of Glucosamine in knee OA Glucosamines vs Placebo: Pain.*

*Adapted from: Towheed et al: Cochrane Database issue 2, 2005

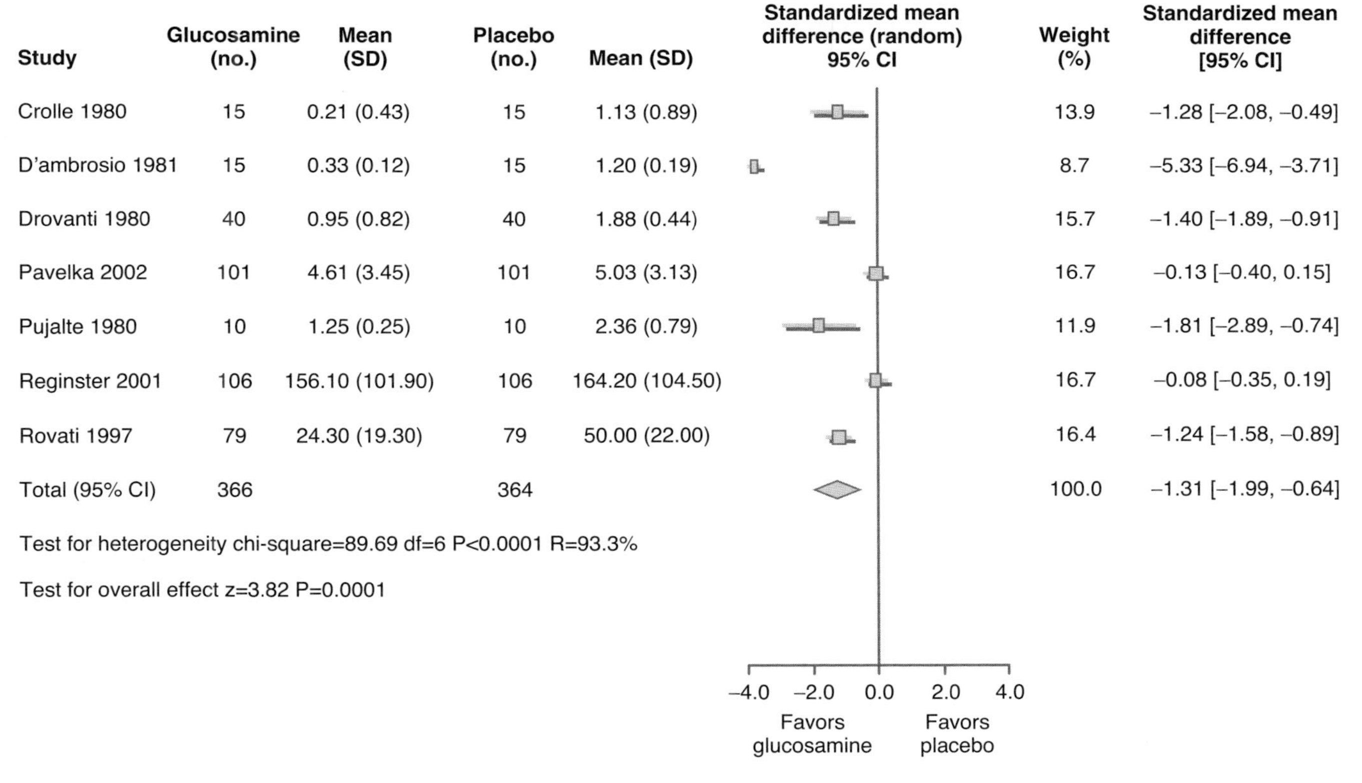

Study	Glucosamine (no.)	Mean (SD)	Placebo (no.)	Mean (SD)	Standardized mean difference (random) 95% CI	Weight (%)	Standardized mean difference [95% CI]
Crolle 1980	15	0.21 (0.43)	15	1.13 (0.89)		13.9	–1.28 [–2.08, –0.49]
D'ambrosio 1981	15	0.33 (0.12)	15	1.20 (0.19)		8.7	–5.33 [–6.94, –3.71]
Drovanti 1980	40	0.95 (0.82)	40	1.88 (0.44)		15.7	–1.40 [–1.89, –0.91]
Pavelka 2002	101	4.61 (3.45)	101	5.03 (3.13)		16.7	–0.13 [–0.40, 0.15]
Pujalte 1980	10	1.25 (0.25)	10	2.36 (0.79)		11.9	–1.81 [–2.89, –0.74]
Reginster 2001	106	156.10 (101.90)	106	164.20 (104.50)		16.7	–0.08 [–0.35, 0.19]
Rovati 1997	79	24.30 (19.30)	79	50.00 (22.00)		16.4	–1.24 [–1.58, –0.89]
Total (95% CI)	366		364			100.0	–1.31 [–1.99, –0.64]

Test for heterogeneity chi-square=89.69 df=6 P<0.0001 R=93.3%

Test for overall effect z=3.82 P=0.0001

FIGURE 17.3. Meta-Analysis of Glucosamine in knee OA Crystalline Glucosamine SO_4 (Rotta) vs Placebo for Pain.*

*Adapted from: Towheed et al: Cochrane Database issue 2, 2005

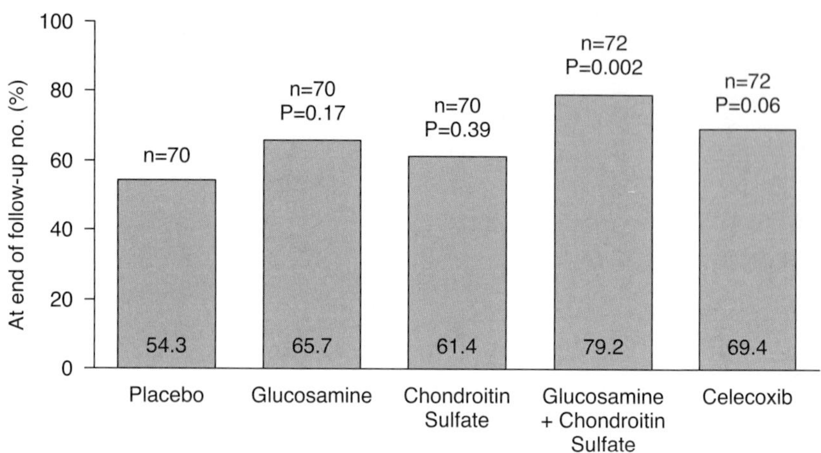

FIGURE 17.4. Patients with Moderate-to-Severe Pain (WOMAC Pain Score 301–400).*
*Adapted from: Clegg et al: NEJM 354:795, 2006.

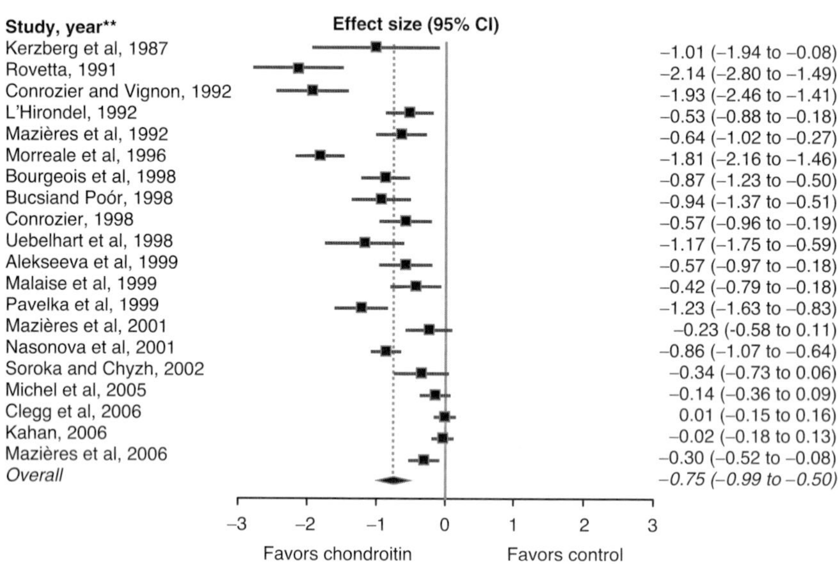

FIGURE 17.5. Forest Plot of 20 Trials Comparing Chondroitin with Control.*
*From: Reichenbach et al: Ann Intern med 146:580, 2007.
**Please refer to the publication for details of the trials in the meta-analysis.

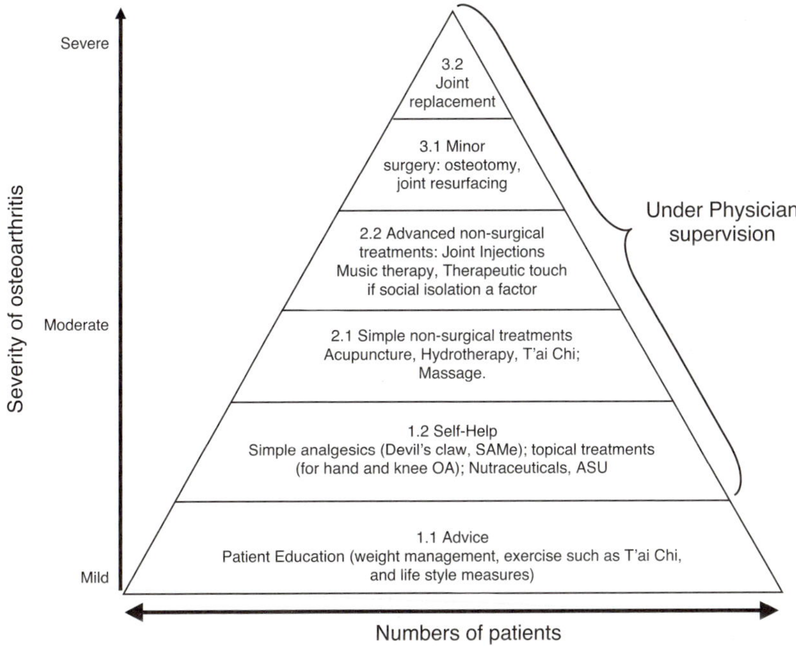

FIGURE 17.6. Suggested treatment protocol for knee OA.

(which could be a result of a placebo response, or even a therapeutic response resulting from limited metabolism of chondroitin), and because no frequent adverse effects have been reported, I generally advise patients to continue taking it as long as they perceive a benefit.

DEVIL'S CLAW

Devil's claw is the common name for 2 perennial plant species, *Harpagophytum procumbens* and *Harpagophytum zeyheri.* Early studies are beset with problems, including subjects with widely diverse medical conditions, a lack of *H. procumbens* extract standardization, and disparate dosing regimens.[38,39] An RCT comparator study by Chantre et al[40] in knee and hip OA indicates that devil's claw appears to be an effective intervention for pain control. A Cochrane review of devil's claw for low back pain found that daily doses, standardized to 50 mg or 100 mg of the compound harpagoside, were better than placebo for short-term improvements in pain and rescue medication.[41] The 1-year follow-up evaluation indicated a tolerance for the H. procumbens extract.[42] Devil's claw may be beneficial for the short-term treatment of pain from OA (8-12 weeks), and may allow for dose reduction of NSAIDs in some patients.

Table 17.6. The evidence for integrative therapies for osteoarthritis at a glance (based on published trial data - see text for details).

Good Scientific Evidence

Integrative Therapy	*Recommendations*	*Comments*
Acupuncture	A course of 1 to 2 treatments per week for a minimum of 8 weeks	May not be beneficial in those already undertaking exercise. Parameters of needling may vary from visit to visit and among different practitioners. Considered very safe in trained hands
Avocado soybean unsaponifiables (ASU)	300mg daily for 3 – 6 months	Up to 3 month delay in effect. No major adverse effects noted
Topical Capsaicin	0.025% to 0.075% cream application	Frequent application required 3-4 times daily. Delay in effect up to 3-4 weeks. Avoid spread to eyes and mouth. Useful in mild symptomatic hand and knee OA
Glucosamine sulfate	1500mg daily	Appears to be safe. Modest effect size in symptomatic knee OA May have better efficacy if used in combination with Chondroitin sulfate
Chondroitin sulfate	1200mg daily	Appears to be safe. Modest effect size if used alone. May have better efficacy if used in combination with Glucosamine sulfate
Devil's Claw	50 to 100mg standardized harpagosides daily for 8-12 weeks	Safety assessments limited. Adverse effects include dyspepsia, lowers arterial blood pressure. Caution if on anti-coagulants Avoid long-term use
SAMe	400mg to 1200mg daily	Has an anti-depressant effect. Delay in onset of action of up to 1 month. Long-term safety data not available

Table 17.6. (Continued)

Conflicting or Inconclusive Scientific Evidence		
Integrative therapy	*Recommendations*	*Comments*
Ashwagandha	Combination products studied	Specific effects unclear in OA trials May cause respiratory depression in large doses
Boswellia	Combination product (Artculin-F) used	Use catiously in patients with pre-existing gastritis or GERD.
Bromelain	Optimal dose unknown	May have potential benefit in mild hand and knee OA
Cat's Claw	Optimal dose unknown	Avoid in patients taking anticoagulant drugs
Magnets	Systematic reviews show no effect	Not recommended based on current evidence
Vitamins (Beta Carotene, vitamin C and E)	Avoid high dose vit C	No convincing evidence for symptomatic benefit or reduced cartilage loss
Trace Minerals	Combination products used	No convincing evidence for symptomatic benefit or reduced cartilage loss
Yoga	Hatha yoga over 8 weeks	Anecdotal reports seem promising. Trial data thus far is sparse. Individualized program under guidance from expert teacher probably the best
Promising Emerging Integrative Therapies		
Integrative therapy	*Recommendations*	*Comments*
Resveratrol (Grape extract)	No dose ranging studies available	Preliminary data in animals promising
Turmeric (Curcumin)	No dose ranging studies available	Available in combination or single herb preparation. Very popular spice in Indian cuisine
Tai Chi/Qigong	Training required under an experienced Tai Chi teacher	Probably useful therapy in sedentary individuals with chronic hip or knee OA
Massage and Therapeutic Touch	Effects	Especially useful in elderly patients with chronic osteoarthritic pain. Further studies needed for cost-effectiveness. May alleviate social isolation

S-ADENOSYLMETHIONINE (SAMe)

S-adenosylmethionine (SAMe) is a naturally occurring compound found in all living cells. It functions as a methyl donor, and is an essential participant in methylation reactions that help produce cartilage proteoglycans. By inference, SAMe may be important in the repair of damaged cartilage. Other mechanisms of action, such as decreasing inflammation and providing analgesia, have also been proposed. SAMe has a serotonergic activity and has been shown to decrease depression, which is another popular use of this compound. A meta-analysis of eleven RCTs comparing SAMe with placebo or NSAIDs in almost 1500 patients with OA (the majority had knee OA) concluded that SAMe was as effective as NSAIDs in reducing pain and improving function.[43] Oral doses ranging from 400 mg to 1200 mg daily were used in the studies. Unfortunately, most of the trials were only 1 month in duration. Besides the absence of long-term data, the authors noted that they could not exclude SAMe's anti-depressant qualities as a factor contributing to its apparent efficacy. SAMe does appear to be as effective in reducing pain (effect size = 0.12) as NSAIDs, regardless of dosage of SAMe or duration of trial. Furthermore, SAMe treated patients were 58% less likely to experience adverse effects than those treated with NSAIDs. A subsequent RCT compared 1200 mg of daily SAMe with celecoxib 200 mg daily in patients with knee OA.[44] SAMe demonstrated similar efficacy as celecoxib; however, SAMe had a slower onset of action, requiring nearly 1 month to achieve the same benefit as celecoxib. Adverse effects of SAMe were mild. One problem encountered in this trial was that the SAMe preparation lost 50% of its potency at one point, and a new batch of SAMe was substituted, allowing the trial to continue. This occurrence highlights the concern about stability of SAMe preparations. As with other dietary supplements, the precise amount of active ingredient contained in commercial preparations can vary widely.

Although the data suggest that SAMe is an effective therapy for OA, further studies are needed to verify this finding in larger trials of longer duration. Clarification of the optimal dose is also necessary.

METHYLSULFONYLMETHANE (MSM)

Methylsulfonylmethane (MSM), the iso-oxidized form of dimethyl-sulfoxide (DSMO), is a common ingredient in many over-the-counter topical preparations and oral dietary supplements sold for a variety of health concerns, including arthritis. Despite multimillion dollar sales and huge popularity in the lay publications, very little evidence is available in the medical literature to evaluate the role of MSM in the treatment of OA. No data are available regarding potential mechanism(s) of action. In a 12-week double-blind placebo-controlled RCT in mild to moderate knee OA (n=118), 500 mg of MSM three times daily, used alone or in combination with 500 mg of glucosamine hydrochloride three times daily, significantly improved pain as measured with the Likert scale and Lequesne index.[45] A more recent report, again in patients with knee OA (n=50), suggested that MSM at a dose of 6 g per day for 12 weeks improved WOMAC pain and function.[46] The authors of this small trial noted that the effect they documented was slight and of questionable clinical significance.[46] The benefits and safety of MSM in managing OA, and of long-term use, cannot be confirmed from these studies.

Other Botanical, Plant and Herbal Preparations

ASHWAGANDHA (*WITHANIA SOMNIFERA*)

Ashwagandha has been used in Ayurvedic medicine for a wide variety of conditions.[47] The active constituents of ashwangandha together are called withanolides, and most studies in humans have used a combination product, so specific conclusions about ashwagandha cannot, therefore, be drawn.[48,49]

BOSWELLIA (*BOSWELLIA SERRATA*)

Resin extracts from the *Boswellia Serrata* tree have been found to inhibit the synthesis of numerous pro-inflammatory mediators, and suggest possible efficacy for OA. High-quality human data are lacking. One early trial used a combination product, so no conclusion can be drawn about Boswellia specifically.[48] Another, more recent, trial in 30 patients with knee OA found improvements in pain and walking distance; however, the descriptions of blinding, randomization and statistical analysis were not well delineated, diminishing the quality of this publication.[50]

BROMELAIN

Bromelain is an aqueous extract obtained from both the stem and fruit of the pineapple plant, which contains many proteolytic enzymes. Brien et al[51] have recently published a review of the evidence of bromelain in the treatment of knee OA. The authors noted several methodological shortcomings of the trials reviewed, including inadequate power, inadequate treatment protocols, and inadequate (or totally absent) follow-up to monitor possible adverse effects of bromelain. Overall, however, bromelain appears to have potential for the treatment of mild symptomatic knee OA, but not in moderate to severe OA.[52] The trials in OA have used bromelain in doses ranging from 540 mg to 1890 mg daily—all with few adverse effects. Further studies are needed to identify the optimal dose over longer periods of time (e.g., 3-4 months) within an RCT.

CAT'S CLAW (*UNCARIA TOMENTOSA, UNCARIA GUIANENSIS*)

Cat's claw, derived from a woody vine native to South America, has been used to treat inflammation, digestive problems, and to promote wound healing. One trial found cat's claw to be beneficial in knee OA;[53] however, data from controlled trials are necessary before cat's claw can be recommended for OA.

GINGER AND TURMERIC

Ginger (*Zingiber officinale*), a rhizome, is popular in Ayurvedic and traditional Chinese medical (TCM) systems as a treatment for rheumatic symptoms. The characteristic aroma of ginger is from ketones, including gingerol, the main extract that has been used in research studies. Ginger extract has potentially important anti-inflammatory properties, and has been shown to inhibit prostaglandin synthesis[54] as well as to inhibit the activation of tumor necrosis factor α and cyclooxygenase-2 expression in in vitro studies of human synoviocytes.[55] These anti-inflammatory effects may potentially benefit patients with OA, since the degenerative process has inflammatory effects at the level of cartilage and subchondral bone. The clinical trials, however, have had mixed results. A large double-blind RCT (n=247) found that ginger reduced the pain of knee OA in the majority of patients,[56] and in a separate crossover study the effect of ginger in OA was significant only in the first period of treatment (i.e., before the crossover).[57] Another small double-blind RCT reported that although placebo was as effective as ginger extract during the first 3 months of the study, by the end of 6 months, the ginger extract group was significantly superior to the placebo group in terms of pain reduction.[58] Because of these conflicting results, there is still uncertainty regarding a role for ginger in the treatment of OA.[59]

Ginger can be consumed as a fresh or dried root. No specific dosing studies have been performed. Adverse effects after ingestion of ginger are uncommon, but they can include mild gastrointestinal effects such as heartburn, diarrhea, and irritation of the mouth. Patients taking anticoagulants such as warfarin (coumadin) should exercise caution when taking ginger, as it has a possibility of affecting fibrinolytic activity. Therefore physicians caring for patients who take warfarin and begin to use high-dose ginger should carefully monitor the International Normalized Ratio (INR) response. Rubbing the oil of ginger into painful joints has been advocated, although this technique has not been studied.

Turmeric is emerging as a potential treatment for inflammatory arthritis, and encouraging data in animal studies was recently published.[60] Data for treatment of OA is lacking; however, it is mentioned here as there is ample "bench" evidence for curcumin, the active component of turmeric, and its anti-inflammatory properties, which would be beneficial in OA.[61,62]

RESVERATROL (GRAPE EXTRACT)

Resveratrol is a polyphenolic compound that is present in various fruits, especially in the skin of red grapes. Recent studies have shown that resveratrol exhibits potent antioxidant properties[63] and is able to exert anti-inflammatory and anticatabolic properties in several cell types.[64] Results confirm that resveratrol is an effective inhibitor of chondrocyte apoptosis in vitro.[65] These findings suggest that this dietary polyphenolic compound may have future applications in the nutraceutical-based therapy of human and animal OA. Animal studies show promising results;[66] however, clinical data in humans are not available as yet.

Topical Therapies

Capsaicin cream: Capsaicin is an alkaloid derived from the seeds and membranes of the nightshade family of plants, which includes the common pepper plant. Capsaicin cream (0.025% to 0.075%) has been shown to be better than placebo in treating hand OA, and knee OA.[67] It does have several mild drawbacks: it is somewhat inconvenient, may be irritating to eyes and mouth, may require 3 to 4 applications per day, and improvement may not occur until 3 to 4 weeks after use. Nevertheless, it is safe and can be used as monotherapy.

Arnica Montana gel applied twice daily for 6 weeks reduced WOMAC scores for pain, stiffness and function in mild to moderate knee OA.[68]

The tolerability of topical arnica was rated "good" by the users. Arnica is approved by the German Commission E as a topical agent for its anti-inflammatory, and analgesic properties. The United States FDA, however, has classified arnica as an unsafe herb.

Anti-Oxidant Vitamins and Trace Minerals

Vitamin C: There has long been recognition that nutritional factors influence the maintenance of bone and joint health, but the evidence to support the use of specific vitamin therapies for OA has not yet been compelling. Nevertheless, vitamin supplements remain among the most frequently used options chosen by patients from the CAM menu. The Framingham OA cohort data suggest that higher vitamin C may reduce OA progression, but not incidence.[69] In this epidemiological study of 640 participants, nutrient intake was calculated from a food frequency questionnaire. Radiographs of the knee joints were taken at baseline and at 8 years. The progression of radiographic knee OA was reduced threefold in those subjects in the middle and highest tertiles of vitamin C intake (highest vs. lowest intake-adjusted odds ratio [OR] = 0.3; 95% CI 0.1–0.6). The patients in the highest tertile of vitamin C intake also had reduced risk of developing knee pain (OR = 0.3; 95% CI 0.1–0.8). However, these results need to be interpreted cautiously because vitamin C was measured only at one time point. Interestingly, high vitamin C intake over 24 months has been shown to have an adverse effect on knee function.[70]

Vitamin E: Several studies have explored the role of vitamin E in the treatment (or prevention) of OA. The above-cited Framingham study found vitamin E to be efficacious in reducing progression of OA, but only in men.[68] Data from the Johnston County Osteoarthritis Project in North Carolina[71] suggested that those with the highest ratios of serum alpha-tocopherol to gamma-tocopherol had half the odds ratio of radiographically verified knee OA in men and African Americans. Wluka et al used MRI to assess whether 500IU of vitamin E affected cartilage volume loss in 117 patients with established knee OA. No significant differences in cartilage loss nor improvement in symptoms were seen, and therefore the authors concluded that there is no clear role for the recommendation of vitamin E.[72] In terms of pain management, vitamin E (alpha-tocopherol 500IU/day for 6 months) appears to have no benefit.[73]

Vitamin D: Vitamin D levels are unrelated to the risk of cartilage loss in knee OA.[74] Lower levels of vitamin D may be associated with osteophytes;[75] however, a causal relationship has not been established between vitamin D and bone turnover in OA.

Beta Carotene: Total daily beta carotene intake and daily retinol equivalent intake do not have any structural or symptomatic benefit in knee OA.[70]

Minerals (Zinc, Selenium, trace minerals, Boron): Little evidence exists for the use of trace minerals for the treatment of symptomatic OA. Zinc, selenium,[76,77] boron, magnesium, and manganese have all been examined in small short-term studies, and no definitive conclusions can be drawn from the published work.

MIND-BODY AND ENERGY MEDICINE (YOGA, TAI-CHI/QIGONG, GUIDED IMAGERY, HYPNOSIS AND REIKI)

Yoga and tai chi, both of which combine physical exercise with a meditative component, are very popular in health clubs across the United States. There is, however, little quality research for these interventions as potential treatments for OA. Two studies of yoga, one in knee OA[78] and another in hand OA,[79] were small, and the results are difficult to extrapolate to the clinical situation. Nevertheless, many patients report benefit with yoga practice, particularly with increased joint function and better muscular strength. If patients want to try yoga, it is recommended to have an individualized program under close supervision of an experienced yoga teacher.

A systematic review of the clinical trial data for tai chi has recently been published.[80] Of published trials, 4 were RCT's and overall there is encouraging evidence suggesting that tai chi improves pain control, balance, and physical functioning.[81–84] The study protocols varied widely, with both group as well as home practice used. Qigong, like tai chi, uses gentle low-impact exercise, as well as breath work, visualization, and meditation.[85] Although no formal trials have been undertaken in OA, in my experience, patients who practice qigong regularly report less joint pain and an overall sense of wellbeing.

Preliminary evidence in small trials of other mind-body techniques such as guided imagery[86] and hypnosis[87] demonstrates the feasibility of these approaches in patients with chronic pain from OA, and may be suitable techniques to consider in individual cases.

OTHER THERAPIES (MAGNETS, MASSAGE, MUSIC THERAPY, AND THERAPEUTIC TOUCH)

Magnet therapy: The use of magnets in the therapy of rheumatic diseases is ancient, yet remains popular. A Cochrane review assessed the available evidence favoring the use of magnets and found it to be limited.[88] Two other reviews found that static magnets did not offer statistically significant short-term pain relief of knee OA relative to placebo.[89,90] No major safety concerns have been raised in relation to magnet therapy. Larger trials that adequately account for patient blinding are needed to confirm whether the positive results in some studies[91] translate to clinically meaningful outcomes for patients.

Massage: Among older adults with OA, massage therapy was found to be most commonly used, followed by chiropractic services.[15] Massage has high patient acceptance and satisfaction, with few side effects.[92] Swedish massage sessions in patients with knee OA reduced WOMAC pain scores and stiffness, as well as "time to walk" indices,[93] with beneficial effects persisting for weeks following treatment cessation. Massage may offer adjunctive therapy to more conventional OA therapies. Further study of massage is required to determine optimal treatment protocols, absolute efficacy, cost-effectiveness, and generalization to other patient groups. Another modality, therapeutic touch, has been found to improve pain and level of function in patients with knee OA;[94] however, it is unknown if this effect is sustained. Finally, in an evaluation of another "sensory" intervention, community-dwelling elderly persons with chronic osteoarthritic pain perceived a reduction in pain using music therapy for 20 minutes daily.[95]

Summary

The randomized trials for integrative modalities in OA show small to moderate effects for most therapeutic interventions, but they are still valuable for patients and clinically relevant for physicians. The results suggest that, for several treatments, the risk-benefit profile is encouraging: acupuncture, several herbal preparations, nutraceuticals, glucosamine and chondrotin sulfate, ASU, and capsaicin cream. For other therapies, the evidence is weak or contradictory: several botanical preparations, MSM, magnet therapy, vitamins and antioxidants, and yoga. And, there are some emerging and promising integrative therapies, including turmeric (curcuminoids) and resveratrol. These may be appropriate in individual situations. The key to successful management involves patients and health professionals working together as a team, in order to develop optimal treatment strategies for the individual. Regular monitoring is important, as the condition will progress in some patients, and different therapeutic approaches may be needed (Table 17.7).

Table 17.7. Key practice points.

Summary points for the management of OA according to clinical severity. A simple method of categorizing patients is suggested to aid the clinician's approach to management.

Category 1: Mild OA

Definition: Modest discomfort and joint stiffness with little or no interference with activities of daily living or participation in life.

Suggested management strategy:

- Advise remaining physically active and lose weight if necessary. Low impact exercise such as Tai Chi/Qi gong may be beneficial
- May not require pharmacological interventions and best to avoid medications in such patients
- Topical treatments may be considered

Category 2: Moderate OA, No comorbidity

Definition: Significant pain and discomfort in joints and/or impairment of joint function that interferes with normal activities and/or those aspects of life considered important to that patient; no major co-morbidity

Suggested management strategy:

- Provide education and assess for need for assistive devices
- Prescribe formal exercise therapy
- Analgesics (Devil's claw or SAMe)
- Topical treatments could be used as adjunctive treatment
- Consider dietary supplements (Nutraceuticals and ASU)
- Acupuncture for symptomatic knee OA

Category 3: Moderate OA, complicated by Comorbid conditions

Definition: Problems with OA as above, complicated by other psychosocial or medical problems such as depression, neurological problems, poor vision and hearing compound mobility on already painful joints

Suggested management strategy:

- As above
- Consider treating the co-morbid conditions may be more effective than treating the OA. This area challenging to discern to what extent problems that may make pain worse like depression or disability (e.g. neurological and sensory problems) are present.
- Avoid NSAID's particularly in older people. Consider SAMe and short term Devil's claw
- Music therapy or therapeutic touch may be helpful

Category 4: Severe OA

Definition: Pain and/or disability that prevents the individual from sleeping, working or engaging in everyday activities of daily living

Suggested Management strategy:

- As above
- Give early consideration to joint replacement surgery in hip and knee OA

REFERENCES

1. Hootman JM, Helmick CG. Projections of US prevalence of arthritis and associated activity limitations. *Arthritis Rheum.* 2006;54(1):226–229.
2. Dillon CF, Rasch EK, Gu Q, Hirsch R. Prevalence of knee osteoarthritis in the United States: arthritis data from the Third National Health and Nutrition Examination Survey 1991–94. *J Rheumatol.* 2006;33(11):2271–2279.
3. Dillon CF, Hirsch R, Rasch EK, Gu Q. Symptomatic hand osteoarthritis in the United States: prevalence and functional impairment estimates from the third U.S. National Health and Nutrition Examination Survey, 1991–1994. *Am J Phys Med Rehabil.* 2007;86(1):12–21.
4. Theis KA, Helmick CG, Hootman JM. Arthritis burden and impact are greater among U.S. women than men: intervention opportunities. *J Womens Health.* 2007;16(4):441–453.
5. Manek NJ, Spector TD. *Genetic Aspects of Osteoarthritis - Evidence for the Inheritance of Osteoarthritis.* In: *Osteoarthritis.* Brandt KD, Doherty M, Lohmander LS, eds. Oxford: Oxford University Press; 2003:25–31.
6. Manek NJ, Hart D, Spector TD, MacGregor AJ. The association of body mass index and osteoarthritis of the knee joint: an examination of genetic and environmental influences. *Arthritis Rheum.* 2003;48:1024–1029.
7. Felson DT, Lawrence RC, Dieppe PA, et al. Osteoarthritis: new insights. Part 1: the disease and its risk factors. *Ann Intern Med.* 2000;133(8):635–646.
8. Felson DT, Lawrence RC, Hochberg MC, et al. Osteoarthritis: new insights. Part 2: treatment approaches. *Ann Intern Med.* 2000;133(9):726–737.
9. Recommendations for the medical management of osteoarthritis of the hip and knee: 2000 update. American College of Rheumatology Subcommittee on Osteoarthritis Guidelines. *Arthritis Rheum.* 2000;43(9):1905–1915.
10. Jüni P, Reichenbach S, Dieppe P. Osteoarthritis: rational approach to treating the individual. *Best Pract Res Clin Rheumatol.* 2006;20(4):721–740.
11. Strand V, Hochberg MC. The risk of cardiovascular thrombotic events with selective cyclooxygenase-2 inhibitors. *Arthritis Rheum.* 2002;47(4):349–355.
12. Hernández-Diaz S, García-Rodríguez LA. Epidemiologic assessment of the safety of conventional nonsteroidal anti-inflammatory drugs. *Am J Med.* 2001;110 Suppl 3A:20S–27S.
13. Quandt SA, Chen H, Grzywacz JG, Bell RA, Lang W, Arcury TA. Use of complementary and alternative medicine by persons with arthritis: results of the National Health Interview Survey. *Arthritis Rheum.* 2005;53(5):748–755.
14. Herman CJ, Allen P, Hunt WC, Prasad A, Brady TJ. Use of complementary therapies among primary care clinic patients with arthritis. *Prev Chronic Dis.* 2004; 1(4):A12.
15. Ramsey SD, Spencer AC, Topolski TD, Belza B, Patrick DL. Use of alternative therapies by older adults with osteoarthritis. *Arthritis Rheum.* 2001;45(3):222–227.

16. Barnes PM, Powell-Griner E, McFann K, Nahin RL. Complementary and alternative medicine use among adults: United States, 2002. *Adv Data.* 2004;(343):1–19.
17. Berman BM, Bausell RB, Lee WL. Use and referral patterns for 22 complementary and alternative medical therapies by members of the American College of Rheumatology: results of a national survey. *Arch Intern Med.* 2002;162(7):766–770.
18. Berman BM, Bausell RB. The use of non-pharmacological therapies by pain specialists. *Pain.* 2000;85(3):313–315.
19. Berman BM, Lao L, Langenberg P, Lee WL, Gilpin AM, Hochberg MC. Effectiveness of acupuncture as adjunctive therapy in osteoarthritis of the knee: a randomized, controlled trial. *Ann. Intern Med.* 2004;141(12):901–910.
20. Vas J, Méndez C, Perea-Milla E, et al. Acupuncture as a complementary therapy to the pharmacological treatment of osteoarthritis of the knee: randomised controlled trial. *BMJ.* 2004;329(7476):1216.
21. Witt C, Brinkhaus B, Jena S, et al. Acupuncture in patients with osteoarthritis of the knee: a randomised trial. *Lancet.* 2005;366(9480):136–143.
22. Scharf HP, Mansmann U, Streitberger K, et al. Acupuncture and knee osteoarthritis: a three-armed randomized trial. *Ann Intern Med.* 2006;145(1):12–20.
23. White A, Foster NE, Cummings M, Barlas P. Acupuncture treatment for chronic knee pain: a systematic review. *Rheumatology.* 2007;46(3):384–390.
24. Foster NE, Thomas E, Barlas P, et al. Acupuncture as an adjunct to exercise based physiotherapy for osteoarthritis of the knee: randomised controlled trial. *BMJ.* 2007;335(7617):436.
25. Berman B. A 60-year-old woman considering acupuncture for knee pain. *JAMA.* 2007; 297(15):1697–1707.
26. Henrotin YE, Deberg MA, Crielaard JM, Piccardi N, Msika P, Sanchez C. Avocado/soybean unsaponifiables prevent the inhibitory effect of osteoarthritic subchondral osteoblasts on aggrecan and type II collagen synthesis by chondrocytes. *J Rheumatol.* 2006;33(8):1668–1678.
27. Blotman F, Maheu E, Wulwik A, Caspard H, Lopez A. Efficacy and safety of avocado/soybean unsaponifiables in the treatment of symptomatic osteoarthritis of the knee and hip. A prospective, multicenter, three-month, randomized, double-blind, placebo-controlled trial. *Rev Rhum Engl Ed.* 1997;64(12):825–834.
28. Maheu E, Mazières B, Valat JP. Symptomatic efficacy of avocado/soybean unsaponifiables in the treatment of osteoarthritis of the knee and hip: a prospective, randomized, double-blind, placebo-controlled, multicenter clinical trial with a six-month treatment period and a two-month followup demonstrating a persistent effect. *Arthritis Rheum.* 1998;41(1):81–91.
29. Appelboom T, Schuermans J, Verbruggen G, Henrotin Y, Reginster JY. Symptoms modifying effect of avocado/soybean unsaponifiables (ASU) in knee osteoarthritis. A double blind, prospective, placebo-controlled study. *Scand J Rheumatol.* 2001;30(4):242–247.
30. Lequesne M, Maheu E, Cadet C, Dreiser RL. Structural effect of avocado/soybean unsaponifiables on joint space loss in osteoarthritis of the hip. *Arthritis Rheum.* 2002;47(1):50–58.

31. Ernst E. Avocado-soybean unsaponifiables (ASU) for osteoarthritis - a systematic review. *Clin Rheumatol.* 2003;22(4-5):285–288.
32. Christensen R, Bartels EM, Astrup A, Bliddal H. Symptomatic efficacy of avocado-soybean unsaponifiables (ASU) in osteoarthritis (OA) patients: a meta-analysis of randomized controlled trials. *Osteoarthritis Cartilage.* 2008;16(4):399–408.
33. Towheed TE, Maxwell L, Anastassiades TP, et al. Glucosamine therapy for treating osteoarthritis. *Cochrane Database Syst Rev.* 2005;18(2):CD002946.
34. Clegg DO, Reda DJ, Harris CL, et al. Glucosamine, chondroitin sulfate, and the two in combination for painful knee osteoarthritis. *N Engl J Med.* 2006;354(8): 795–808.
35. McAlindon TE, LaValley MP, Gulin JP, Felson DT. Glucosamine and chondroitin for treatment of osteoarthritis: a systematic quality assessment and meta-analysis. *JAMA.* 2000;283(11):1469–1475.
36. Michel BA, Stucki G Frey D, et al. Chondroitins 4 and 6 sulfate in osteoarthritis of the knee: a randomized, controlled trial. *Arthritis Rheum.* 2005;52(3):779–786.
37. Reichenbach S, Sterchi R, Scherer M, et al. Meta-analysis: chondroitin for osteoarthritis of the knee or hip. *Ann Intern Med.* 2007;146(8):580–590.
38. Denner SS. A review of the efficacy and safety of devil's claw for pain associated with degenerative musculoskeletal diseases, rheumatoid, and osteoarthritis. *Holist Nurs Pract.* 2007;21(4):203–207.
39. Brien S, Lewith GT, McGregor G. Devil's Claw (Harpagophytum procumbens) as a treatment for osteoarthritis: a review of efficacy and safety. *J Altern Complement Med.* 2006;12(10):981–993.
40. Chantre P, Cappelaere A, Leblan D, Guedon D, Vandermander J, Fournie B. Efficacy and tolerance of Harpagophytum procumbens versus diacerhein in treatment of osteoarthritis. *Phytomedicine.* 2000;7(3):177–183.
41. Gagnier JJ, van Tulder MW, Berman B, Bombardier C. Herbal medicine for low back pain: a Cochrane review. *Spine.* 2007;32(1):82–92.
42. Gagnier JJ, Chrubasik S, Manheimer E. Harpgophytum procumbens for osteoarthritis and low back pain: a systematic review. *BMC. Complement Altern Med.* 2004;4:13.
43. Soeken KL Lee WL, Bausell RB, Agelli M, Berman BM. Safety and efficacy of S-adenosylmethionine (SAMe) for osteoarthritis. *J Fam Pract.* 2002;51(5): 425–430.
44. Najm WI, Reinsch S, Hoehler F, Tobis JS, Harvey PW. S-adenosyl methionine (SAMe) versus celecoxib for the treatment of osteoarthritis symptoms: a double-blind cross-over trial. [ISRCTN36233495]. *BMC Musculoskelet Disord.* 2004;5:6.
45. Usha PR, Naidu MU. Randomised, Double-Blind, Parallel, Placebo-Controlled Study of Oral Glucosamine, Methylsulfonylmethane and their Combination in Osteoarthritis. *Clin. Drug Investig.* 2004;24(6):353-363.
46. Kim LS Axelrod LJ, Howard P, Buratovich N, Waters RF. Efficacy of methylsulfonylmethane (MSM) in osteoarthritisain of the knee: a pilot clinical trial. *Osteoarthritis Cartilage.* 2006;14(3):286–294.
47. Mishra LC, Singh BB, Dagenais S. Scientific basis for the therapeutic use of Withania somnifera (ashwagandha): a review. *Altern Med Rev.* 2000;5(4):334–346.

48. Kulkarni RR, Patki PS, Jog VP, Gandage SG, Patwardhan B. Treatment of osteoarthritis with a herbomineral formulation: a double-blind, placebo-controlled, cross-over study. *J Ethnopharmacol.* 1991;33(1-2):91–95.
49. Chopra A, Lavin P, Patwardhan B, Chitre D. A 32-week randomized, placebo-controlled clinical evaluation of RA-11, an Ayurvedic drug, on osteoarthritis of the knees. *J Clin Rheumatol.* 2004;10(5):236–245.
50. Kimmatkar N, Thawani V, Hingorani L, Khiyani R. Efficacy and tolerability of Boswellia serrata extract in treatment of osteoarthritis of knee–a randomized double blind placebo controlled trial. *Phytomedicine.* 2003;10(1):3–7.
51. Brien S, Lewith G, Walker A, Hicks SM, Middleton D. Bromelain as a Treatment for Osteoarthritis: a Review of Clinical Studies. *Evid Based Complement Alternat Med.* 2004;1(3):251–257.
52. Brien S, Lewith G, Walker AF, Middleton R, Prescott P, Bundy R. Bromelain as an adjunctive treatment for moderate-to-severe osteoarthritis of the knee: a randomized placebo-controlled pilot study. *QJM.* 2006;99(12):841–850.
53. Piscoya J, Rodriguez Z, Bustamante SA, Okuhama NN, Miller MJ, Sandoval M. Efficacy and safety of freeze-dried cat's claw in osteoarthritis of the knee: mechanisms of action of the species Uncaria guianensis. *Inflamm Res.* 2001;50(9):442–448.
54. Grzanna R, Lindmark L, Frondoza CG. Ginger–an herbal medicinal product with broad anti-inflammatory actions. *J Med Food.* 2005;8(2):125–132.
55. Frondoza CG, Sohrabi A, Polotsky A, Phan PV, Hungerford DS, Lindmark L. An in vitro screening assay for inhibitors of proinflammatory mediators in herbal extracts using human synoviocyte cultures. *In Vitro Cell Dev Biol Anim.* 2004; 40(3-4):95–101.
56. Altman RD, Marcussen KC. Effects of a ginger extract on knee pain in patients with osteoarthritis. *Arthritis Rheum.* 2001;44:2531–2538.
57. Bliddal H, Rosetzsky A, Schlichting P, et al. A randomized, placebo-controlled, cross-over study of ginger extracts and ibuprofen in osteoarthritis. *Osteoarthritis Cartilage.* 2000;8(1):9–12.
58. Wigler I, Grotto I, Caspi D, Yaron M. The effects of Zintona EC (a ginger extract) on symptomatic gonarthritis. *Osteoarthritis Cartilage.* 2003;11:783–789.
59. Marcus DM, Suarez-Almazor ME. Is there a role for ginger in the treatment of osteoarthritis? *Arthritis Rheum.* 2001;44:2461–2462.
60. Funk JL, Frye JB, Oyarzo JN. et al. Efficacy and mechanism of action of turmeric supplements in the treatment of experimental arthritis. *Arthritis Rheum.* 2006;54: 3452–3464.
61. Aggarwal BB, Sundaram C, Malani N, Ichikawa H. Curcumin: the Indian solid gold. *Adv Exp Med Biol.* 2007;595:1–75.
62. Shishodia S, Sethi G, Aggarwal BB. Curcumin: getting back to the roots. *Ann N Y Acad Sci.* 2005;1056:206–217.
63. Khanna D, Sethi G, Ahn KS, et al. Natural products as a gold mine for arthritis treatment. *Curr Opin Pharmacol.* 2007;7(3):344–351.
64. Shakibaei M, John T, Seifarth C, Mobasheri A. Resveratrol inhibits IL-1 beta-induced stimulation of caspase-3 and cleavage of PARP in human articular chondrocytes in vitro. *Ann N Y Acad Sci.* 2007;1095:554–563.

65. Csaki C, Keshishzadeh N, Fischer K, Shakibaei M. Regulation of inflammation signalling by resveratrol in human chondrocytes in vitro. *Biochem Pharmacol.* 2008;75(3):677-687.
66. Elmali N, Esenkaya I, Harma A, Ertem K, Turkoz Y, Mizrak B. Effect of resveratrol in experimental osteoarthritis in rabbits. *Inflamm Res.* 2005;54(4):158–162.
67. Zhang WY, Li Wan Po A. The effectiveness of topically applied capsaicin. A meta-analysis. *Eur J Clin Pharmacol.* 1994;46(6):517–522.
68. Knuesel O, Weber M, Suter A. Arnica montana gel in osteoarthritis of the knee: an open, multicenter clinical trial. *Adv Ther.* 2002;19(5):209–218.
69. McAlindon TE, Jacques P, Zhang Y, et al. Do antioxidant micronutrients protect against the development and progression of knee osteoarthritis? *Arthritis Rheum.* 1996;39(4):648–656.
70. Wang Y, Cicuttini FM, Vitetta L, Wluka AE. What effect do dietary antioxidants have on the symptoms and structural progression of knee osteoarthritis over two years? *Clin Exp Rheumatol.* 2006;24(2):213–214.
71. Jordan JM, De Roos AJ, Renner JB. A case-control study of serum tocopherol levels and the alpha- to gamma-tocopherol ratio in radiographic knee osteoarthritis: the Johnston County Osteoarthritis Project. *Am J Epidemiol.* 2004;159:968–977.
72. Wluka AE, Stuckey S, Brand C, Cicuttini FM. Supplementary vitamin E does not affect the loss of cartilage volume in knee osteoarthritis: a 2 year double blind randomized placebo controlled study. *J Rheumatol.* 2002;29(12):2585–2591.
73. Brand C, Snaddon J, Bailey M, Cicuttini F. Vitamin E is ineffective for symptomatic relief of knee osteoarthritis: a six month double blind randomised, placebo controlled study. *Ann Rheum Dis.* 2001;60:946–949.
74. Felson DT, Niu J, Clancy M. et al. Low levels of vitamin D and worsening of knee osteoarthritis: results of two longitudinal studies. *Arthritis Rheum.* 2007;56: 129–136.
75. Hunter DJ, Hart D, Snieder H, Bettica P, Swaminathan R, Spector TD. Evidence of altered bone turnover, vitamin D and calcium regulation with knee osteoarthritis in female twins. *Rheumatology.* 2003;42:1311–1316.
76. Hill J, Bird HA. Failure of selenium-ace to improve osteoarthritis. *Br J Rheumatol.* 1990;29:211–213.
77. Canter P, Wider HB, Ernst E. The antioxidant vitamins A, C, E and selenium in the treatment of arthritis: a systematic review of randomized clinical trials. *Rheumatology.* 2007;46:1223–1233.
78. Kolasinski SL, Garfinkel M, Tsai AG, Matz W, Van Dyke A, Schumacher HR. Iyengar yoga for treating symptoms of osteoarthritis of the knees: a pilot study. *J Altern Complement Med.* 2005;11(4):689–693.
79. Garfinkel MS, Schumacher HR Jr, Husain A, Levy M, Reshetar RA. Evaluation of a yoga based regimen for treatment of osteoarthritis of the hands. *J Rheumatol.* 1994;21(12):2341–2343.
80. Lee MS, Pittler MH, Ernst E. Tai chi for osteoarthritis: a systematic review. *Clin Rheumatol.* 2008; 27(2):211–218.

81. Hartman CA, Manos TM, Winter C, Hartman DM, Li B, Smith JC. Effects of T'ai Chi training on function and quality of life indicators in older adults with osteoarthritis. *J Am Geriatr Soc.* 2000;48(12):1553–1559.
82. Fransen M, Nairn L, Winstanley J, Lam P, Edmonds J. Physical activity for osteoarthritis management: a randomized controlled clinical trial evaluating hydrotherapy or Tai Chi classes. *Arthritis Rheum.* 2007;57(3):407–414.
83. Brismée JM, Paige RL, Chyu MC. Group and home-based tai chi in elderly subjects with knee osteoarthritis: a randomized controlled trial. *Clin Rehabil.* 2007;21(2):99–111.
84. Song R, Lee EO, Lam P, Bae SC. Effects of tai chi exercise on pain balance, muscle strength, and perceived difficulties in physical functioning in older women with osteoarthritis: a randomized clinical trial. *J Rheumatol.* 2003;30(9):2039–2044.
85. Manek NJ, Lin C. *Qigong.* In: Yuan C, Bieber EJ, Bauer B, eds. *Textbook of Complementary and Alternative Medicine.* Boca Raton, FL: Taylor & Francis; 2003:199–210.
86. Baird CL. Sands L. A pilot study of the effectiveness of guided imagery with progressive muscle relaxation to reduce chronic pain and mobility difficulties of osteoarthritis. *Pain Manag Nurs.* 2004;5(3):97–104.
87. Gay MC, Philippot P, Luminet O. Differential effectiveness of psychological interventions for reducing osteoarthritis pain: a comparison of Erikson [correction of Erickson] hypnosis and Jacobson relaxation. *Eur J Pain.* 2002;6(1):1–16.
88. Hinman MR, Ford J, Heyl H. Effects of static magnets on chronic knee pain and physical function: a double-blind study. *Altern Ther Health Med.* 2002;8(4):50–55.
89. Bjordal JM, Johnson MI, Lopes-Martins RA, Bogen B, Chow R, Ljunggren AE. Short-term efficacy of physical interventions in osteoarthritic knee pain. A systematic review and meta-analysis of randomised placebo-controlled trials. *BMC Musculoskelet Disord.* 2007;8:51.
90. Pittler MH, Brown EM, Ernst E. Static magnets for reducing pain: systematic review and meta-analysis of randomized trials. *CMAJ.* 2007;177(7):736–742.
91. Wolsko PM, Eisenberg DM, Simon LS, et al. Double-blind placebo-controlled trial of static magnets for the treatment of osteoarthritis of the knee: results of a pilot study. *Altern Ther Health Med.* 2004;10(2):36–43.
92. Cameron, M. Is manual therapy a rational approach to improving health-related quality of life in people with arthritis? *Australas Chiropr Osteopathy.* 2002;10(1): 9–15.
93. Perlman AI, Sabina A, Williams AL, Njike VY, Katz DL. Massage therapy for osteoarthritis of the knee: a randomized controlled trial. *Arch Intern Med.* 2006;166(22):2533–2538.
94. Gordon A, Merenstein JH, D'Amico F, Hudgens D. The effects of therapeutic touch on patients with osteoarthritis of the knee. *J Fam Pract.* 1998;47(4):271–277.
95. McCaffrey R, Freeman E. Effect of music on chronic osteoarthritis pain in older people. *J Adv Nurs.* 2003;44:517–524.

18

Integrative Rheumatology in the Pediatric Patient

DEBORAH JANE POWER, DO

KEY CONCEPTS

- Until recently, little research has been published on integrative medicine in pediatric rheumatology or in the area of complementary and alternative medicine (CAM) use in pediatric rheumatology.
- The utilization of CAM with the current conventional treatment paradigms in pediatric rheumatology appeals to parents because of the perceived low risk of long/short-term side effects and the absence of detrimental effects on growth and development.
- Given the frequent lack of effective pain control with current pharmaceutical therapy, CAM provides an opportunity to improve quality of life in pediatric rheumatology patients.
- Specific CAM practices with potential benefit in juvenile idiopathic arthritis (JIA) include medicinal products/herbs and supplements, massage therapy, chiropractic treatment, osteopathic manipulative treatment, acupuncture, biofeedback/hypnosis, and cognitive areas such as hope, coping skills, and listening.
- Areas of active research in integrative pediatric rheumatology include treatment of pain without pharmaceuticals, the avoidance (or low dose) of corticosteroids, nutrition to support growth and development, anti-inflammatory treatments, and attention to positive self image.

■

Introduction

The use of complementary and alternative medicine (CAM) has gained popularity in adult rheumatology,[1,2] and there has also been an increase in the use of these modalities within the field of pediatric rheumatology. Use of complementary and alternative modalities in young children, regardless of diagnosis, has been estimated at 11–21% in general pediatric clinics, while in children with chronic diseases, the rates are much higher at 64%–80%.[3] This reflects a marked increase from a 1996 Medical Expenditure Panel Survey, a national survey of non-institutionalized children younger than 18, which found CAM use at only 1.8% for the US population.[4] However, very little published information exists regarding the efficacy and safety of these methods in the pediatric rheumatology population.[5] Also absent from the medical literature is a description of how to integrate CAM into the traditional model of pediatric rheumatology.

Integrative Medicine (IM) has been defined as an approach utilizing active and effective elements from traditional fields of medicine (e.g., traditional Chinese medicine (TCM) or Ayurvedic medicine), demonstrating their effectiveness through modern scientific research, and educating the professional and public community about the appropriate use of CAM therapies.[2] CAM encompasses a variety of modalities including (but not limited to): acupuncture, biofeedback, chiropractic care, exercise therapies, herbal therapies, massage therapy, nutritional counseling, prayer, spiritual healing, tai chi, Qigong and yoga.

Pediatric rheumatology involves the treatment of patients from 6 months to age 16, and includes over 100 different medical conditions. Juvenile idiopathic arthritis (JIA, formerly called juvenile rheumatoid arthritis), systemic lupus erythematosus (SLE), juvenile dermatomyostitis, juvenile vasculitis, juvenile scleroderma and juvenile spondyloarthropathy syndromes are some of the more common conditions seen in the pediatric rheumatology clinic (see Table 18.1).

There are currently fewer than 200 practicing board-certified pediatric rheumatologists in the United States—an extreme shortage according to a 2004 report to Congress by the U.S. Department of Health Services, Health Resources and Services Administration.[6] A 75% increase in the number of practicing pediatric rheumatologists is necessary to fully address the needs of U.S. pediatric patients. Until that level is met, other medical professionals will be called upon to treat pediatric patients with these conditions. Given the increasing use of CAM, many medical staff members dealing with children with rheumatologic conditions will benefit with CAM knowledge.

Table 18.1. Pediatric Rheumatology – Commonly Seen Conditions.

Juvenile Idiopathic Arthritis
Pediatric Systemic Lupus Erythematosus
Spondylitis – seen with Inflammatory Bowel disease, Reactive Arthritis, Psoriasis, Behcet's Syndrome
Antiphospholipid Syndrome
Kawaski's disease
Sjogren's Syndrome
Vasculitis – Wegner's Granulomatosis, Chrug-Straus, Polyarteritis Nodosa, Microscopic Polyangiitis, Takaysu's Arteritis
Scleroderma (Systemic Sclerosis), limited scleroderma (morphea)
Mixed Connective Tissue Disease
Sarcoidosis
Lyme Disease
Henoch-Schonlein purpura
Serum sickness
Fibromyaglia Syndrome
Erythromelalgia
Raynaud's disease
Growing pains
Iritis and other inflammatory eye disease
Low bone mineral density

*Adapted from Cassidy & Petty 2005

The most common form of juvenile rheumatologic disease, JIA, affects 148 to 167 children per 100,000; it is the most common chronic disease in children under 17, and is the most common cause of disability in children.[5] While the overall prevalence of pediatric rheumatic disease is relatively low, collectively these conditions are among the most common chronic illnesses of childhood and involve considerable disease burden and disability.[7]

Unique Treatment Needs of Pediatric Rheumatology Patients

Growth disturbances and nutritional considerations are associated with the pain and inflammation of JIA. Children with JIA have a caloric intake less than 50% of their estimated needs. They have been shown to have decreased lean muscle mass, and increase in fat mass. Elevated levels of interleukin-1 and tumor necrosis factor–alpha are implicated in the increased resting energy expenditure seen in patients with JIA. Generalized growth delay is common in patients with JIA, and is believed to be multifactorial. Corticosteroid treatment is known to have a suppressive effect on osteoblasts, thereby slowing growth. Inflammation can destroy the growth center, accelerate bone maturation, or cause premature closure of the growth plate. Overgrowth of the bones can occur in response to the increased blood flow from chronic inflammation. In addition, both active disease and glucocorticoid therapy can result in decreased bone mineral density, which increases the risk of fracture.[8]

Treatment of JIA is initiated in order to control inflammation and pain, maintain physical function, and promote normal development, growth and wellbeing.[8] Medications used in children include nonsteroidal anti-inflammatory drugs (NSAIDs), disease-modifying or slow-acting antirheumatic drugs, glucocorticoids, cytotoxic or immunosuppressive agents, and biologic response modifiers.[5] These medications have been shown to control the inflammation of JIA, but may have negative side effects which may limit their use. Biologic response modifiers have been used in the treatment of JIA since 2000, when Lovell and colleagues reported the initial outcomes of therapy with etanercept. Patients with polyarticular JIA who had failed to respond to (or tolerate) methotrexate showed dramatic response to, and marked decrease in inflammation with, etanercept within 3–4 injections. Treatment with anti-tumor necrosis factor agents, including infliximab and adalimumab, has been associated with increased risks of infection including tuberculosis, serious infections, and malignancy. The risk of malignancy associated with biologic agents is complicated by the increased incidence of malignancy in children with rheumatic disease.[5]

Parents of children afflicted with JIA struggle with the risks associated with conventional treatments versus the long-term consequences of a deforming, debilitative condition. They look to unconventional remedies as an alternative to potentially toxic treatment options. However, many unconventional therapies may pose a risk to children and adolescents.[9]

Use of unconventional remedies has been reported in 70% of patients with juvenile arthritis.[10] Many experts suggest that it is better to let parents try remedies which are innocuous, to caution them about potentially dangerous treatments such as megavitamins, and to tell them to refrain from participating in such approaches as bee-sting therapy.[5] By carefully choosing available, tested approaches to specific aspects of disease management, a practitioner can make thoughtful recommendations to pediatric patients and their parents.

The Use of CAM in Pain Management

Even with advances in the use of biologic therapies to treat patients with JIA, SLE, and other pediatric rheumatologic conditions, the majority of children still experience pain.[11,12] A growing body of research in pediatric rheumatic disease such as JIA, and idiopathic pain syndromes such as juvenile primary fibromyalgia syndrome (JPFS), highlights the importance of environmental and cognitive behavioral influences in the child—emotional distress, daily stress, and mood, as well as alterations in self-image, development, and coping techniques.[13] Some of these changes are due to the chronic nature of the condition, and others are the result of side effects from treatment medications.[5] The use of prednisone (either for life-threatening complications of rheumatic conditions, or to decrease pain, swelling and/or stiffness), with the resulting side effects of weight gain, cushingoid facies, hirsuitism and striae, can negatively impact a child's self-image.

A review of CAM therapies for management of acute pediatric pain found that cognitive-behavior interventions, relaxation techniques, breathing exercises, transcutaneous electric nerve stimulation (TENS), biofeedback, and acupuncture can supplement pharmacological methods of pain management in children.[14] Sensory and procedural information, combined with behavioral techniques such as progressive muscle relaxation, breathing techniques, and imagery can be used to divert attention away from pain and to decrease muscle tension, pain, and anxiety. Children are also highly susceptible to the power of suggestion, making useful the "magic glove" technique, in which an imaginary glove is placed on a child's hand, finger by finger, and the child is told that the glove will help to lessen the discomfort of a medical procedure. With more widespread pain, a magic blanket may cover the painful area. Guided imagery, using sights and sounds in a child's imagination to help the child feel good and less afraid (for example, children imagining being in their favorite place and the sights, sounds, and smells of that place) has been effective. Older children can imagine doing their favorite activity, and the sensations of experiencing the activity. These techniques not only provide distraction, but also enhance relaxation. Documented physiologic responses include decreased oxygen consumption, blood pressure, heart rate, and tonic muscle tension.[14] The use of such techniques may enable the practitioner to greatly decrease the dosage of pharmacologic agents required for adequate pain control.

The Use of CAM in Pediatric Populations

Kemper[15] noted that approximately 20%–30% of general pediatric patients had used one or more CAM therapies, while use among adolescents ranged from 50%–75%. Rates among patients with chronic, recurrent, or incurable conditions, such as those with rheumatoid arthritis, cancer, asthma, and cystic fibrosis range from 30%–70%. Still, only a minority of patients and families talk with their physicians about their use of CAM treatments. A Danish study found that 53% of patients seen in a 2-week period in a general pediatric clinic had used CAM at least once, while 2% of the total pediatric population used CAM instead of conventional medicines.[16] The fact that the term CAM encompasses a wide range of different therapies, based on diverse philosophies, beliefs, assumptions and practices, makes comparisons difficult (see Table 18.2). For example, visits with a homeopathic practitioner may typically be lengthy and focus on taking an extensive history, while chiropractic appointments may be brief and concentrate on physical examination and adjustment procedures.

More research on the use of CAM in pediatric populations is necessary, especially for those children with conditions that impose a heavy burden of suffering both on the patients and their families. Attention should be focused

Table 18.2. Unconventional Treatment Use by Parents.

Acupuncture
Nutritional advice or lifestyle diets
Massage therapy
Herbal remedies purchased
Biofeedback training
Training or practice of meditation, imagery or relaxation techniques
Homeopathic treatment
Spiritual healing or prayer
Hypnosis
Traditional medicine, such as Chinese, Ayurvedic, American Indian, etc.
Other treatment

*Davis & Darden, 2003

on conditions for which CAM therapies offer a reasonable likelihood of being helpful; for example, chronic and severe pain syndromes, and rheumatic and autoimmune disorders. Also, research priorities should focus on those CAM therapies already widely used by children and families, which include nutritional supplements such as vitamins, minerals and herbal remedies. Much research has been conducted on adult populations, but important questions remain about safety and toxicity in pediatric groups.[17]

A survey of families of children with special health care needs in southern Arizona found that 64% of the families reported using CAM for their child, and 48% had used such therapies within the past 6 months. The most common CAM therapies were spiritual healing/prayer/blessings, followed by massage, oral herbs, and special diets. The least frequently used were acupuncture and self-hypnosis. Use of CAM for the child was strongly related to the use of CAM in the past by the family member answering the survey.[18] These data on most frequently used CAM therapies contrast with another study,[19] which found that the most common methods were chiropractic, homeopathic, naturopathic, and acupuncture, accounting for 84% of CAM use in that population. Various studies reporting CAM utilization list different CAM therapies, resulting in different percentages of each type used. Also, the fact that these studies were done in different geographical areas may reflect the differing availability of the various modalities, or the ethnic backgrounds and religious beliefs of the study population. Spigelblatt surveyed a French-speaking Canadian population, while the Arizona study community contained primarily white and Hispanic subjects.

One study looked at the prevalence of CAM pediatric patients seen in a rheumatology clinic and reported the type of CAM therapy used.[20] CAM for this study was defined as any supplement, therapy, or remedy use by a patient which was not prescribed by the rheumatologist, other physician, or registered dietician, excluding multivitamins and meal-replacement products. Alternative therapies also included consultations with alternative health care practitioners such as naturopaths, homeopaths, or chiropractors. Two-thirds of the patients had used at least one form of CAM in the past 12 months, while half had used more than one form of CAM. Vitamins and minerals were the most frequently used form of CAM (Vitamin C, D, E, A, and B6). Relaxation techniques, copper bracelets or rings, and herbal remedies were also commonly used. The research found that those children who had more than one diagnosis were more likely to have used CAM approaches. It was recommended that all practitioners ask patients and their parents about the use of CAM, and to even assume that if children have more than one diagnosis, they will be using more than one form of CAM.[20]

An early study looked at patients who attended arthritis youth camps.[10] Between 1 and 8 "unconventional remedies" (mean 2.6) had been used by 70%

of the patients. The most commonly used alternative remedies were copper bracelets (68%), diet (43%), and supplements (38%), including shellfish and seaweed extracts, cod liver oil, megavitamins, and herbal remedies. The use of specific dietary restrictions is a potentially serious problem in children whose growth is already compromised by the chronic arthritis process. Some factors contributing to the use of CAM by adults—including chronic pain, the cyclical nature of the illness, and inadequate education about the disease—may be equally applicable to children and parents of children with chronic disease.

Recent work addressed the perceptions of parents of patients with JIA regarding conventional and CAM therapies. Of the 92% of patients who had used CAM, 54% had used massage, 54% utilized vitamins and other supplements, 35% avoided food that worsened pain, and 33% had used stress management techniques. Parents reported therapies that were most helpful included biologic medications, methotrexate, naproxen, wheelchairs, orthotics, heat, vitamin C & D, music, support groups, and prayer. Zero median side effects from CAM use were reported.[21]

Specific CAM Practices for Use in Pediatric Rheumatology

NONPHARMACEUTICAL MEDICINAL PRODUCTS (HERBS, DIETARY SUPPLEMENTS, VITAMINS, AND HOMEOPATHY)

The categories of herbs, dietary supplements, and homeopathy often overlap. Herbal products are regulated as dietary supplements under the Dietary Supplement Health and Education Act of 1994 (DSHEA). But when the same products are diluted and prepared according to the Homeopathic Pharmacopoeia of the United States, they become pharmaceutical products according to the 1938 Food Drug and Cosmetic Act and are regulated by the Food and Drug Association (FDA). Details of homeopathic approaches are found in Chapter 13.

Recent national surveys indicate that more than 20%–40% of all children have used dietary supplements, of which vitamins and minerals are most common. Outpatient clinical surveys reported that children and adolescents with chronic medical conditions were more likely to use dietary supplements. In a survey of postoperative pediatric patients, 29.5% indicated they had used one or more CAM therapies in the year before surgery, and 12.8% had used herbal remedies before surgery. In a preoperative pediatric survey, 42% had used some form of vitamins, nutritional supplements, herbs, or homeopathy. The most prevalent dietary supplement given to children presenting for elective surgery was Echinacea.[22] This can present problems, in that immunostimulatory herbal supplements, such as echinacea, may exacerbate preexisting autoimmune disease (such as SLE) or precipitate autoimmune disease in children genetically predisposed to such disorders.[23]

Parents gave their children dietary supplements or used homeopathic remedies for many reasons, including maintaining health, preventing disease, and treating a chronic or acute disease.[24]

MASSAGE

A 1997 study of pediatric massage therapy (MT) looked at children with a diagnosis of JIA.[25] These children were found to have mild functional limitations with age-appropriate activities of daily living; those with severe limitations were excluded. Random assignments were made to massage therapy for 15 minutes daily for 30 days by a parent, or to relaxation therapy with a 15-minute relaxation session with a parent every evening for 30 days. Assessments of pain by the pediatric rheumatologist, the parents' perception of the pain, and the child's assessment were recorded. Behavior observation of anxiety and salivary cortisol levels were measured.

The findings demonstrated reduced anxiety levels in children who received massage therapy, based on behavioral observations and lower salivary cortisol levels. In addition, the results suggested decreased pain and fewer reports of severe pain. The physician's assessment led the authors to suggest a lesser degree of pain and less morning stiffness by the end of the month of massage therapy. They did not speculate on the underlying mechanism for the massage therapy–pain reduction relationship, but concluded that massage is a cost-effective therapy for children with JIA. Further research was recommended to compare the relative effectiveness and costs/benefits of these therapies in different age groups, as well as any long-term effects.

In a more general 2007 overview of pediatric MT, the authors[26] searched for relevant pediatric massage studies and separated them into two sections: proven effects, and promising effects of MT. Pediatric MT was defined as the "manual manipulation of soft tissue intended to promote health and well-being in children and adolescents." In a previous review[27] of 24 randomized control trials of pediatric MT for children between 2 and 19, multiple-dose effects, including improvements in anxiety, muscle tone, and arthritis, were found to be significant. The review also found support for reduced pain in children who had JIA.

Emphasizing that the general rule for MT and musculoskeletal conditions is that massage during the acute phase should be avoided, but that subacute and chronic injuries may be addressed, investigators showed that MT has promising effects for reducing pain in children with JIA, especially in the subacute phases, with improved joint mobility.[25] Clinicians have also noted that children with ankylosing spondylitis may benefit from MT to improve joint mobilization, muscle strength, and flexibility.[28]

MT is seen as a component, along with relaxation techniques, hypnosis, guided imagery, biofeedback, and acupuncture, of a comprehensive chronic pain management approach in children. A caution is advised in the use of MT, however, with the use of analgesics and muscle relaxants. Because analgesics reduce pain sensation, there is an alteration in tissue response, which can then alter the temperature, blood flow, and muscle-guarding of the child. Therapists must be extremely conservative with their treatment design to assure there is no undue injury. Muscle relaxants can interfere with muscle reflexes. Thus, deep tissue work, range of motion exercises, and excess stretching should be avoided while the child is being treated with muscle relaxants.

A current challenge in offering pediatric MT to children with serious medical conditions is that US massage school graduates often have little or no education in pediatric MT, and few continuing education programs exist. Canadian programs tend to include education in pediatric MT, but massage for children with special health care needs is not necessarily covered. In summary, it appears that MT may be safely recommended for pediatric patients when provided by qualified, trained massage therapists working as part of an interdisciplinary medical team.[26]

CHIROPRACTIC TREATMENT

Doctors of chiropractic (DCs) are the most frequently consulted CAM providers in the US, and are licensed in all 50 states. Considerable numbers of children and adolescents seek chiropractic care. According to a 1994 survey, DCs were the alternative practitioners most often consulted by pediatric patients.[19] While most adults consult DCs for musculoskeletal conditions, children frequently visit DCs for respiratory problems, ear, nose and throat problems, and general preventive care. Randomized controlled clinical trials of chiropractic conditions are rare, and there are none in the area of pediatric rheumatology.

A survey of DCs in the Boston area in 1998 indicated that children and adolescents constituted 11% of total patient visits.[29] On average, those DCs surveyed had been treating pediatric patients for 12 years. Two-thirds of them reported training in pediatric medicine, including pediatric courses in chiropractic colleges, postgraduate elective courses, or national conference workshops. Most DCs (79%) reported that they routinely modify their therapeutic techniques for children. Pediatric techniques included using light force, using an activator device to deliver gentle torque, performing adjustments on a child-sized adjustment table, performing adjustments on the mother's lap, and familiarizing children with the adjustment by performing techniques on an animal or doll.

Almost 75% of those surveyed recommended herbal/nutritional supplements, with half dispensing the supplements in the office. While pediatricians may be unfamiliar with chiropractic care, the fact that families are using these therapies needs to be acknowledged. Doctors should inquire about all therapies that pediatric patients use, including chiropractic care, as well as herbal remedies, acupuncture, meditation, and other CAM therapies. National studies are needed to assess the safety and efficacy of pediatric chiropractic care.[29] In addition, the practitioner's level of education and experience in the use of herbal and nutritional supplements needs to be scrutinized.

OSTEOPATHIC MANIPULATIVE MEDICINE

Osteopathic manipulative treatment (OMT) is the therapeutic application of manually guided forces by an osteopathic physician to alleviate somatic dysfunction through a variety of techniques. Some osteopathic physicians practice OMT exclusively and do not prescribe medications, while others utilize a variety of treatment options. Research on adults in family practice clinics demonstrated OMT was more likely to be performed in conjunction with medication treatment rather than in avoidance of medication.[30] OMT is based upon the osteopathic philosophy:[31]

1. The body is a unit.
2. The body has self-regulatory mechanisms.
3. Structure and function are reciprocally interrelated.
4. Rational osteopathic treatment is based upon these principles.

Osteopathic medical students are taught to apply manipulation of the musculoskeletal system to reestablish normal anatomic relationships and subsequent physiologic function.[32] The key diagnostic finding in OMT is somatic dysfunction, defined as impaired or altered function of the somatic (body framework) system; it is diagnosed through physical examination. The osteopathic physician looks for tissue texture changes, asymmetry, restriction, and tenderness, which are then treated with a variety of techniques based upon the individual patient's needs.[33]

Review of the literature demonstrates the use of OMT in the pediatric population has been shown to be more effective than placebo in the treatment of asthma, acute otits media, and colic, and has also demonstrated benefit in children with cerebral palsy.[34–37] A retrospective study in 2006 reviewed the medical records of over 500 pediatric patients and found that no treatment-associated complications from OMT were documented. Thirty-one (9%) of patients had documented treatment-associated aggravations.[38] Data in the adult population is promising for the treatment of low back pain[39] and acute ankle sprains,[40] which supports the need for research in the treatment of pediatric musculoskeletal conditions. Osteopathic techniques have been demonstrated to restore functional anatomy and decrease edema, two conditions frequently present in JIA.[40]

ACUPUNCTURE

Most chronic pain clinics, including more than 30% of pediatric pain clinics in the United States, offer acupuncture therapy.[41,42] Acupuncture, as defined by the National Center for Complementary and Alternative Medicine (NCCAM), describes a family of procedures involving stimulation of specific anatomic locations on the skin by a variety of techniques. The most studied stimulation method involves penetration of the skin by hair-thin, solid, metallic needles, manipulated manually or by electrical stimulation (see Chapter 10 for further information). The aim is to restore health by correcting an imbalance in *qi* (vital energy). Recent systematic reviews of acupuncture for specific pain conditions have demonstrated evidence of effectiveness, but there is a lack of data in the pediatric population. Some suggest that this may be due to the perception of fear of needles in children, which can be a barrier to acceptance of acupuncture in the pediatric population. Some studies indicate that children are often open to acupuncture, especially for chronic illnesses, and that fear may be overcome by careful explanation and demonstration before acupuncture is administered.

One study of children treated with acupuncture (lower back, hip and lower-extremity complaints, 41%; abdomen pain, 24%; or headache, 15%) found that in addition to reduced pain scores, the children experienced an "overall improvement of wellbeing" during treatment.[43] Patients in other studies have reported increased school attendance, improved sleep patterns, and the ability to participate in more extracurricular activities. No side effects or complications related to treatment were reported. Unfortunately, these studies did not include randomization or control subjects.[41,43,44]

Another study of 28 children with chronic pain (myofascial and migraine headaches, 46%; abdominal pain, 21%; fibromyalgia, 11%; and type I complex regional pain syndrome of an extremity, 11%) examined effectiveness and acceptance of acupuncture and hypnotherapy. Over a 6-week period, 94% of the children accepted acupuncture along with a 20-minute hypnotherapy session; only two children refused. Reports of pain-associated disability from the children and parents, and the children's pain ratings, were assessed before and after each of the 6 weekly sessions. The subjects experienced an average of 46% reduction in pain and a 32% reduction in pain-related disability, without any adverse events or withdrawals from the study due to negative effects of treatment. An interesting finding was the improvement in the correlation between the parent and child ratings of pain following the CAM interventions. This study was limited, in that acupuncture and hypnotherapy were not evaluated individually, and there was no control group.[45]

While there is an increase in high-quality studies demonstrating the usefulness and safety of acupuncture in adults, the same is not true in the pediatric acupuncture literature.[41] Acupuncture is appealing as a treatment modality for children, given the lack of associated side effects and the potential reduction in pain and fatigue levels and improvement in quality of life, and should be considered as adjunctive therapy.[41,46]

BIOFEEDBACK / HYPNOSIS

Biofeedback has been defined as a process that allows for the reporting (feedback) of information to the patient about certain physiologic processes, in an effort to teach self-modulation. Patients are able to appreciate the response of their body to certain stimuli, and alter behavior in order to modulate that response. Biofeedback has been studied in the pediatric population.[47,48,49] Much of the published literature addresses the use of biofeedback in children with headache, anxiety/stress disorders, sleep disorders, Raynaud's disease, reflex sympathetic dystrophy, asthma, and a variety of cognitive-based conditions.[47] While relaxation and self-hypnosis were found to be well-established treatment options for recurrent headache, thermal biofeedback was deemed probably effective.[48]

Self-hypnosis allows for the narrowing of attention or consciousness in an effort to decrease stress and pain. Types of relaxation/self-hypnosis techniques amenable to pediatric patients include deep breathing, progressive muscle relaxation, guided imagery, and self-hypnosis. These techniques have been demonstrated as effective within the pediatric population, but have not been studied specifically in pediatric rheumatology.[48,49] The combination of biofeedback with relaxation/self-hypnosis has been utilized in a variety of treatment strategies. This blend of modalities helps lower sympathetic tone, develops a sense of control, and reinforces awareness of mind/body connections.[47]

HOPE

One interesting study was conducted to assess family functioning and hope in patients with juvenile arthritis. Sixty-eight children with the diagnosis of juvenile arthritis, aged 8 to 12 years, were given a number of questionnaires to complete. One family member per child was also selected to complete the same questionnaire. Analysis of the responses showed a negative correlation between family functioning and children's hope. When the parent reported greater dissatisfaction with family functioning, the child's level of hope was lower. Hope was not found to be related to parent or child ratings of the patient's quality of life.[50]

COPING SKILLS

The ability to adapt to a chronic illness such as JIA is associated with positive benefits. Unique to pediatric rheumatology is the complex interplay between the child and the family/caregiver(s). Chronic illness affects the emotional health and behavior of the child, and the ability of the caregiver(s) to function well. It can also cause emotional strain on the caregiver.[51] Summer camps for patients with pediatric rheumatologic conditions are a positive intervention, resulting in an increased sense of control and improved self-esteem.[52]

Since summer camps at present do not allow for parental/caregiver interaction, family retreats have been developed. These retreats are designed from a family systems model, and typically involve all members of a household. They offer comprehensive, multidisciplinary treatment in a single therapeutic event. The sessions focus on improving functional capacities, enhancing coping skills, and facilitating family functioning in the major domains of living. A study was conducted with families who attended a Louisiana family retreat. The results demonstrated improvements for caregivers in several areas related to coping with the stress of having a child with a rheumatologic condition. Caregivers reported a decrease in their children's internalizing behavior problems (e.g., emotional distress) 6 months following the retreat. The retreat also decreased the emotional and social isolation of having a child with a relatively rare condition.[51]

After assessment of the relationship between health-related quality of life and the experience of pain (as well as coping strategies) in children with JIA, results indicated that the children were experiencing mild disability, and children reported the highest level of problems in the area of physical functioning. Parents most frequently identified problem solving and self-efficacy as their coping strategies. Children with JIA had more problems with physical functioning than healthy children, more emotional problems, more difficulty with peer relationships, and more problems with schooling. Children with JIA had difficulty communicating with health professionals about their problems.

Adequate training in the skills needed to interview children is necessary, and it is important to obtain information from both the patient and the parents/caregiver(s), as there appeared to be differing perceptions of pain intensity and pain coping strategies between the two groups.[53]

LISTENING

Listening to the patient is one of the components of health care which can be overlooked in a busy clinical practice. Sir William Osler wrote, "Listen to the patient and he will tell you his diagnosis." Yet, many articles indicate that physicians allow their patients to speak for an average of 11 seconds before interrupting.[54] An important feature of communication includes listening well, with an open mind and heart. "Our patient's opinions about what they want are pivotal to any decision making," according to Dykes. Ian McWhinney, considered the founder of family medicine, on listening to patients, stated, "If we could just learn to listen, everything would fall in to place. Listening is the key to being patient-centered."[55] Experience in the pediatric rheumatology clinic highlights the importance of listening effectively to both the parents/caregivers and children, to improve treatment outcomes.

In a national survey of parents with children younger than 3 years old, parents wanted more information and support about child-rearing concerns, and felt that physicians often failed to discuss nonmedical questions.[56]

Open and compassionate communication between the clinician and the parents and children, especially in the case of life-altering or life-threatening conditions, is important. The time invested in building rapport and trust with the child and the family increases the reporting of the actual reason for the clinic visit. Parents feel they need more (and clearer) information about the health status of the child, and additional information about the child's condition, treatment options, and long-term implications of the condition. (Levetown, 2008).[57] There are moral, ethical, and developmental obligations to

Table 18.3. Strategies to Engage Children in the Outpatient Setting.

Speak with the child; not at or to him or her
Speak in a private setting
Determine whom the child would like to be present
Begin with a nonthreatening topic
Listen actively
Pay attention to body language and tone of voice
Use drawings, games, or other creative communication tools
Elicit fears and concerns by reference to self or a third party
Ask the child what he or she would do with 3 wishes or a magic wand

*Levetown et al, 2008

communicate directly with the child. Involving children openly in the health care process improves their skills in making decisions in the future, and begins the transition process to self-determination as an adult. Strategies to facilitate direct communication with the child are listed in Table 18.3. The need for children to have useable information, to be given choices (including the desired level of involvement) and to be asked their opinion provides a sense of control, which allows for less fear and a reduction in the negative effects of the illness or injury.[57]

Conclusion

Until recently there was little published research on the use of CAM in pediatric rheumatology. The use of CAM in the pediatric patient has gained popularity, however, as parents face the challenges of easing pain and discomfort while limiting the potential side effects posed by frequently prescribed pharmaceutical agents. In spite of the increased use of CAM, there is limited data on the safety and efficacy of these modalities in pediatric rheumatology. With an extreme shortage of practicing pediatric rheumatologists, it is even more important that other health care providers become knowledgeable in CAM methods.

While there have been advances in the treatment of juvenile idiopathic arthritis (JIA), systemic lupus erythematosus (SLE), and other pediatric rheumatologic conditions, pain remains a significant symptom for the majority of patients. Most of the published studies have focused upon pain relief, and cognitive methods of dealing with a long-term medical condition. Many CAM modalities suitable to the pediatric patient have demonstrated positive impacts on pain; these include relaxation techniques, breathing exercises, guided imagery, acupuncture, and biofeedback with self-hypnosis. CAM is attractive to many parents, and to the patients themselves, as a means of avoiding the nutritional and developmental complications of corticosteroids, as well as other pharmaceuticals used to address pain.

One unique aspect of the care of the pediatric patient is the need to address the concerns and desires of the parents. Much effort has been directed at improving clinicians' listening skills, in an effort to allow the parents' concerns to become an integral part of the healing process.

Continued research into the use of complementary and alternative medicine in pediatric rheumatology is needed. Shifting the use of potentially toxic agents to the use of safer interventions is crucial. In addition, the use of modalities that support the child and the family unit may improve long-term outcomes in these chronic conditions. Future studies that elucidate the immunological processes of pediatric rheumatologic conditions will allow CAM researchers to specifically target inflammation, allowing for safer alternatives to conventional pharmaceuticals.

REFERENCES

1. Berman BM, Bausell RB, Lee WL. Use and referral patterns for 22 complementary and alternative medical therapies by members of the American College of Rheumatology: results of a national survey. *Arch Intern Med.* 2002;162(7):766–770.
2. Moss D, McGrady AV, Davies TC, Wickramasekera I. *Handbook of mind-body medicine for primary care.* Thousand Oaks, CA: Sage Publications, Inc.; 2003.
3. Sibinga EM, Ottolini MC, Duggan AK, Wilson MH. Parent-pediatrician communication about complementary and alternative medicine use for children. *Clin Pediatr.* 2004;43(4):367–373.
4. Davis MP, Darden PM. Use of complementary and alternative medicine by children in the United States. *Arch Pediatr Adolesc Med.* 2003;157(4):393–396.
5. Cassidy JT, Petty RE, Laxter RM, Lindsley CB. *Textbook of Pediatric Rheumatology. 5th ed.* Philadelphia, PA: W.B. Saunders Company; 2005.
6. Health Resources and Services Administration (HRSA). The pediatric rheumatology workforce: A study of the supply and demand for pediatric rheumatologists. Report to Congress. 2007; http://bhpr.hrsa.gov/healthworkforce/reports/ped_rheumatology. Accessed on July 2, 2008.
7. Mayer ML, Sandborg CI, Mellins ED. Role of pediatric and internist rheumatologists in treating children with rheumatic diseases. *Pediatrics.* 2004;113(3 Pt 1):173–181.
8. Weiss JE, Ilowite NT. Juvenile idiopathic arthritis. *Rheum Dis Clin North Am.* 2007;33(3):441–470.

9. Ernst E. Serious adverse effects of unconventional therapies for children and adolescents: a systemic review of recent evidence. *Eur J Pediatr.* 2003;162(2):72–80.
10. Southwood TR, Malleson PN, Roberts-Thomson PJ, Mahy M. Unconventional remedies used for patients with juvenile arthritis. *Pediatrics.* 1990;85(2):150–154.
11. Schanberg LE, Anthony KK, Gil KM, Maurin EC. Daily pain and symptoms in children with polyarticular arthritis. *Arthritis Rheum.* 2003;48(5):1390–1397.
12. Anthony KK, Schanberg LE. Pain in children with arthritis: a review of the current literature. *Arthritis Rheum.* 2003;49(2):272–279.
13. Anthony KK, Schanberg LE. Pediatric pain syndromes and management of pain in children and adolescents with rheumatic disease. *Pediatr Clin North Am.* 2005;52(2):611–635.
14. Rusy LM, Weisman SJ. Complementary therapies for acute pediatric pain management. *Pediatr Clin North Am.* 2000;47(3):589–599.
15. Kemper KJ. Complementary and alternative medicine for children: Does it work? *Arch Dis Child.* 2001;84(1):6–9.
16. Madsen H, Andersen S, Nielsen RG, Dolmer BS, Høst A, Damkier A. Use of complementary/alternative medicine among paediatric patients. *Eur J Pediatr.* 2003;162(5):334–341.
17. Kemper KJ, Cassileth B, Ferris T. Holistic pediatrics: a research agenda. *Pediatrics.* 1999;103(4 Pt 2):902–909.
18. Sanders H, Davis MF, Duncan B, Meaney FJ, Haynes J, Barton LL. Use of complementary and alternative medical therapies among children with special health care needs in southern Arizona. *Pediatrics.* 2003;111(3):584–587.
19. Spigelblatt L, Laîne-Ammara G, Pless IB, Guyver A. The use of alternative medicine by children. *Pediatrics.* 1994;94(6 Pt 1):811–814.
20. Hagen LEM, Schneider R, Stephens F, Modrusan D, Feldman BM. Use of complementary and alternative medicine by pediatric rheumatology patients. *Arthritis Rheum.* 2003;49(1):3–6.
21. Rouster-Stevens K, Nageswaran S, Arcury TA, Kemper KJ. How do parents of children with juvenile idiopathic arthritis (JIA) perceive their therapies? *BMC Complement Altern Med.* 2008;8:25.
22. Everett LL, Birmingham PK, Williams GD, Brenn BR, Shapiro JH. Herbal and homeopathic medication use in pediatric surgical patients. *Paediatr Anaesth.* 2005;15(6):455–460.
23. Lee AN, Werth VP. Activation of autoimmunity following use of immunostimulatory herbal supplements. *Arch Dermatol.* 2004;140(6):723–727.
24. Gardiner P, Riley DS. Herbs to homeopathy-medicinal products for children. *Pediatr Clin North Am.* 2007;54:859–874.
25. Field T, Hernandez-Reif M, Seligman S, et al. Juvenile rheumatoid arthritis: benefits from massage therapy. *J Pediatr Psychol.* 1997;22(5):607–617.
26. Beider S, Moyer CA. Randomized control trials of pediatric massage: a review. *Evid Based Complement Alternat Med.* 2007;4(1):23–34.
27. Beider S, Mahrer NE, Gold JI. Pediatric massage therapy: an overview for clinicians. *Pediatr Clin North Am.* 2007;54(6):1025–1041.

28. Salvo S. *Mosby's pathology for massage therapists*. St. Louis: Elsevier Mosby; 2004.
29. Lee ACC, Li DH, Kemper KJ. Chiropractic care for children. *Arch Pediatr Adolesc Med*. 2000;154(4):401–407.
30. Licciardone JC et al. Osteopathic manipulative treatment of somatic dysfunction among patients in the family practice clinic setting: a retrospective analysis. *J Am Osteopath Assoc*. (2005).
31. Leleszi JP, Lewandrowski JG. Managing pain in patients at the end of life. *J Am Osteopath Assoc*. 2007;107(Supp 4):ES3–9.
32. Kuchera ML. *Osteopathic perspectives: Medical history*. Monograph, Kirksville College of Osteopathic Medicine. 1993;1–37.
33. Kuchera ML. *Medical History: Osteopathic Perspectives*. Kirksville, MO: KCOM Press; 1994.
34. Educational Council on Osteopathic Principles. *Glossary of osteopathic terminology*. In: Ward RC, ed. *Foundations of osteopathic medicine. 2nd ed*. Baltimore, MD: Lippincott Williams & Wilkins; 2003:1229–1253.
35. Guiney PA, Chou R, Vianna A, Lovenheim J. Effects of osteopathic manipulative treatment on pediatric patients with asthma: a randomized controlled trial. *J Am Osteopath Assoc*. 2005;105(1):7–12.
36. Mills MV, Henley CE, Barnes LL, Carreiro JE, Degenhardt BF. The use of osteopathic manipulative treatment as adjuvant therapy in children with recurrent acute otitis media. *Arch Pediatr Adolesc Med*. 2003;157(9): 861–866.
37. Davis MT, Worden K, Clawson D, Meaney FJ, Duncan B. Confirmatory factor analysis in osteopathic medicine: fascial and spinal motion restrictions as correlates of muscle spasticity in children with cerebral palsy. *J Am Osteopath Assoc*. 2007;107(6):226–232.
38. Duncan B, Barton L, Edmonds D, Blashill BM. Parental perceptions of the therapeutic effect from osteopathic manipulation or acupuncture in children with spastic cerebral palsy. *Clin Pediatr*. 2004;43(4):349–353.
39. Hayes NM, Bezilla TA. Incidence of iatrogenesis associated with osteopathic manipulative treatment of pediatric patients. *J Am Osteopath Assoc*. 2006;106(10): 605–608.
40. Licciardone JC, King HH, Hensel KL, Williams DG. Osteopatthic health outcomes in chronic low back pain: The osteopathic trial. *Osteopath Med Prim Care*. 2008;2:5.
41. Eisenhart AW, Gaeta TJ, Yens DP. Osteopathic manipulative treatment in the emergency department for patients with acute ankle injuries. *J Am Osteopath Assoc*. 2003;103(9):417–421.
42. Kundu A, Berman B. Acupuncture for pediatric pain and symptom management. *Pediatr Clin North Am*. 2007;54(6):885–899.
43. Lee AC, Highfield ES, Berde CB, Kemper KJ. Survey of acupuncturists: practice characteristics and pediatric care. *West J Med*. 1999;171(3):153–157.
44. Lin YC, Ly H. Acupuncture and needlephobia: The pediatric patient's perspective. *Medical Acupuncture*. 2003;14(3):15–16.

45. Lin YC, Bioteau A, Lee AC. Acupuncture for the management of pediatric pain: a pilot study. *Medical Acupuncture.* 2002;14(1):45–6.
46. Zeltzer LK, Tsao JC, Stelling C, Powers M, Levy S, Waterhouse M. A phase I study of the feasibility and acceptability of an acupuncture/hypnosis intervention for chronic pediatric pain. *J Pain Symptom Manage.* 2002;24(4):437–446.
47. Chaudhuri M. Acupuncture Treatment for an adolescent with chronic fatigue syndrome. *Medical Acupuncture.* 2008;20(1):61-62.
48. Culbert TP, Kajander RL, Reaney JB. Biofeedback with children and adolescents: clinical observations and patient perspectives. *J Dev Behav Pediatr.* 1996;17(5): 342–350.
49. Holden EW, Deichmann MM, Levy JD. Empirically supported treatments in pediatric psychology: recurrent pediatric headache. *J Pediatr Psychol.* 1999;24(2):91–100.
50. Walco GA, Sterling CN, Conte PM, Engel RG. Empirically supported treatments in pediatric psychology: disease-related pain. *J Pediatr Psychol.* 1999;24(2):155–167.
51. Connelly TW Jr. Family functioning and hope in children with juvenile rheumatoid arthritis. *MCN Am J Matern Child Nurs.* 2005;30(4):245–250.
52. Hagglund KJ, Doyle NM, Clay DL, Frank RG, Johnson JC, Pressly TA. A Family retreat as a comprehensive intervention for children with arthritis and their families. *Arthritis Care Res.* 1996;9(1):35–41.
53. Steff ME, Shear ES, Levinson JE. Summer camps for juveniles with rheumatic disease: do they make a difference? *Arthritis Care Res.* 1989;2(1):10–15.
54. Sawyer MG, Whitham JN, Roberton DM, Taplin JE, Varni JW, Baghurt PA. The relationship between health-related quality of life, pain and coping strategies in juvenile rheumatoid arthritis. *Rheumatology.* 2004;42(3):325–330.
55. Dykes JR. Learning to listen. *Fam Med.* 2005;37(3):161–2.
56. Kelly L. Listening to patients: A lifetime perspective from Ian McWhinney. *Can J Rural Med.* 1998;3(3):168–169.
57. Young KT, Davis K, Schoen C, Parker S. Listening to parents: A national survey of parents with young children. *Arch Pediatr Adolesc Med.* 1998;152(3):255–262.
58. Levetown M and the Committee on Bioethics. Communicating with children and families: From everyday interactions to skill in conveying distressing information. *Pediatrics.* 2008;121(5): e1441–e1460.

19

The Patient Perspective

KAREN M. COOPER, RN, BSN, MA

KEY CONCEPTS

- Patients find value and empowerment in the blending of conventional western medicine with complementary and alternative medicine.
- Patient-centered care begins with mindful listening.
- When you empower the patient they are more likely to begin and maintain healthy self-care behaviors.
- Learn to use online resources and technology to help direct your patients.
- Practice your own self care.[1]

"The small room with the patient waiting on the examining table is its own kind of universe—a place where fears and hopes intersect with the precision of medical science. This can be a place of contraction or expansion; a place of aloneness or connection, a place of routine or discovery. What really matters is having the courage to be fully present to what is happening in that moment."

The Institute for Study of Health and Illness at Commonweal (ISHI) (2008)

Introduction

As I reflect upon how and why I became one of those patients who believe in the power of Integrative Medicine, the eternal question that sages have pondered for centuries comes up: Who Am I?

When it comes to receiving health care, I am either the dream patient, or the source of mystification for today's medical doctor. Like 40% to 62% of contemporary Americans (depending on which source you use), and more than 60% of rheumatology patients, I see alternative practitioners more often than my primary care provider, don't always reveal the complementary and alternative medicine (CAM) modalities that I use, and frequently avail myself to the advice of friends and the internet to search for information regarding health care products and solutions.[3–6]

I maintain a degree of cynicism mixed with hopeful trust when it comes to our healthcare system. I ask questions, am well-educated, and have experienced a wide range of healing approaches, from the Native American sweat lodge to polarity therapy with a tuning fork. I expect an intelligent conversation with my health care practitioners about what might be helpful or harmful when it comes to my health and wellbeing, and that they will be skillful in taking a comprehensive history and assessment in order to arrive at an accurate diagnosis. Since the literature suggests that the best outcomes are achieved when patients and physicians are equal partners,[2,6–8] I assume that they will listen and include me in decision-making for my own plan of care. I am frequently disappointed.

Unfortunately, there is much to be said (too much for this chapter) regarding the way HMOs and healthcare systems in the United States require physicians to reduce their time with patients to the proverbial 10-minute visit in order to maintain a salary. I don't place the entire blame on the system either; as a Registered Nurse, I appreciate efficiency, and serving people in need in a timely fashion. And, I must admit, there are times when I find myself at the urgent care clinic seeking a "quick fix," such as an antibiotic to alleviate a sinus infection, and would genuinely like to be on my way after only 10 minutes. Alas, as a patient, even with a "ten minute" visit I am required to be there 15 minutes early to help the receptionist populate computer fields before being herded into a cold room to sit on crinkly paper, left with the feeling of being "processed." In this instance, the dictionary definition of *patient* is fitting: "One who endures trying circumstances…" At our best we rise up to meet the rest of the proviso, "…to persevere calmly when faced with difficulties."[9] This is, however, a challenging edict when one is suffering at the mercy of the health care system, protected only by a flimsy gown and our willingness to be a "good patient."

The Good Patient is the Unsung hero of the Clinic[10]

"People often discuss what makes a good or bad doctor. A good doctor, for example, must be knowledgeable, technically adept, compassionate, patient, kind, trustworthy, morally sound, and a great communicator...There is a striking similarity between the virtues of the good doctor and those of the good patient. Good patients are at once compassionate towards fellow patients and overworked hospital staff, tolerant when awaiting their turn and answering oft repeated questions, kind when communicating with others, trustworthy when reporting facts or taking their medicine, and, above all, understanding of the limitations and fallibility of medicine...Whereas the good doctor must exercise these virtues and qualities while under pressure from bickering patients, anxious relatives, and limited time, the good patient must apply them in times of physical or emotional pain." (Sokol, 2004)

The Patient Perspective

The importance of the patient perspective can no longer be ignored, as consumers are voting with their pocketbooks.[3,11–13] The use of CAM therapies continues to rise, and consumers pay for these services out of pocket. This popularity persists despite a lack of well developed evaluation standards,[14] poor study designs,[15] and even despite a consensus definition of CAM. Many researchers arbitrarily consider CAM to include meditation, diet, prayer, exercise, or dietary supplements, whereas others do not.

Patients often find value and empowerment in blending what is known to be effective in conventional Western medicine with healing modalities from other traditions, philosophies, approaches, and cultures. A growing number of patients decry parochial attitudes among conventional practitioners; they resent being patronized and excluded in formulating treatment decisions. As a result, they are doing what makes sense to them, and seeking alternatives.[16]

What drives patients to more alternative practitioner visits than primary care, and why are they willing to spend out-of-pocket money to integrate CAM practices and products? Surveys show that only about 20% of users think that alternative medicine therapies are superior to conventional therapies (Figure 19.1),[12] so what are patients getting from these providers that are not received from conventional practitioners? And why do 60% of rheumatology patients, in particular, use CAM?[5,17]

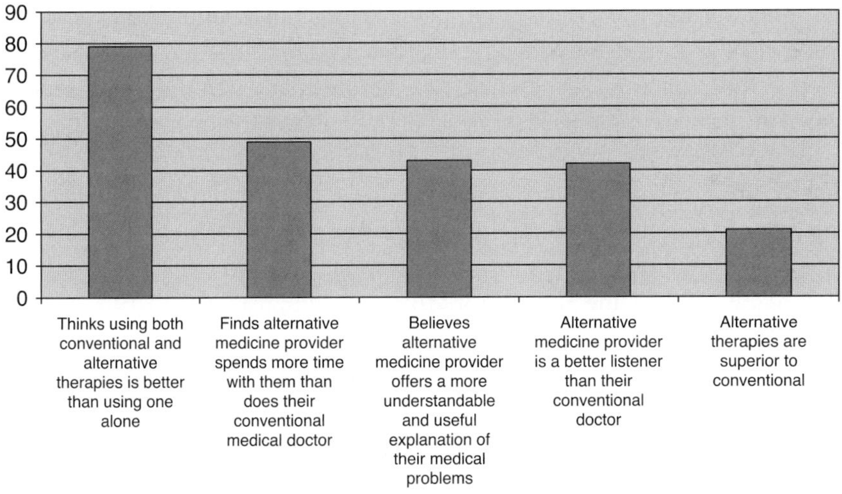

FIGURE 19.1. Patient Comparison of CAM and Conventional Health Care.
Adapted from HPDP, 2005; p. 57.

One of the answers is presented in an *Arthritis Today* interview by Judith Horstman[8] with Dr. James McKoy:

> "Integrative medicine provides what most people with a chronic ailment yearn for: a feeling that your practitioner has a personal interest in you as an individual, not just your disease and statistics."

This ties in with a foundational concept of healing medicine, beneficence. Patients believe that this is as fundamental to their care as the provider's medical knowledge about their disease.

> *"...All healthcare professionals have a duty not only to avoid harm but also a positive duty to do good—that is, to act in the patient's best interest[s]. This duty of beneficence takes precedence over any self-interest."*
>
> -The Federation of State Medical Boards "Model Guidelines for the Use of Complementary and Alternative Therapies in Medical Practice 2002" (HPDP, 2005, p. 298).

It is commonly assumed that patients don't tell physicians about their integrative practices out of fear of being reprimanded,[7,18] but this is erroneous.[2,19,20] To the chagrin of such conventional thinkers, patients use CAM without regard to their physician's approval; this phenomenon transcends a "don't ask, don't tell" policy. While it's true that some patients forget to mention their CAM use while in a fog of pain, published reports state that most rheumatology patients purposefully conceal CAM use due to a disagreement with the health professional regarding symptoms, the impact of disease, and treatment outcomes.[2,7]

Patients often assume that providers don't query them regarding CAM use due to time constraints, or a lack of knowledge of the subject.[21] More likely is the lack of a genuine listening presence on the part of the provider. This is a reflection of quality, rather than quantity of time. The Bravewell Collaborative,[22] an Integrative Medicine philanthropic organization, reaffirms this:

> *"As odd as it may seem to need to remind healthcare providers to put their patients at the center of the care they give, we do. As practitioners feel greater pressure to see more patients in less time, care has become centered not on the needs of patients, but around the needs of the system itself."*

If an integrated approach is what patients are seeking, how can the practitioner use his/her skills to meet that demand?

The Integrative Rheumatologist

> *"Integrative Medicine reaffirms the importance of the relationship between practitioner and patient, focuses on the whole person, is informed by evidence, and makes use of all appropriate therapeutic approaches, healthcare approaches, and disciplines to achieve optimal health and healing."*
> (Consortium of Academic Health Centers for Integrative Medicine, 2004.)

In my perspective as the patient, there are two key concepts for the practice of integrative rheumatology. In addition to having knowledge and experience in both conventional and alternative therapies, you also need the skills and the time to become adept at nonjudgmental listening, and in communicating understandable and meaningful information. It is to your advantage to engage your patients as participants in their own care. Focusing upon the development of superb listening skills, along with the ability to empower a patient in their quest for healing, is key.

> *"The patient's story is the human voice in medicine."*
> (Childress & Mohmann, 2002"

DEVELOPING THE SKILLS: HEARING THE STORY

The patient uses story to describe and interpret what's happening to her or him—the reason why they are there to see you. Story reveals what the patient hopes to derive from the visit; it defines the desired health outcomes for the patient (and by the patient). Hearing the story is valuable for physicians because through the telling, patients expose and are forced to examine their own assumptions, biases, and conflicting behaviors—e.g., "I want to have more vitality, and be without so much pain" and "I would never go to water aerobics"—thus providing a real opportunity to work towards aligning the competing elements, and developing effective therapeutic options.

The story provides an opportunity for truthful dialogue; with truthful dialogue the practitioner can provide the guidance needed to help patients understand and accept that the choices they make are *their* responsibilities, made in collaboration with a knowledgeable health professional.[25] By listening closely to patients' stories, the practitioner's perspective is broadened; the ability to organize and integrate complex situations is enhanced; a greater understanding of the many self-management decisions a chronically ill person must make daily is gained;[26] and, perhaps, to see better solutions for rheumatology patients.

The importance of listening is addressed by the writings of renowned philosopher and spiritual teacher, the late Jiddu Krishnamurti, who emphasized listening as one of the greatest arts in life, saying:

> *"Listening is an art not easily come by, but in it there is beauty and great understanding. To listen there must be an inward quietness, a freedom from the strain of acquiring, a relaxed attention. This alert yet passive state is able to hear what is beyond the verbal conclusion."*[27]

In practicing such alert and full listening, the practitioner cultivates non-judgment and acquires what many patients sense is missing from much of conventional medicine: the practitioner hearing the voice of the patient, even though "it is the voice of medicine that you record in the chart."[28]

WHO HAS TIME TO LISTEN?

Physicians interrupt patients an average of 21 seconds after asking, "What brings you to clinic today?"[29] I would prefer instead that they actually listen after asking me that question, and that they hear how this problem creates conflict in my cultural, spiritual, mental, and relational spheres. These aspects aren't easily measurable, but intrinsically have value because they relate to my ability to be independent in activities of daily living, to my quality of life, and to what degree I am able to follow their prescription. The same studies show that it actually does *not* take more time to let the patient first tell their story; in fact, 80% of the time you will get the information you need in just two minutes![30] The difference is that the patient leaves feeling satisfied, and is therefore more likely to be compliant with the plan of care.

It may seem impossible to listen well to a patient who sounds unfocused and rattles off a litany of events that seem unrelated to their symptoms. I've experienced this myself as a nurse during the triage process: I catch the less developed part of myself thinking, "I wish they would just get to the point." It takes practice to hear the words with compassion, to observe body language, and to mindfully guide the patient towards identifying their goals as related to chief complaint; but when you do, you can usually reach a point of mutuality in the plan of care, and it's more efficient in the long term.

Nurse researchers D.R. Lauver, B. Owen, J. Egan, et. al.,[31] demonstrate that provider–practitioner interactions correlate with patients' preventive behaviors, and the desired outcome of controlling chronic conditions. With practiced listening and communication techniques, the practitioner is able to individualize recommendations using focused communication and messages tailored for concepts of beliefs, affect, and external barriers. With this approach, patients showed an increase in compliance for health screening and follow-up (even in brief encounters).

Do interactions between practitioners and rheumatology patients correspond in a similar fashion? It appears to be so. In 2008, Sleath and colleagues examined whether patients of 23 rheumatologists at universities and private practice clinics were more likely to tell their physicians about their CAM use if the rheumatologist had a participatory decision-making style. Their findings suggest that engaging patients when making treatment decisions leads to a greater likelihood that patients will disclose their use of CAM.

EMPOWERING THE PATIENT

When a patient is engaged in making decisions regarding his own care, he is more likely to maintain self-care behaviors and make healthier long-term lifestyle changes.[32] The patient becomes comfortable enough to reveal his use of CAM, and the degree to which he is able to comply with prescribed conventional (or CAM) treatments.

Michael Weiss[33] describes the empowerment approach as one that acknowledges how patients incorporate changes into their lives, and honors that the patient has the ultimate power to reject the suggestions and recommendations of the other team members. In this way, healthcare practitioners gain the most accurate information and are able to determine the most effective therapies to suggest, whether they are CAM modalities or conventional, because trust is established.

Pearls for Practice: 10 Ways to Engage, Educate and Empower your Patients

1. *Listen.* True for any practitioner, particularly when working with populations who have chronic problems. Two of the most highly rated items on patient satisfaction questionnaires are "treated me with respect" and "respected my feelings."[31] Nonjudgmental listening to your patients conveys respect and may help to clarify issues that lie beneath the surface of the initial presentation.
   - *To listen requires being present mentally.* Slow down your breathing and relax your jaw and shoulders as you look at the patient while hearing his/her story, without jumping ahead to solutions, judgments or explanations. It takes practice!
2. *Ask the question.* Remember that most patients don't mention their use of CAM unless the interviewer asks.
   - *Be precise: what is considered alternative to you may seem common to the patient.* Include specifics on an assessment form, or pose questions such as, "Are you using any supplements, vitamins, sports powders…anything else?" Often patients do not think to include herbals, over-the-counter and home remedies, or things such as plants or medicinal teas that he uses for vitality and general well being.
   - *Determine the amount of time, money and energy your patient is spending on CAM, as a tool for weighing pros and cons of various therapies.* This can serve as a reality check for the patient, and helps you to recognize the value he places on the products he is using.
3. *Identify an individual's receptivity to CAM,* and obstacles to better health that the patient encounters by asking questions such as:
   - "What, if anything, have you tried in the past that worked to "help you feel better?" "have you heard about and wondered whether it might work for you?", or "Are you interested in learning about ways to reduce stress?" CAM is not for everyone; in this way, you

can assess your patient's level of knowledge, values, hopes and fears, and direct him/her to accessible, reliable resources and modalities that may be of interest.

4. *Engage and empower your patients.* Some ideas:
    - *Clarify and have patients write down their short-term and long-term health goals; guide them from passive to active* (see Chapter 20). For example, they say they would like to travel, or feel safe enough to be able to walk in the woods independently, on an uneven surface; or get down on the floor and have fun playing with the grandkids (goals based on intrinsic values). Alas, they can't because their knees hurt too much when they walk or get down on the floor, they are fearful of tripping on a root, or it is too embarrassing to need help getting up (obstacles). You suggest a list of movement modalities (e.g., tai chi, water aerobics, Feldenkrais method, yoga) and benefits regarding how they improve strength and balance, and negotiate ways the patients might meet their goals by progressing from the less threatening massage, to the slightly more challenging water walking or tai chi.
    - *Ask patients to do homework.* Encourage them to take notes in a notebook, exercise log book, digital device or journal. Hold them accountable for reporting back their experiences, what they tried, or obstacles they encountered. This means you may need to flag the chart to remind you or a staff member to ask them to identify their progress; often small improvements over time lead them closer to their desired stated goals.
5. *Help patients detect whether products, practices, or websites are probably fraudulent or potentially fruitful by giving them a resource list.* If you don't have time to develop one of your own, direct them to resources and ask them to report back what they learned, appreciated, or didn't like, on the next visit. **(See resources in Appendix B).** To save time during the visit, ask for "the one or two things that really made a difference."
    - *Get to know referral sources.* Try out CAM practitioners yourself, either group classes or individuals. To respect and encourage professionalism, either pay for the service or offer an exchange. Exchanges of service or knowledge are a great way to develop a deeper understanding of practices and "shared patients."
    - *Provide a "favorites" list of local practitioners* that patients and staff contribute to, rather than a brochure or advertisement **(see Appendix A).** These are not recommendations or direct referrals,

they are akin to the bookstore that displays "staff favorites" to capture the attention of consumers. Items and questions on the list are designed to stimulate thought about how to choose a provider, and can include aspects that influence their decision.

6. *Become a "Netizen."* Defined as "somebody who has access to and uses the Internet frequently."[9] Multiple sources show that your patients are already there. Use this to your advantage.
   - *Consider a membership to Internet sources* such as consumerlab.com or Natural Medicine Comprehensive Database (www.natural-database.com), to update your general knowledge about specific herbs and supplements and to see brand names that have been tested for purity and their prices (not the same as Consumer Reports, although that may be another resource).
   - *Direct patients to free sources* (or access yourself) such as:
     - PDRhealth.com, scholar.google.com, medlineplus.org, the Cochrane Collaboration (www.cochrane.org)
     - The Arthritis Foundation (www.arthritis.org), Lupus Foundation of America, Inc. (www.lupus.org), the National Fibromyalgia Association (www.fmaware.org) and other nationally recognized organizations for evidence-based literature and links of comprehensive web sites.

   The national associations in particular may be especially helpful to young bloggers who feel isolated (although misconceptions and questions may result, as content is not necessarily moderated by health professionals).
   - *Look at blogs yourself* to get an idea of the patient experience.
   - *Query your patients* who have "grown up" with computers and the Internet for sites they find valuable – they are a great resource and it will save you time and trouble compared to random searches. It can facilitate conversation related to determining harmful vs. helpful sites at future visits.
   - *If you are already internet-savvy, create your own web site.* Make it senior friendly, which will welcome patients of any age, even those baby boomers with limited Internet experience, who are likely to be a large cohort with arthritis (see National Institute on Aging link in Appendix). Include links to studies or articles that you have written or screened specifically related to rheumatologic conditions.
7. *Familiarize yourself with the most recent studies*; reviews are an efficient way to do this. See free resources above.

8. *See through the eyes of your patients.*
   - The next time you are browsing through the shelves of your local bookstore or library, investigate areas your patients may be drawn to, such as Alternative, Complementary or Holistic Medicine; Self-Help, Self Improvement, Health (men and women's), Nursing or Medicine, Nutrition or Diet, Fitness and Exercise, or disease-specific topics, to see what influences the mass market has on your patients.
   - Search the Internet with an objective eye to see how people are influenced, and read the information on sites before recommending them to patients.
9. *It's okay to start small.* If you have limited time or knowledge and aren't sure whether you want a totally integrative practice, choose one or two new CAM therapies to focus on for the year or next 6 months.
   - *Consider how you might integrate this data into your practice.* For example, you might start by writing a brief critique or summary of studies related to tai chi for arthritis, select a book or Internet site as a resource to post in your wait area, explore local offerings, and ask patients for feedback about the practice and the instructor after they've tried it for a month. Or, you may have a particular condition or person, such as a fibromyalgia patient, in mind, so you investigate local classes and find ones to recommend that offer an active style of yoga which also incorporates stress-reducing breathing and meditation practices.
10. *Practice self-care, become more self-aware.* Experience CAM yourself. Attend a class or private sessions with some local instructors. I recommend trying something for several sessions before making a judgment, and keeping a journal of your experiences, both objective and subjective. As is true with some conventional medications, it may take 3 to 6 weeks for a practice to take effect; it might be that it was just an unusual day for the CAM therapist, or your own mood created a less-than-effective treatment session. It may take trying a few different modalities or teachers to find one that resonates with your needs, style, and values.

Conclusion

I admit that as someone who has a higher education, including nursing and Holistic Health degrees, I am privileged. I am able to use a critical eye to evaluate research studies in both CAM and conventional medicine, and to appreciate the value of the various therapies. On the surface, it seems so much easier to pop a pill rather than establish a daily practice for the rest of my life...until the side effects of NSAIDs begin to eat at my stomach lining or my pocketbook. Or, until I find myself swallowing pills with disdain, resenting dependency on a substance, dependency on insurance coverage and people in white coats, mourning the loss of my own free will and spontaneity because I must always be aware of where the pill bottle is, lest I not be able to function well on a given day without it.

Lisa Fraenkel and colleagues[34] report that rheumatology patients are willing to use something less effective than a known, proven treatment (NSAIDs). This, too, is true for me, if I can have a better quality of life in the process. In other words, it gives me more peace of mind to stoically get by without, or to use something other than the prescription or over-the-counter medication, if the side effects lower my ability to function or reduce my clarity of thinking.

This is the profile of many CAM users as reported in the 2005 Complementary and Alternative Medicine in the United States report by the Board on Health Promotion and Disease Prevention.[2]

It should come as no surprise that those of us with conditions such as arthritis, chronic pain, and other persistent conditions use CAM the most, for here is where conventional medicine, even with some improvements over time, has failed us.[2,18] There are no instant fixes, no "magic bullet" when it comes to chronic health problems—no glory or glamour, and a lot of complexity. It takes a practitioner with a brilliant and creative mind, a keen eye, a compassionate heart, and an ability to patiently puzzle through mystery to deal with the rheumatologic patient. Finding such practitioners is a common, although often elusive, goal of most patients.

Thus, patients are coming up with their own creative ways to cope, to be involved in their own care, to bring relief and get back to living a full life again. If it doesn't appear to be harmful, doesn't cost too much, and may be helpful, what have we got to lose?

REFERENCES

1. Institute for the Study of Health and Illness at Commonweal (ISHI). Is there room for your heart in the practice of medicine?" CME/CEU programs brochure. 2008. Available at: http://www.commonweal.org/ishi/programs/index.html. Accessed on Box 19.1.
2. Committee on the Use of Alternative Medicine by the American Public Board on Health Promotion and Disease Prevention (HPDP). Complementary and alternative medicine in the United States. pp. 1, 45–57, 298–302, and Appendix E.

Washington, D.C: National Academies Press; 2005. Available at: http://books.nap.edu/openbook. Accessed on March 20, 2010.

3. National Center for Complementary and Alternative Medicine (NCCAM), website. The Use of Complementary and Alternative Medicine in the United States. Accessed March 1, 2010 at http://nccam.nih.gov/news/camstats/2007/camsurvey_fs1.htm 4/1/2010.
4. Eisenberg DM, Davis RB, Ettner SL, et al. Unconventional medicine in the U.S.: prevalence, costs, and patterns of use. *JAMA*. 1998;290:1569–1575.
5. Rao JK, Mihaliak K, Kroenke K, Bradley H, Tierney WM, Weinberer M. Use of complementary therapies for arthritis among patients of rheumatologists. *Ann Inter Med*. 1999;131:409–416.
6. Jacobi C, Boshuizen HC, Rupp I, Dinant HJ, van den Bos GA. Quality of rheumatoid arthritis care: the patient's perspective. *Int J Qual Health Care*. 2004;16(1):73–81.
7. Cauffield JS. The psychosocial aspects of complementary and alternative medicine. *Pharmacotherapy*. 2000;20(11):1289–1294.
8. Horstman J. 2001. Some rheumatologists are changing their approach: using "integrative medicine," they treat the whole patient. Arthritis Today More than Medicine. Obtained from http//ww.2.arthritis.org/resources/arthritistoda/2001_archives on September 18, 2007.
9. Encarta® World English Dictionary©. Microsoft Corporation. New York: Bloomsbury Publishing Plc.;1999.
10. Sokol D. How (not) to be a good patient. *BMJ*. 2004;328(7437):471.
11. Astin JA. Why patients use alternative medicine: results of a national study. *JAMA*. 1998;279:1548–1553.
12. Eisenberg DM, Kessler RC, Vanompay MI, et al. Perceptions about complementary therapies relative to conventional therapies among adults who use both: results from a national survey. *Ann Intern Med*. 2001;135(5):344–351.
13. NCCAM. website, http://nccam.nih.gov/; accessed March 20, 2008.
14. McDowell J. Complementary and alternative medicine: a qualitative study of beliefs of a small sample of Rocky Mountain area nurses. *Medsurg Nurs*. 2004;13(6):383–390.
15. Barnes PM, Powell-Griner E, McFann K, Nahin RL. Complementary and alternative medicine use among adults: United States 2002. *Adv Data*. 2004;27(343):1–19.
16. American Medical Student Association (AMSA). EDCAM-CAM and medical education report 2007. Available at: http://www.amsoa/org/humed/CAM/mededreport.cfm. Accessed on March, 20, 2008.
17. Hagen LE, Schneider R, Stephens D, Modrusan D, Feldman BM. Use of complementary and alternative medicine by pediatric rheumatology patients. *Arthritis Rheum*. 2003;49(1):3–6.
18. Marcus DM. Alternative medicine and the Arthritis Foundation. *Arthritis Rheum*. 2002;47(1):5–7.
19. Gordon MM, Capell HA, Madhok R. The use of the Internet as a resource for health information among patients attending a rheumatology clinic. *Rheumatology*. 2002;41(12):1402–1405.

20. Sleath B, Callahan LF, Devellis RF, Beard A. Arthritis patients' perceptions of rheumatologists' participatory decision-making style and communication about complementary and alternative medicine. *Arthritis Rheum*. 2008;59(3):415–421.
21. Ahlmen M, Nordensiold U, Archenholtz I, et al. Rheumatology outcomes: the patient's perspective. A multicentre focus group interview study of Swedish rheumatoid arthritis patients. *Rheumatology*. 2005;44:105–110.
22. Bravewell Collaborative. 2008. Web site. Available at: http://www.bravewell.org. Accessed on March 20, 2010.
23. Consortium of Academic Health Centers for Integrative Medicine. 2004. Web site. Available at: http://www.ahc.umn.edu/cahcim/about/home.html. Accessed on March 20, 2010. Box 19.4
24. Childress M.D. Mohmann M.E. The importance of medicine I: narrative medicine. University of Virginia Health Science Center catalog, September. 2002. [box 19.5]
25. Angelmar, R., Berman, P.C. Patient empowerment and efficient health outcomes. Presention at Financing Sustainable Healthcare Europe: New Approaches for Better Outcomes Conference: Heilsinki Feb. 2007. Available at: http://www.sustainhealthcare.org/Report_3.pdf. Accessed on March 20, 2010.
26. Funnell MM, Anderson RM. Empowerment and self-management of diabetes. *Clin Diabetes*. 2004;22(3):123–127.
27. Lee RE. The Arts of Listening, Looking and Learning. USA Journal of the Krishnamurti Schools. May 2000. Available at: http://www.journal.kfionline.org/article.asp?issue=4&article=2. Accessed on March 20, 2010.
28. Janisse T. Medical Ethics: stories tell us what we need to know: perspective for ethical dilemmas. *Perm J*. 2004;8(1):98–99.
29. Lussier M.T, Richard, C. Doctor-patient communication: time to talk. *Can Fam Physician*. 2006;52:1401–1402.
30. Langewitz W, Denz M. Keller A, Ruttimann S, Wossmer B. Spontaneous talking time at start of consultation in outpatient clinic:cohort study. *BMJ*. 2002;325(7366):682–683.
31. Lauver DR, Owen B, Egan J, Lovejoy LS, Henriques JB. Relationships of practitioner communications and characteristics with women's mammography use. *Patient Educ Couns*. 2003;51:65–74.
32. Lauver DR, Settersten L, Kane JH, and Henriques JB. Tailored messages, external barriers and women's utilization of professional breast cancer screening over time. *Cancer*. 2003;97(11):2724–2735.
33. Weiss M. Empowerment: A patient's perspective. *Diabetes Spectr*. 2006;19(2): 116–118.
34. Fraenkel L. Bogardus S. Concato Wittink D. Treatment options in knee osteoarthritis: The patient's perspective. *Arch Intern Med*. 2004;164:1299–1304.

Appendix A – Patient "CAM Favorites" Survey

The following item is a tool that you may copy or adapt to fit your current practice. It is a way to engage your patients through the use of survey participation, while gaining information about local CAM practitioners that may be worth investigating. The questions are also designed to stimulate thought as to what kinds of things participants should look for when they are seeking services. You may want to keep the results in a notebook for your patients to peruse.

[YOUR LETTER HEAD HERE]

Cam Favorites

Here you will find brief surveys completed by patients in our practice. They rate various aspects of local practitioners who offer CAM (Complementary & Alternative Medicine) services and promote the integration of CAM with conventional medicine. These surveys are not a complete list, nor do they address all aspects that you may wish to consider; they are simply a tool to help you reflect on what might work best for you in terms of educational classes, specific providers, and specific types of therapies.

You are welcome to complete a survey yourself and return it to us to be included in "CAM Favorites." To avoid bias, please do not write your name on the form. Although the completed forms are property of this practice and may not be copied or used by any other person or practice, you are welcome to share the blank ones.

To ensure that patients receive the safest, most effective, and complete care, we encourage you to discuss any interest in CAM modalities and providers with your primary care provider and nurses, with members of our staff, and with any other health care practitioners providing your care.

DISCLAIMER: As these are not referrals, anyone reading the contents of these surveys and choosing to receive services from the listed providers assumes total and complete responsibility for his/her selection, agrees that their participation with said providers shall be undertaken at her/his sole risk, and that the individual or practice on this letterhead shall not be liable for any injuries or any damage to her/him or her/his property, or be subject to any claim, demand, injury, action, or causes of action, or for any damages whatsoever. Any surveys received will be the sole property of the person or practice listed on this letterhead, and we reserve the right to discard any surveys that we deem inappropriate, dishonest, harmful, or submitted by the provider themselves or relatives or employees of providers.

Integrative Practitioner Feedback Form

Fill out as much as you want (or have time for) and give to receptionist.

Submitted by: ☐ Staff ☐ Patient Date of Service/Treatment/Class: ______
Practitioner/Teacher Name and title: ______________________________
Business Name and type of service:______________________________
Street Address:____________________City: ___________Zip:_________
Phone:________________Email:_______________Website:___________

Rheumatological Condition treated: ______________________________

Overall Impression

1.	With this service I felt:	☐ Better	☐ Worse	☐ No change
	☐ Immediately	☐ Within 2–3 days	☐ Within 2 weeks	☐ After several appointments
2.	I would recommend this person for other rheumatology patients:	☐ Yes	☐ No	
	• If no, I might try this type of therapy, but with a different practitioner:	☐ Yes	☐ No	
3.	This didn't help my rheumatic condition specifically, but I would recommend it for general health and well-being.	☐ Yes	☐ No	
4.	Compared to others offering this type of therapy, class or service, I would rate this person and service:	☐ Low	☐ Average	☐ High
5.	Cost:	$ ________		
	Amount of time or number of sessions required:	________		

Accessibility and Efficiency

1.	How easy was it to make an appointment?	☐ Easy	☐ Average	☐ Difficult
2.	Appointments can be made by:	☐ Phone	☐ Web	☐ Walk-in
3.	How easy was the building to find?	☐ Easy	☐ Average	☐ Difficult
4.	Parking was: ☐ Did not use	☐ Easy	☐ Average	☐ Difficult
5.	☐ Provided for the physically challenged		☐ Free	☐ Safe
6.	The reception/check-in was efficient & friendly:	☐ Yes	☐ No	☐ No waiting
7.	Bathroom was accessible:	☐ Yes	☐ No	☐ Don't know
8.	My appointment was completed in the time I expected	☐ Yes	☐ No	

Aesthetics and Comfort

1.	How comfortable was the reception/waiting area?	☐ Comfortable	☐ Uncomfortable	
2.	The general ambience felt healing to me.	☐ Yes	☐ No	
3.	Temperature and light levels were acceptable or adjusted to my needs:	☐ Yes	☐ No	☐ Not Sure
4.	Please rate how the design and décor affected you:			
5.	Color:	☐ Negative	☐ Neutral or didn't notice	☐ Positive
6.	Artwork:	☐ Negative	☐ Neutral or didn't notice	☐ Positive
7.	Furniture and other objects:	☐ Negative	☐ Neutral or didn't notice	☐ Positive
8.	Noises (including quiet or music):	☐ Negative	☐ Neutral or didn't notice	☐ Positive
9.	Were scents of any kind present in the air or used in products without your prior consultation? (including essential oils, air fresheners, flowers, lotions, candles, others)		☐ Yes	☐ No
10.	If Yes, the aroma was:	☐ Negative	☐ Neutral or didn't notice	☐ Positive

Communication – please check all that apply.

☐ Privacy–I felt that my information and physical privacy were maintained.
☐ I was called by my preferred name.
☐ I was encouraged to ask questions or tell them my needs anytime during the session.
☐ They asked about my physical and medical history and current medications.
☐ They asked me about CAM modalities I am using, have tried, or was interested in.
☐ We discussed the potential effects of integrating my CAM and conventional medicine treatments, including today's session.
☐ Practitioner was professional yet approachable.
☐ The practitioner or teacher was knowledgeable about my condition.
☐ Practitioner has experience working with rheumatology patients.
☐ Was the practitioner credentialed, certified, licensed, and /or registered with a professional organization? ☐ Yes ☐ No ☐ Don't know
☐ The way they talked with me was warm and encouraging.
☐ I felt rushed or that they were in a hurry.
☐ I was asked about aspects affecting my well-being other than my rheumatic condition (such as lifestyle, career or school, friends and family, spiritual practices, beliefs and values, fears, finances).

Follow Up – Please check all that apply

☐ I was encouraged to call with questions
☐ They provided valid resources, or told me how & where to get more information
☐ I was provided the opportunity to schedule another appointment
☐ We discussed after-care/possible effects of the treatment

Appendix B – Resources for an Integrative Practice Helpful Websites Related to CAM, Rheumatology and to Help Patients Detect Health Frauds and Scams

- Alternative Therapies in Health and Medicine
  http://www.alternative-therapies.com
  Forum for sharing information concerning the practical use of alternative therapies in preventing and treating disease, healing illness, and promoting health. This is a peer-reviewed healthcare journal indexed since 1996 in the National Library of Medicine.
- Arthritis Foundation
  http://www.arthritis.org/alternatives.php
  General overview and articles about CAM; "Seven Danger Signs About a Therapist": http://www.arthritis.org/seven-danger-signs.php
- Consortium for Academic Health Centers for Integrative Medicine
  http://www.imconsortium.org/
  Comprised of thirty nine academic medical centers promoting rigorous studies, innovative educational programs and integrative medicine; some offer clinical services; only refer to their members for integrative medicine; has FAQ link.
- Council of Better Business Bureaus (CBBB)
  www.bbb.org
  The BBB reports and accepts complaints on businesses, including charity and nonprofits. Provides links by zip codes to state regulating agencies; not CAM-specific, but their Resource Library is good for the Internet novice as it includes information about protecting against online identity theft, phishing, and shopping online.
- Food and Drug Administration (FDA)
  http://www.fda.gov
  FDA can tell you whether they have taken action against a product or its marketer. You may also call to alert the FDA about a potentially illegal product to prevent others from falling victim to health fraud. See: "FDA Consumer Magazine Nov–Dec 1999 Vol 33, No. 6 "How to Spot a Health Fraud."
- Federal Trade Commission (FTC)
  www.ftc.gov
  Offers tips on avoiding health fraud online. See "Diet, Health & Fitness, Consumer Protection, Facts for Consumers"
  http://www.ftc.gov/bcp/edu/pubs/consumer/health/hea07.shtm

- Institute of Noetic Sciences
  http://www.noetic.org/
  Nonprofit membership organization that conducts and sponsors leading-edge research in conscious-awareness
- National Center for Complementary and Alternative Medicine (NCCAM)
  www.nccam.nih.gov
  The site has many FAQs and sections related to CAM, and a search box for specific disease conditions, products and other terms. Downloadable PDF versions for easy printing for your patients, many available in Spanish. See:
  - "10 things to know about evaluating medical resources on the web" http://nccam.nih.gov/health/webresources/
  - "Selecting a CAM Practitioner" http://nccam.nih.gov/health/practitioner/
- National Clearinghouse for CAM (NCCAM)
  http://nccam.nih.gov/health/clearinghouse/
  The public's point of contact for scientifically based information on CAM and for information about NCCAM. Most extensive rheumatology-related information is for therapies related to rheumatoid arthritis.
- National Council Against Health Fraud
  http://www.ncahf.org
  This site appears to be updated to 2004; has some helpful links to other organizations.
- National Institute of Arthritis and Musculoskeletal and Skin Diseases (NIAMS; a division of National Institutes of Health, Department of Health and Human Services (NIH,DHHS))
  www.niams.nih.gov
  Government-designated National Arthritis, Musculoskeletal and Skin Diseases Information Clearinghouse; has limited information re. CAM, primarily on Glucosamine/the GAIT trail, Osteoarthritis, and some articles about projects related to CAM studies.
- National Institutes of Health Office of Dietary Supplements
  http://ods.od.nih.gov
  Provides information about informed decision-making; "Tips for Older Supplement Users"; articles pertaining to specific supplements and some rheumatic disease conditions
- National Institute on Aging (NIA); National Institute on Aging Information Center
  www.nia.gov; www.niapublications.org

Information and tips on healthy aging, care giving, medications, dietary supplements, diseases, and "Making Your Web Site Senior Friendly". Resources available in both English and Spanish. Copies also provided in PDF format and print versions.

- www.nihseniorhealth.gov is a senior-friendly website from the National Institute on Aging and the National Library of Medicine with simple-to-use website features and popular health topics for older adults. Has large type and a "talking" function.
- Quackwatch, Inc.
  www.quackwatch.org
  Consumer advocacy group offers tips on avoiding health fraud.

20

The Future of Rheumatology Is Integral

DANIEL MULLER, MD, PhD

We are on the verge of a breakthrough in the practice of medicine: *integral medicine*. Time will tell exactly how close we are to experiencing widespread incorporation of these ideas and methods into the majority of practices—optimistically, the next few years; pessimistically, perhaps the next few lifetimes. What are these new ideas and modalities on the horizon? Although there are so many topics that could be covered here, from mind-body medicine to the newest biologics, we will instead focus on planting the seeds of possibilities. Here, we discuss some of the more philosophical ideas that could change the way we interact with patients.

In this book, readers may have noticed many areas of overlap across chapters, reflecting the art and science of integrative rheumatologic care. What runs through these chapters is a theme, largely unspoken. Ultimately, our goal is to ask, "How do we better take care of ourselves so that we can better take care of our patients?" In this final chapter, we will touch on 6 seed topics:

Active Healing
Integrative versus Integral Medicine
Wisdom and Compassion
Lenses
Creativity
Dropping Attachment to Outcomes

Active Healing

One of the most important new concepts in medicine, this movement asks: how do we move from more invasive and passive methods of healing, where a practitioner takes care of a patient, to more active methods of healing where that person is active in creating her own path to health? What modalities can we use, initially, to help a patient? Then, subsequently, what can we suggest for the patient so that she takes the responsibility for her own health?

Table 20.1 shows general methods and modalities, moving roughly from passive to active. Our goal is to use these more passive methods to help an individual move toward self-sustaining, active methods of healing—and, indeed, toward personal evolution and growth of consciousness. For example, if we start a patient on an antidepressant, we'll also develop the next steps to take after the antidepressant is tapered. We might use herbals or supplements with fewer side effects to help in tapering the medications. If a patient with osteoarthritis is suffering from pain, we might give medication on a short-term basis, but then we'll move her towards exercise, and perhaps mind-body therapies. We'll plant seeds for further active methods, so the patient is equipped to take over the task of creating her own path for health, and happiness.

We realize that some individuals will need medication for the rest of their lives. But for many others, symptoms are indicators that lifestyle changes are needed. Often a patient needs a path on which to grow in both physical and conscious ways. And we, the practitioners, also must be on our own paths of development in order to better guide others.

Table 20.1. Methods of Healing from Passive to Active.

Surgery >	*Injection* >	*Insertion* >	*Ingestion* >	*Manipulation* >
	Drugs	Acupuncture	Foods	Physical therapy
			Herbs	Chiropractic
			Homeopathy	Bodywork
			Drugs	Massage

Bioenergetic >	*Talk/Prayer* >	*Movement* >	*Meditation*
Chanting	Psychotherapy	Dance	Visualization
Guided visualization	Hypnosis	Qigong/TaiChi	Self-hypnosis
Shamanic	Spiritual	Alexander	Journaling
Drumming		Feldenkrais	Art therapy
Music		Aikido	Mandela art
Theraputic touch		Karate	Biofeedback
		Any Exercise done mindfully!	**Any Awareness Practice!**

Integrative versus Integral Medicine

An older term for "integrative medicine" was holistic medicine, looking at the "whole" patient. Others have written about the integration of complementary and alternative medicine (CAM) with allopathic medicine.[1] But CAM is a constantly moving target. Once these CAM modalities are incorporated into routine allopathic care, and taught in our training programs, they are no longer considered "complementary" or "alternative." Integrative medicine is still a helpful term, and it is currently the one that many use. When there are good double-blinded studies, we are able to make evidence-based decisions for care. When these studies aren't available, we must use our knowledge and intuition to balance risk and benefit, as well as economics, to find the best paths with our patients. For example, there may not be powerful evidence for the efficacy of omega-3 fatty acids in osteoarthritis, but we know it has some good anti-inflammatory effects in rheumatoid arthritis, relieves signs of dyslipidemia, and is inexpensive, so we might use it in osteoarthritis anyway. When we explore options *with* our patients, we are moving into "Integral Medicine."

Integral medicine is where we realize we are as much affected by our interaction with patients as our patients are affected by their interaction with us. The term "integral medicine" comes from the work of a truly remarkable modern philosopher, Ken Wilber. He developed over the past 30 years a proposed four-quadrant "theory of everything" (Figure 20.1).[2,3] In this model, there are levels (Figure 20.2) and lines (Figure 20.3) of development, encompassing the inner and outer states of both individuals and society – including *everything*. These figures and our discussion here are greatly simplified, but for the complete theory see his works.[2,3]

The **Upper Right** portion of this figure describes most of what we currently teach in basic science education. In this model, we start with the building blocks—amino acids, nucleic acids, sugars. We then think about the next level, the polymeric nature of proteins, DNA, and complex sugars and interactions between these molecules within a cell, DNA replication, regulatory systems, intracellular physiology, cellular biology, and secretion mechanisms. The next level would include interactions between cells—membrane biology, signaling. The function and structure of organs follows, along with systems interactions of endocrine biology, immunology, and neurobiology. Note that each higher level includes all of the levels below. For example, in the evolution of the neural system you cannot have cortical function without having a limbic system. We can directly, and *objectively*, observe processes and outward behavior in this quadrant.

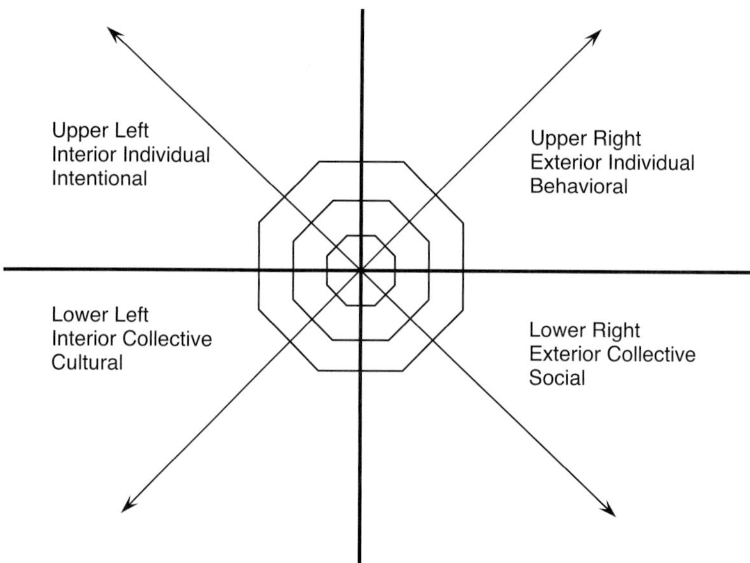

FIGURE 20.1. Ken Wilber's 4-Quadrant "Theory of Everything".

One important part of this model is the explanation of where the psychological and social aspects of medicine fit into this broad view (Figure 20.2). The **Upper Left** portion of this figure focuses on the psychological (and higher) interior development of the individual. This aspect can be inferred through observing behavior—but not directly observed. You must ask if a person is a Democrat or a Republican, as you cannot know this by looking inside the person's head with an MRI, and she can lie. The **Lower Right** of the figure outlines the external, observable social aspects of our society. The **Lower Left** of the figure outlines the development of the inner cultural aspects of society.

Sometimes we observe that patients and physicians have difficulty communicating with each other. A physician who does not believe that any CAM therapy could be worthwhile, and a patient who is not comfortable with allopathic therapy, are operating in different quadrants. The patient might be operating largely from the perspective of the interior quadrant **Upper Left,** while the physician might be largely operating out of the exterior quadrant of the **Upper Right**. If each cannot see that both quadrants are important, then, using completely different sets of assumptions about the world, they will find themselves speaking different languages. Many CAM practitioners who don't have allopathic training use terms that overlap with scientific terms but may have vastly different, often metaphoric, meanings. For example the terms

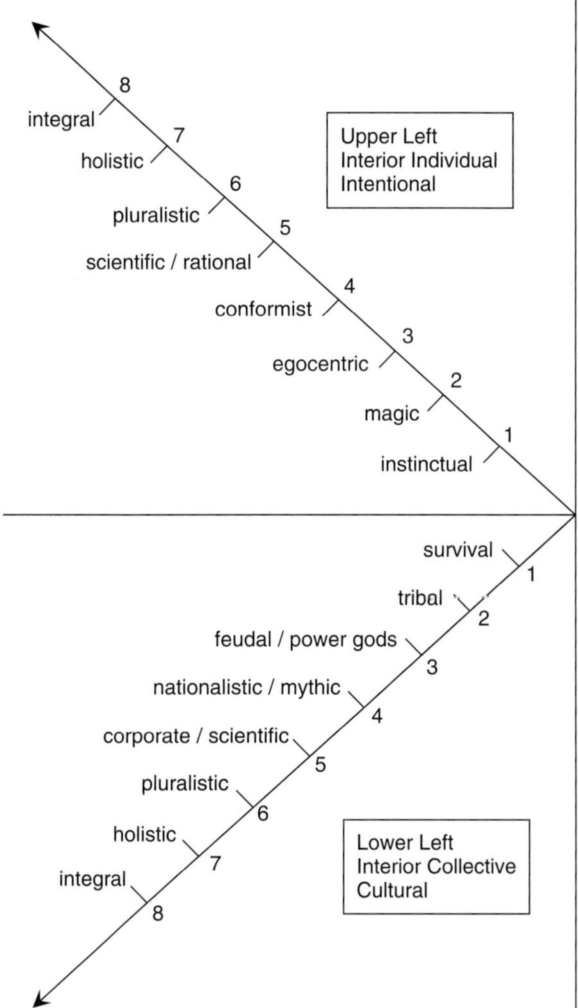

FIGURE 20.2. Levels of Development for the Interior Quadrants: the Upper Left Individual and Lower Left Collective.

kidney, *liver*, and *spleen* in traditional Chinese medicine have very different meanings from our organ-specific descriptions in allopathic medicine. Some CAM practitioners speak about parasites and chronic yeast infections in patients who clearly do not have the types of infections we diagnose as allopathic practitioners.

These types of miscommunications aren't limited to clinical medicine. Mental health practitioners can speak from the upper left quadrant (i.e., psychoanalysis) or the upper right quadrant (i.e., biological psychiatry). In a similar

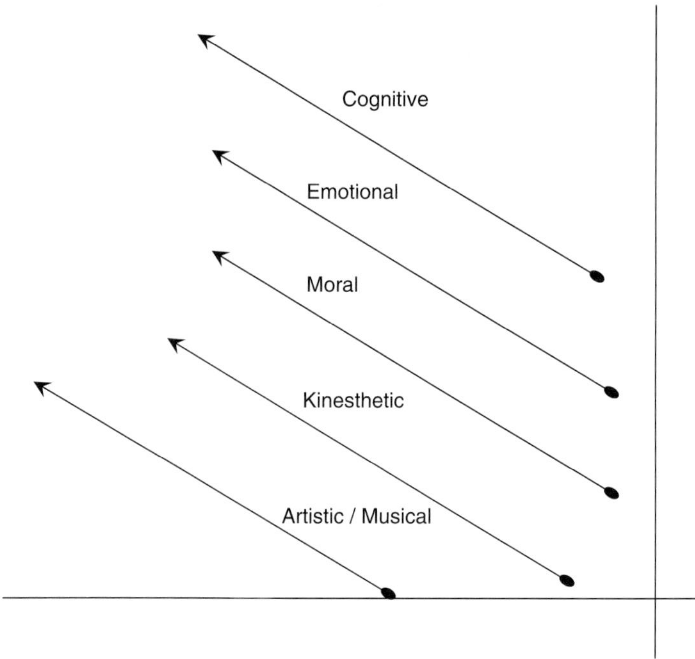

FIGURE 20.3. Each Level of Development in the Left Upper Quadrant has Multiple "Intelligences" or Lines of Development.

manner, some scientists have difficulty talking to other scientists when they are operating within the paradigms of different quadrants.

The **Upper Left** also focuses on the psychological development of the individual. There are different "levels" of development. Again, each transition from one level to the next higher level *transcends* that lower level and yet also *includes* that lower level. These levels are also reflected in the lower 2 quadrants of social and cultural levels. For example, in medical school we operate at the **Scientific-Rational** level. However, if we have a member of a gang in our clinic, they might be operating at the **Tribal** level. This would be important to keep in mind for proper communication. Remembering that in this model we transcend and include, therefore, we can see their worldview, if we are aware; however, they cannot see or understand our worldview.

How can you tell at which level someone is operating? It can be simple, since with each level an individual considers a larger number of the people around them "family." At the tribal level, for instance, a gang member considers only the members of his gang, and perhaps his relatives, as "family." At the nationalistic level, it is "my country, right or wrong." At a pluralistic level, someone might want to be as inclusive as possible, but cannot accept those who willfully pollute the environment. At the highest integral levels, the realization arises that every individual is exactly where she needs to be at that moment, and is deeply respected for her ability to function at her current level. At your own Integral level, it is your duty to help everyone who wishes to rise to a higher level of consciousness. Yet, you have no duty to do so for any one individual. A paradox is characteristic of this Integral level. There is no truth without its opposite.[4] (Wilber, Engler, Brown, 1986, pp 225, 259).

The interior cultural levels and exterior social levels are at the mean, or mode level of its inhabitants. If you are at a lower than average level, the average tends to pull you up toward the mean. But higher levels may seem strange or even dangerous from that perspective. If you are at a higher level, you may feel as though you are in a difficult position, since in order to operate in the world at that level, you may need to act as though you were at a lower level. The average of that level pulls you down toward the mean.

In a truly integral medicine model, our intake history would outline and consider the impact of all 4 quadrants on a patient's life. Then the physician would help the patient design a program that would include methods for balancing and growing her functioning in each quadrant.

The 4-quadrant theory is only a model, and therefore reductionistic. A map helps us *visualize* the territory, but now, let's *explore* the territory.

Wisdom and Compassion

In the context of integral medicine, wisdom is the process of gaining information about ourselves.[2,3] This wisdom can help us rise above the needs and worries that interfere with our ability to listen deeply to patients, and helps in the development of intuition. Compassion is bringing what we have learned through wisdom practice to the practical interaction we have with others in the world. If our minds are not preoccupied with the future or the past, we can be present with our patients, listening deeply to what they say. If we listen carefully, we can better make diagnoses and develop the treatment plans needed.

Wisdom can be developed through meditative or contemplative practice, but there is no "meditation prescription." Christian contemplative practice, Jewish meditative practice, and Buddhist meditation are simply different boats to the same place. However, there are a few good methods that can help start a meditation program. Many swear by Kabat-Zinn's Mindfulness Based Stress Reduction course.[5] Dr. Utzinger's chapter in this book (Chapter 12) provides further recommendations.

After much practice, we have found that patients feel better and report greater emotional intuition. When you feel truly stuck, seek guidance from a psychologist, if possible, one who can work with dreams.

Lenses

Practicing wisdom involves learning about ourselves, but the lenses we usually wear sometimes blind us to seeing clearly. What are these lenses? Some of them develop from staying exclusively within the quadrants where we are comfortable. If we operate only at the **Scientific-Rational** level we may not be able to see the role of anything other than the highest technologies of surgery and medication for helping our patients. If we cannot accept patients as whole individuals, and see their positive characteristics as well as their harmful habits, then we may be unable meet them where they need to be. For example, if a physician practices from the **Right Upper** quadrant alone, she might dismiss someone with fibromyalgia from her clinic for "just being too fat." If we're unable to explore the psychological and social factors that have led to this weight gain and pain syndrome, we will be unable to help this person find the next steps she needs to take. Sometimes, we can only plant seeds for treatments the patient can follow later. But sometimes we come up with an explanation of the origin of a patient's problem that resonates with the patient, and what we think are impossible changes really do occur. For further ideas about listening to patients, see Cooper's chapter (19) on the patient's perspective.

The 4-quadrant Integral Model is just one set of lenses with which to see the world. There are other models that may be helpful, such as David Keirsey's *Please Understand Me II.*[6] This temperament-sorter is based the Myers-Briggs test, and therefore Jung's work, and is particularly helpful for those feeling like they are in unknown territory. For a complementary take on personalities, read Helen Palmer's *The Enneagram,*[7] and for a more advanced treatment of the enneagram read Almass' *Facets of Unity.*[8]

To learn about the borderline between modern psychology and personal transformation, we recommend John Welwood's *Toward a Psychology of Awakening*[9](2000) and David Richo's *How to be an Adult in Relationships.*[10] (2002). For readings at the edges of psychology and healing, look for Anondea Judith's *Eastern Body, Western Mind*[11] (2004), Edward Tick's *The Practice of Dream Healing,*[12] and Bert Hellinger's *Love's Hidden Symmetry.*[13]

Finally, to really stretch the interface of science, psychology, and consciousness, read Lynne McTaggart's *The Field* (2002)[14] and *The Intention Experiment* (2007),[15] Edward and Emily Kelly's *Irreducible Mind* (2007).[16] Subscribe to *Explore: The Journal of Science and Healing* (Elsevier), and also read all of the past editorials by Dr. Larry Dossey.

Creativity

Water, food, shelter, sleep, and sex are considered the basics of life—but we would add one more; creativity. Often, when creative urges arise we will sacrifice sex, sleep, food, water, until we are exhausted. But all too often in our modern society we allow "passive" activity such as television, shopping, substances, and even surfing the Internet to rule our lives. Fine in small amounts, or when needed, these passive activities can be devastating to our happiness and health when they become addictions. It's important, every once in a while, to allow our natural creative urges room and space to take over.

Dropping Attachment to Outcomes

At the highest levels of understanding, we as medical practitioners see that the patient in front of us is absolutely perfect. And letting her know that, can be a way to start the healing. At the same time, we know that change sometimes has to occur. The practitioner's responsibility is to combine her rational allopathic knowledge and reasoning with highly intuitive knowing, along with the patient's intrinsic knowledge and drive to heal, to help guide that individual onto the next steps on their path.

Part of this understanding is a loosening of our attachment to outcome. Our conventional medical training teaches us that we need to fix people who are broken, and sometimes we start to develop an ego from feeling important and powerful. But our egos can get in the way of being the best healers we can be. When we grasp too hard, we may crush the one we are trying to save. Hold the patient and their outcome gently, like a butterfly; too hard a grasp will crush it. No need to push it away, either. And remember that what has worked for one patient may not work for someone else.

Most people get attached to the path they have used for success, and perhaps think everyone should take the same path. Dropping this attachment to outcome will allow your intuition to become clear.

Summary

Remember that these are only a few ways to think about the future of medicine. Our craft is in constant evolution. The Integral model can be helpful, and it can be a guide. But it is only a map, not the territory. We must go out there and walk the territory by practicing both the art and science of medicine.

Just as we ask our patients to be creative and forge their own paths, we must forge our own.

The keys to the personal evolution of consciousness are already present. Let us work on our own evolution at the same time that we are helping our patients work on theirs.

REFERENCES

1. Faass N. *Integrating Complementary Medicine into Health Systems.* Gaithersburg, MD: Aspen; 2001.
2. Wilber K. *A Brief History of Everything*. Boston: Shambhala; 1996.
3. Wilber K. *Integral Spirituality*. Boston: Integral Books; 2006.
4. Wiber K, Engler J, Brown D. *Transformations of Consciousness: Conventional and Contemplative Perspectives on Development*. Boston: Shambhala; 1986.
5. Kabat-Zinn J. *Full Catastrophe Living: Using the Wisdom of Your Body and Mind to Face Stress, Pain, and Illness*. New York: Delta; 1990.
6. Keirsey D. *Please Understand Me II: Temperament, Character, Intelligence*. DelMar, CA: Prometheus Nemesis; 1998.
7. Palmer H. *The Enneagram: Understanding Yourself and Others in Your Life*. New York: HarperCollins; 1998.
8. Almass A. *Facets of Unity. The 8 of Holy Ideas.* Boston: Shambhala; 1998.
9. Welwood J. *Toward a Psychology of Awakening: Buddhism, Psychotherapy, and the Path of Personal and Spiritual Awakening.* Boston: Shambhala; 2000.
10. Richo D. *How to be an Adult in Relationships: The Five Keys to Mindful Loving.* Boston: Shambhala; 2002.
11. Judith A. *Eastern Body Western Mind: Psychology and the Chakra System as a Path to the Self.* Berkeley: Celestial Arts; 2004.
12. Tick E. *The Practice of Dream Healing: Bringing Ancient Greek Mysteries into Modern Medicine*. Wheaton, IL: Quest; 2001.
13. Hellinger B. *Love's Hidden Symmetry: What makes Love Work in Relationships.* Phoenix: Zeig Tucker; 1998.
14. McTaggart L. *The Field.* New York: HarperCollins; 2002.
15. McTaggart L. *The Intention Experiment.* New York: Free Press; 2007.
16. Kelly E, Kelly E, Crabtree A, Gauld A, Grossa M, Greyson B. *Irreducible Mind: Toward a Psychology for the 21st Century.* Lanham, MD: Rowman and Littlefield; 2007.

INDEX

Note: Page numbers followed by "*f*" and "*t*" denote figures and tables, respectively.

H

I

R

S